Pharmacogenomics and Personalized Medicine

Pharmacogenomics and Personalized Medicine

Editors

Erika Cecchin
Gabriele Stocco

MDPI • Basel • Beijing • Wuhan • Barcelona • Belgrade • Manchester • Tokyo • Cluj • Tianjin

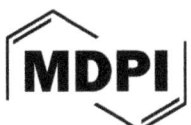

Editors
Erika Cecchin
Experimental and Clinical
Pharmacology, Centro di
Riferimento Oncologico di
Aviano (CRO), IRCCS
Italy

Gabriele Stocco
Department of Life Sciences,
University of Trieste
Italy

Editorial Office
MDPI
St. Alban-Anlage 66
4052 Basel, Switzerland

This is a reprint of articles from the Special Issue published online in the open access journal *Genes* (ISSN 2073-4425) (available at: https://www.mdpi.com/journal/genes/special_issues/Pemed).

For citation purposes, cite each article independently as indicated on the article page online and as indicated below:

LastName, A.A.; LastName, B.B.; LastName, C.C. Article Title. *Journal Name* **Year**, *Article Number*, Page Range.

ISBN 978-3-03936-730-6 (Hbk)
ISBN 978-3-03936-731-3 (PDF)

© 2020 by the authors. Articles in this book are Open Access and distributed under the Creative Commons Attribution (CC BY) license, which allows users to download, copy and build upon published articles, as long as the author and publisher are properly credited, which ensures maximum dissemination and a wider impact of our publications.

The book as a whole is distributed by MDPI under the terms and conditions of the Creative Commons license CC BY-NC-ND.

Contents

About the Editors vii

Erika Cecchin and Gabriele Stocco
Pharmacogenomics and Personalized Medicine
Reprinted from: *Genes* **2020**, *11*, 679, doi:10.3390/genes11060679 1

Matteo Dugo, Andrea Devecchi, Loris De Cecco, Erika Cecchin, Delia Mezzanzanica, Marialuisa Sensi and Marina Bagnoli
Focal Recurrent Copy Number Alterations Characterize Disease Relapse in High Grade Serous Ovarian Cancer Patients with Good Clinical Prognosis: A Pilot Study
Reprinted from: *Genes* **2019**, *10*, 678, doi:10.3390/genes10090678 7

Zulfan Zazuli, Leila S. Otten, Britt I. Drögemöller, Mara Medeiros, Jose G. Monzon, Galen E.B. Wright, Christian K. Kollmannsberger, Philippe L. Bedard, Zhuo Chen, Karen A. Gelmon, Nicole McGoldrick, Abhijat Kitchlu, Susanne J.H. Vijverberg, Rosalinde Masereeuw, Colin J.D. Ross, Geoffrey Liu, Bruce C. Carleton and Anke H. Maitland-van der Zee
Outcome Definition Influences the Relationship between Genetic Polymorphisms of *ERCC1*, *ERCC2*, *SLC22A2* and Cisplatin Nephrotoxicity in Adult Testicular Cancer Patients
Reprinted from: *Genes* **2019**, *10*, 364, doi:10.3390/genes10050364 23

Yingqi Xu, Shuting Lin, Hongying Zhao, Jingwen Wang, Chunlong Zhang, Qun Dong, Congxue Hu, Desi Shang, Li Wang and Yanjun Xu
Quantifying Risk Pathway Crosstalk Mediated by miRNA to Screen Precision drugs for Breast Cancer Patients
Reprinted from: *Genes* **2019**, *10*, 657, doi:10.3390/genes10090657 41

Laith N. AL-Eitan, Ayah Y. Almasri and Rame H. Khasawneh
Impact of *CYP2C9* and *VKORC1* Polymorphisms on Warfarin Sensitivity and Responsiveness in Jordanian Cardiovascular Patients during the Initiation Therapy
Reprinted from: *Genes* **2018**, *9*, 578, doi:10.3390/genes9120578 59

Marianna Lucafò, Gabriele Stocco, Stefano Martelossi, Diego Favretto, Raffaella Franca, Noelia Malusà, Angela Lora, Matteo Bramuzzo, Samuele Naviglio, Erika Cecchin, Giuseppe Toffoli, Alessandro Ventura and Giuliana Decorti
Azathioprine Biotransformation in Young Patients with Inflammatory Bowel Disease: Contribution of Glutathione-S Transferase M1 and A1 Variants
Reprinted from: *Genes* **2019**, *10*, 277, doi:10.3390/genes10040277 73

Neha S. Bhise, Abdelrahman H. Elsayed, Xueyuan Cao, Stanley Pounds and Jatinder K. Lamba
MicroRNAs Mediated Regulation of Expression of Nucleoside Analog Pathway Genes in Acute Myeloid Leukemia
Reprinted from: *Genes* **2019**, *10*, 319, doi:10.3390/genes10040319 85

Carin A. T. C. Lunenburg, Linda M. Henricks, André B. P. van Kuilenburg, Ron H. J. Mathijssen, Jan H. M. Schellens, Hans Gelderblom, Henk-Jan Guchelaar and Jesse J. Swen
Diagnostic and Therapeutic Strategies for Fluoropyrimidine Treatment of Patients Carrying Multiple *DPYD* Variants
Reprinted from: *Genes* **2018**, *9*, 585, doi:10.3390/genes9120585 97

Rossana Roncato, Lisa Dal Cin, Silvia Mezzalira, Francesco Comello, Elena De Mattia, Alessia Bignucolo, Lorenzo Giollo, Simone D'Errico, Antonio Gulotta, Luca Emili, Vincenzo Carbone, Michela Guardascione, Luisa Foltran, Giuseppe Toffoli and Erika Cecchin
FARMAPRICE: A Pharmacogenetic Clinical Decision Support System for Precise and Cost-Effective Therapy
Reprinted from: *Genes* **2019**, *10*, 276, doi:10.3390/genes10040276 111

Cathelijne H. van der Wouden, Paul C. D. Bank, Kübra Özokcu, Jesse J. Swen and Henk-Jan Guchelaar
Pharmacist-Initiated Pre-Emptive Pharmacogenetic Panel Testing with Clinical Decision Support in Primary Care: Record of PGx Results and Real-World Impact
Reprinted from: *Genes* **2019**, *10*, 416, doi:10.3390/genes10060416 125

Cristina Lucía Dávila-Fajardo, Xando Díaz-Villamarín, Alba Antúnez-Rodríguez, Ana Estefanía Fernández-Gómez, Paloma García-Navas, Luis Javier Martínez-González, José Augusto Dávila-Fajardo and José Cabeza Barrera
Pharmacogenetics in the Treatment of Cardiovascular Diseases and Its Current Progress Regarding Implementation in the Clinical Routine
Reprinted from: *Genes* **2019**, *10*, 261, doi:10.3390/genes10040261 141

Sonja Pavlovic, Nikola Kotur, Biljana Stankovic, Branka Zukic, Vladimir Gasic and Lidija Dokmanovic
Pharmacogenomic and Pharmacotranscriptomic Profiling of Childhood Acute Lymphoblastic Leukemia: Paving the Way to Personalized Treatment
Reprinted from: *Genes* **2019**, *10*, 191, doi:10.3390/genes10030191 167

About the Editors

Erika Cecchin is a pharmacologist of the Clinical and Experimental Pharmacology Unit of CRO-Aviano, where she works in the field of the pharmacogenetic research for the optimization of chemotherapeutic treatment in cancer. She is a co-author of more than 80 full-length publications in international peer-reviewed journals and chapters in international books. She is part of the Board of Teachers of the PhD School in Biotechnology and Biomedical Sciences at the University of Udine-Italy. Since 2015, she has been an active member of the Ubiquitous Pharmacogenomics Consortium (www.upgx.eu) with the aim to implement pharmacogenomics in clinical practice across Europe. She is also a member of the Pharmacogenetics and Pharmacogenomics Section (PGx Section) of the International Union of Basic and Clinical Pharmacology (IUPHAR).

Gabriele Stocco has been Associate Professor in Pharmacology at the University of Trieste since 2019. His research interest focuses on translational studies on pharmacogenetics and therapy personalization of antimetabolites and biologics used in chronic and oncologic pediatric diseases. Gabriele Stocco has a degree in Medicinal Chemistry with honors from the University of Trieste, a PhD in Pharmacology from the University of Trieste, and received doctoral and post-doctoral training from St. Jude Children's Hospital in Memphis, USA. His scientific effort is evident in his more than 80 scientific publications.

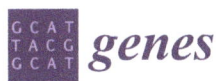

Editorial

Pharmacogenomics and Personalized Medicine

Erika Cecchin [1,*] and Gabriele Stocco [2,*]

1. Experimental and Clinical Pharmacology, Centro di Riferimento Oncologico di Aviano (CRO) IRCCS, 33081 Aviano, Italy
2. Department of Life Sciences, University of Trieste, 34127 Trieste, Italy
* Correspondence: ececchin@cro.it (E.C.); stoccog@units.it (G.S.); Tel.: +39-04-3465-9667 (E.C.); +39-04-0558-8634 (G.S.)

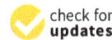

Received: 3 June 2020; Accepted: 18 June 2020; Published: 22 June 2020

Abstract: Pharmacogenomics is one of the emerging approaches to precision medicine, tailoring drug selection and dosing to the patient's genetic features. In recent years, several pharmacogenetic guidelines have been published by international scientific consortia, but the uptake in clinical practice is still poor. Many coordinated international efforts are ongoing in order to overcome the existing barriers to pharmacogenomic implementation. On the other hand, existing validated pharmacogenomic markers can explain only a minor part of the observed clinical variability in the therapeutic outcome. New investigational approaches are warranted, including the study of the pharmacogenomic role of the immune system genetics and of previously neglected rare genetic variants, reported to account for a large part of the inter-individual variability in drug metabolism. In this Special Issue, we collected a series of articles covering many aspects of pharmacogenomics. These include clinical implementation of pharmacogenomics in clinical practice, development of tools or infrastructures to support this process, research of new pharmacogenomics markers to increase drug efficacy and safety, and the impact of rare genetic variants in pharmacogenomics.

Keywords: pharmacogenomics; personalized medicine; human genetics; pharmacology

---

Precision medicine has the ultimate goal of exactly matching each therapeutic intervention with the patient's molecular profile. Over the last twenty years, the study of human genetics has been fueled by cutting-edge sequencing technologies leading to a deeper understanding of the relationship between genetic variation and human health [1]. The study of genetics has been widely applied in precision medicine, and one of the emerging applications is pharmacogenomics-informed pharmacotherapy, tailoring drug selection and dosing to the patient's genetic features. To date, pharmacogenomic variation has an established role in drug efficacy and safety, enabling the creation of treatment guidelines by international scientific consortia aimed at creating medical guidance for the clinical application of pharmacogenomics. Specifically, the Clinical Pharmacogenetics Implementation Consortium (CPIC) and the Dutch Pharmacogenetics Working Group (DPWG) have developed validated guidelines for several drug-gene interactions that are made freely available as an on-line resource (www.pharmgkb.org) [2]. However, the uptake of pharmacogenomics into routine clinical care remains limited. A range of major barriers has been identified, spanning from basic pharmacogenomics research through implementation. The study of previously neglected rare genetic variants and the validation of their functional and clinical impact through the development of pre-clinical models and in silico tools is warranted to improve pharmacogenomic knowledge. On the other hand, ongoing international coordinated efforts set up to overcome the existing barriers to pharmacogenomic implementation will provide new tools and insights into the clinical application of pharmacogenomics, thus helping to pave the way for widespread adoption [3]. In this Special Issue, eleven papers are published, covering different aspects of research and clinical application in the field of pharmacogenomics.

Six papers report original results on the discovery of new genetic markers of the outcome of a pharmacological treatment in terms of either efficacy or toxicity. Two papers focus on the pharmacogenomics of platinum derivatives. Dugo and colleagues [4] report the results of the bioinformatic revision of a dataset of radically resected ovarian cancer patients from TCGA, treated with an adjuvant platinum-based treatment. They focus on tumor tissue genetic alterations and specifically on somatic copy number alteration, highlighting a significantly different pattern of genomic amplification in platinum resistant patients versus platinum sensitive. The paper underscores the importance of considering the tumor tissue genome when approaching the issue of pharmacogenomics in cancer treatment. Moreover, it points out the great opportunity offered by the large amount of genomic data produced by international consortia like TCGA that could be mined to highlight innovative pharmacogenomic markers. The research paper by Zazuli and colleagues [5] addresses the issue of predictive markers of nephrotoxicity due to cisplatin treatment. They attempt to validate some previously investigated genetic polymorphisms in *SLC22A2* and *ERCC2*. Quite interestingly, they aim to define whether different clinical definitions of nephrotoxicity (adjusted-AKI or CTCAE-AKI designation) could have contributed to previous inconsistent results on the predictive role of the analyzed variants. They report that the association with the polymorphisms was only significant when considering the nephrotoxicity definition according to CTCAE v4.03. This paper raises the important issue of the definitions of clinically relevant outcomes in pharmacogenomics, which may have hindered the generation of solid and reproducible data among various studies in the field. More generally, heterogeneity in ethnicity, demographic characteristics and treatment modalities (dose or co-treatment) could affect comparability among studies. Yanqui Xu and colleagues [6] describe an original analysis of publicly available data investigating effective drugs for breast cancer using a system approach. The analysis is focused on identifying molecules effective in particular breast cancer subtypes by considering the impact of potentially effective drugs on the pathway crosstalk mediated by miRNAs. In their integrated analysis, the authors point out, for example, sorafenib as a medication potentially effective on the basal subtype, or irinotecan for Her2-positive subtype. Al-Eitan and colleagues [7] evaluate the association between a panel of seven polymorphic variants in the well-established candidate genes *CYP2C9* (three variants) and *VKORC1* (four variants) and warfarin anticoagulant effects, in a cohort of unrelated Jordanian-Arab patients with cardiovascular disease. Warfarin response was evaluated in terms of the achievement of a coagulation level in the therapeutic range during therapy and of the drug dose required by the patient. Variants of both genes were associated with warfarin effects and dose requirement. Interestingly, the haplotype derived by the combination of the variants of each gene were also associated with the effects of warfarin, confirming the relevance of the multilocus *CYP2C9/VKORC1* genotype to improving warfarin therapy for Arab patients also. Lucafò and colleagues [8] evaluated the contribution of a panel of candidate genetic variants on the efficacy and pharmacokinetics and of azathioprine in a cohort of young Italian patients with inflammatory bowel disease. These variants included those well established in *TPMT*, but also in two highly polymorphic glutathione transferase enzymes, in particular the *GST-A1* and *GST-M1* isoforms. Interestingly, all variants affected azathioprine efficacy in this cohort. In particular, *TPMT* polymorphisms, associated with reduced enzymatic activity, determined improved response to azathioprine, due to reduced inactivation of the drug. On the other hand, variants determining reduced activity of *GST-A1* or *GST-M1* determined reduced azathioprine efficacy, likely because of a lower drug activation. The effect on azathioprine metabolite concentration and dose was confirmed for *GST-M1* and *TPMT*. Bise and colleagues [9] evaluate the potential involvement of miRNAs in determining the variation in expression levels of drug transporters or enzymes involved in the activation or inactivation of cytarabine and other analogs, an important mechanism potentially determining drug resistance. The authors evaluate miRNA and gene-expression levels of cytarabine metabolic pathway genes in 8 AML cell lines and the TCGA database, demonstrating that miR-34a-5p and miR-24-3p regulate DCK, an enzyme involved in activation of cytarabine, and DCTD, an enzyme involved in metabolic inactivation of cytarabine expression, respectively. The authors also confirmed the binding of these mRNA–miRNA pairs on the basis of gel shift assays.

Three papers report the results of research work aimed at investigating how to improve pharmacogenomic implementation in clinical practice. The work of Lunenburg and colleagues [10] approached the theme of rare genetic profiles that are not included in the current version of pharmacogenomic guidelines, and the importance of integrating phenotyping strategies into genotyping in these cases. Specifically, they investigated seven cases of rare occurrence of *DPYD* compound heterozygosity for two of the four *DPYD* genetic polymorphisms with a validated effect on fluoropyrimidines safety. The most difficult task in these cases is the phasing of the genotypes in order to obtain a proper translation of genotype to phenotype. Since currently available phasing strategies are difficult to translate into a diagnostic routine, the authors point out the necessity in these sporadic cases of performing DPD phenotyping based on the measurement of DPD activity, in order to define the real enzymatic capacity of each individual. The paper by Roncato et al. [11] describes the development of FARMAPRICE, an IT-based clinical decision support system (CDSS) for the user-friendly application of existing pharmacogenomic guidelines in the clinical practice of drug prescription in Italy. The lack of dedicated IT tools is an acknowledged barrier to the implementation of pharmacogenomics. Even if the usability of electronic health records must be greatly improved in order to allow an effective translation of genetic information into routine drug prescription in Italy, the development of tools like FARMAPRICE can be helpful in facilitating the process. Another paper by Van Der Wouden and colleagues [12] investigated the up-take of a similar tool in a different European health care system. A pharmacogenomic CDSS is currently in use in the Netherlands and is fully integrated with patients' electronic health records. Specifically, the study reports the results of the uptake of this tool within a prospective pilot study with community pharmacies (the Implementation of Pharmacogenetics into Primary care Project (IP3) study). Two hundred patients were pre-emptively genotyped for eight pharmacogenes, and the genotypes were embedded in the electronic health records. The data were used by pharmacists and general practitioners for the purposes of drug prescription. The approach was demonstrated to be feasible in the context of primary care and manageable for pharmacists and general practitioners. Almost all of the patients had the opportunity to re-use their genetic data more than once and about one fourth of the patients had at least one actionable piece of information in their pharmacogenetic passport.

This special issue also includes two outstanding literature reviews. Davila-Fajardo's [13] revision is focused on implementation/cardiology. Indeed, drugs used in this clinical setting have a huge interindividual variability, which is reflected in highly impactful under- or over-treatment, which severely affects the safety of the patients. The choice of the drug and the dose is often critical, and strict clinical monitoring is required to adjust the treatment, as in the case of warfarin. Many gene–drug interactions are available that have been validated by large prospective clinical trials with the opportunity to integrate clinical and genetic information in predictive pharmacogenetic algorithms. Cost-effectiveness studies were also conducted supporting the application of PGx information in the dose adjustment. In conclusion, PGx tests for clopidogrel in high-risk patients and warfarin in patients including all indications could begin to be implemented in daily clinical practice, similar to simvastatin tests. Acenocoumarol should be limited to patients who do not reach the INR after a certain period of treatment. The algorithm could improve acenocoumarol dosage selection for patients who will begin treatment with this drug, especially in extreme-dosage patients. Further studies are necessary to confirm that the PGx test for acenocoumarol is ready for use. Pavlovic and colleagues [14] summarized the contribution of high-throughput technologies, including microarrays and next-generation sequencing, to the pharmacogenomics and pharmacotranscriptomics of pediatric acute lymphoblastic leukemia (ALL). Emerging molecular markers responsible for the efficacy, adverse effects and toxicity of the drugs commonly used for pediatric ALL therapy, i.e., glucocorticoids, vinka alkaloids, asparaginase, anthracyclines, thiopurines and methotrexate are presented in the review. For instance, among the most promising, the authors describe *CEP72* rs924607 TT genotype and its association with vincristine induced neuropathy. The authors underline that while a significant amount of data has been generated using high-throughput technologies, the clinical implementation of these findings is still limited. To increase clinical implementation of this outstanding research, the authors discuss the relevance of data analysis and of designing prediction models using bioinformatics, machine learning algorithms and artificial intelligence.

In conclusion, the studies collected in this volume underline the potential of innovative molecular approaches, including multilocus genotyping, sequencing of rare variants and epigenetic features, in identifying genetic determinants of interindividual variability in the effects of drugs in several important clinical settings, including chemotherapy of breast cancer and leukemia and anticoagulant therapy for cardiovascular diseases. The integration of multiple layers of pharmacological information, including variation in gene expression and function of drug targets, pharmacokinetic profiles, also obtained through innovative statistical and bioinformatic approaches, holds the potential of explaining the predictable sources of interpatient variability in drug effects, which properly implemented will bring to precision therapy.

Author Contributions: E.C. and G.S., conceptualization, writing, review and editing. All authors have read and agreed to the published version of the manuscript.

Funding: This research received no external funding.

Acknowledgments: The Editors would like to thank all the authors and reviewers for their contributions to this issue.

Conflicts of Interest: The authors declare no conflict of interest.

References

1. Van Der Wouden, C.H.; Bohringer, S.; Cecchin, E.; Cheung, K.-C.; Davila-Fajardo, C.L.; Deneer, V.H.M.; Dolzan, V.; Ingelman-Sundberg, M.; Jonsson, S.; O Karlsson, M.; et al. Generating evidence for precision medicine: Considerations made by the Ubiquitous Pharmacogenomics Consortium when designing and operationalizing the PREPARE study. *Pharmacogenet. Genom.* **2020**. [CrossRef] [PubMed]
2. Relling, M.V.; Klein, T.E.; Gammal, R.S.; Whirl-Carrillo, M.; Hoffman, J.M.; Caudle, K.E. The Clinical Pharmacogenetics Implementation Consortium: 10 Years Later. *Clin. Pharmacol. Ther.* **2019**, *107*, 171–175. [CrossRef] [PubMed]
3. Chenoweth, M.J.; Giacomini, K.M.; Pirmohamed, M.; Hill, S.L.; Van Schaik, R.H.N.; Schwab, M.; Shuldiner, A.R.; Relling, M.V.; Tyndale, R.F. Global Pharmacogenomics Within Precision Medicine: Challenges and Opportunities. *Clin. Pharmacol. Ther.* **2019**, *107*, 57–61. [CrossRef] [PubMed]
4. Dugo, M.; Devecchi, A.; De Cecco, L.; Cecchin, E.; Mezzanzanica, D.; Sensi, M.; Bagnoli, M. Focal Recurrent Copy Number Alterations Characterize Disease Relapse in High Grade Serous Ovarian Cancer Patients with Good Clinical Prognosis: A Pilot Study. *Genes* **2019**, *10*, 678. [CrossRef] [PubMed]
5. Zazuli, Z.; Otten, L.S.; Drogemoller, B.; Medeiros, M.; Monzon, J.G.; Wright, G.E.B.; Kollmannsberger, C.K.; Bedard, P.L.; Chen, Z.; Gelmon, K.A.; et al. Outcome Definition Influences the Relationship Between Genetic Polymorphisms of ERCC1, ERCC2, SLC22A2 and Cisplatin Nephrotoxicity in Adult Testicular Cancer Patients. *Genes* **2019**, *10*, 364. [CrossRef] [PubMed]
6. Xu, Y.; Lin, S.; Zhao, H.; Wang, J.; Zhang, C.; Dong, Q.; Hu, C.; Desi, S.; Wang, L.; Xu, Y. Quantifying Risk Pathway Crosstalk Mediated by miRNA to Screen Precision drugs for Breast Cancer Patients. *Genes* **2019**, *10*, 657. [CrossRef] [PubMed]
7. Al-Eitan, L.N.; Almasri, A.Y.; Khasawneh, R.H. Impact of CYP2C9 and VKORC1 Polymorphisms on Warfarin Sensitivity and Responsiveness in Jordanian Cardiovascular Patients during the Initiation Therapy. *Genes* **2018**, *9*, 578. [CrossRef] [PubMed]
8. Lucafo, M.; Stocco, G.; Martelossi, S.; Favretto, D.; Franca, R.; Malusa, N.; Lora, A.; Bramuzzo, M.; Naviglio, S.; Cecchin, E.; et al. Azathioprine Biotransformation in Young Patients with Inflammatory Bowel Disease: Contribution of Glutathione-S Transferase M1 and A1 Variants. *Genes* **2019**, *10*, 277. [CrossRef] [PubMed]
9. Bhise, N.S.; Elsayed, A.H.; Cao, X.; Pounds, S.; Lamba, J.K. MicroRNAs Mediated Regulation of Expression of Nucleoside Analog Pathway Genes in Acute Myeloid Leukemia. *Genes* **2019**, *10*, 319. [CrossRef] [PubMed]

10. Lunenburg, C.; Henricks, L.M.; Van Kuilenburg, A.B.P.; Mathijssen, R.H.J.; Schellens, J.H.M.; Gelderblom, H.; Guchelaar, H.-J.; Swen, J.J. Diagnostic and Therapeutic Strategies for Fluoropyrimidine Treatment of Patients Carrying Multiple DPYD Variants. *Genes* **2018**, *9*, 585. [CrossRef] [PubMed]
11. Roncato, R.; Cin, L.D.; Mezzalira, S.; Comello, F.; De Mattia, E.; Bignucolo, A.; Giollo, L.; D'Errico, S.; Gulotta, A.; Emili, L.; et al. FARMAPRICE: A Pharmacogenetic Clinical Decision Support System for Precise and Cost-Effective Therapy. *Genes* **2019**, *10*, 276. [CrossRef]
12. Van Der Wouden, C.H.; Bank, P.C.D.; Ozokcu, K.; Swen, J.J.; Guchelaar, H.-J. Pharmacist-Initiated Pre-Emptive Pharmacogenetic Panel Testing with Clinical Decision Support in Primary Care: Record of PGx Results and Real-World Impact. *Genes* **2019**, *10*, 416. [CrossRef] [PubMed]
13. Dávila-Fajardo, C.L.; Díaz-Villamarín, X.; Antúnez-Rodríguez, A.; Fernández-Gómez, A.E.; García-Navas, P.; Martinez-Gonzalez, L.; Dávila-Fajardo, J.A.; Barrera, J.C. Pharmacogenetics in the Treatment of Cardiovascular Diseases and Its Current Progress Regarding Implementation in the Clinical Routine. *Genes* **2019**, *10*, 261. [CrossRef] [PubMed]
14. Pavlovic, S.; Kotur, N.; Stankovic, B.; Zukic, B.; Gasic, V.; Dokmanovic, L. Pharmacogenomic and Pharmacotranscriptomic Profiling of Childhood Acute Lymphoblastic Leukemia: Paving the Way to Personalized Treatment. *Genes* **2019**, *10*, 191. [CrossRef] [PubMed]

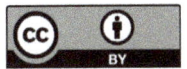

© 2020 by the authors. Licensee MDPI, Basel, Switzerland. This article is an open access article distributed under the terms and conditions of the Creative Commons Attribution (CC BY) license (http://creativecommons.org/licenses/by/4.0/).

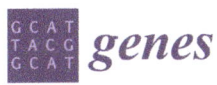

Article

Focal Recurrent Copy Number Alterations Characterize Disease Relapse in High Grade Serous Ovarian Cancer Patients with Good Clinical Prognosis: A Pilot Study

Matteo Dugo [1,*,†], Andrea Devecchi [1,†], Loris De Cecco [1], Erika Cecchin [2], Delia Mezzanzanica [3], Marialuisa Sensi [1] and Marina Bagnoli [3,*]

1   Platform of Integrated Biology, Department of Applied Research and Technological Development, Fondazione IRCCS Istituto Nazionale dei Tumori, 20133 Milan, Italy
2   Experimental and Clinical Pharmacology Unit, Centro di Riferimento Oncologico, IRCCS National Cancer Institute, 33081 Aviano, Pordenone, Italy
3   Molecular Therapy Unit, Department of Research, Fondazione IRCCS Istituto Nazionale dei Tumori, 20133 Milan, Italy
*   Correspondence: matteo.dugo@istitutotumori.mi.it (M.D.); marina.bagnoli@istitutotumori.mi.it (M.B.)
†   Equally contributing authors.

Received: 12 July 2019; Accepted: 2 September 2019; Published: 5 September 2019

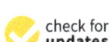

Abstract: High grade serous ovarian cancer (HGSOC) retains high molecular heterogeneity and genomic instability, which currently limit the treatment opportunities. HGSOC patients receiving complete cytoreduction (R0) at primary surgery and platinum-based therapy may unevenly experience early disease relapse, in spite of their clinically favorable prognosis. To identify distinctive traits of the genomic landscape guiding tumor progression, we focused on the R0 patients of The Cancer Genome Atlas (TCGA) ovarian serous cystadenocarcinoma (TCGA-OV) dataset and classified them according to their time to relapse (TTR) from surgery. We included in the study two groups of R0-TCGA patients experiencing substantially different outcome: Resistant (R; TTR ≤ 12 months; n = 11) and frankly Sensitive (fS; TTR ≥ 24 months; n = 16). We performed an integrated clinical, RNA-Sequencing, exome and somatic copy number alteration (sCNA) data analysis. No significant differences in mutational landscape were detected, although the lack of BRCA-related mutational signature characterized the R group. Focal sCNA analysis showed a higher frequency of amplification in R group and deletions in fS group respectively, involving cytobands not commonly detected by recurrent sCNA analysis. Functional analysis of focal sCNA with a concordantly altered gene expression identified in R group a gain in Notch, and interferon signaling and fatty acid metabolism. We are aware of the constraints related to the low number of OC cases analyzed. It is worth noting, however, that the sCNA identified in this exploratory analysis and characterizing Pt-resistance are novel, deserving validation in a wider cohort of patients achieving complete surgical debulking.

Keywords: ovarian cancer; platinum resistance; focal copy number alterations; whole exome sequencing

---

1. Introduction

High grade serous ovarian cancer (HGSOC) is the most common and lethal epithelial ovarian cancer (EOC) subtype, causing 70–80% of ovarian cancer deaths worldwide [1]. Due to the lack of specific symptoms it is generally diagnosed at advanced stages when it has diffusely metastasized into the peritoneal cavity. Standard treatment includes aggressive primary debulking surgery (PDS) followed by platinum (Pt)-based therapy; but, despite the improvement of surgical approaches and drug development, survival rate has changed little in the last decades [2].

Pt-based therapy remains the cornerstone treatment type and, currently, BRCA1/2 mutation status is the only biomarker that allows up-front identification of patients with Pt-sensitive or resistant disease [3]. As a consequence, around 30% of patients undergoing Pt-based chemotherapy do not respond to treatment. Also, around 80% of those patients achieving complete response will relapse with a median progression-free survival of 18 months, developing a disease that progressively becomes Pt-resistant, a largely incurable state [2,3].

The opportunity to effectively treat and control HGSOC progression is limited by tumor heterogeneity and genomic instability. HGSOC following p53 mutation undergo multiple sequential mutational processes that shape a complex genome, strongly dominated by somatic copy number aberrations (sCNA). As a result, HGSOC like other CNA driven tumors, as esophageal cancer, non-small-cell lung cancer and triple negative breast cancer, have a low frequency of recurrent oncogenic mutations and a few recurrent sCNA [4]. These multiple mutational forces acting on HGSOC cause difficulties in the identification of targetable genetic lesion(s).

At present, no residual tumor (R0) after PDS is the most important prognostic factor for survival in advanced stage disease [2]. Analyzing clinical data of The Cancer Genome Atlas (TCGA) ovarian serous cystadenocarcinoma (TCGA-OV) we observed that in the group of patients experiencing early relapse were included also those who received optimal clinical treatment (Pt-based therapy and no residual disease after PDS) supporting the notion that intrinsic characteristic(s) of the tumor play a major role in the lack of responsiveness.

The aim of the present pilot study is to decipher the genomic landscape characterizing the highly selected cohort of HGSOC patients who experienced an early relapse, in spite of their expected favorable outcome as assessed by clinical parameters.

2. Materials and Methods

2.1. Data Source and Samples Selection

Mutational and copy number data of TCGA-OV samples were downloaded from the Broad Institute Firehose web portal (https://gdac.broadinstitute.org/) with data version 2016_01_28. Clinical data were obtained from the ovarian cancer landmark paper [5]. RNA-Seq raw counts data were obtained from the Genomic Data Commons data portal (https://portal.gdc.cancer.gov/) with accession date 12th March 2019.

For genomic analyses we selected patients with: (i) no residual disease (R0) after PDS; (ii) whole-exome sequencing data available; (iii) sCNA data available; (iv) a follow-up time $\geq$ 12 months. Forty-eight patients having these characteristics were then classified according to their time to relapse (TTR). Since the time of end-of-treatment was not recorded, the disease-free interval was calculated from the date of surgery. Patients were categorized on the basis of disease-free period length and we identified two subgroups having very different TTR: the refractory/resistant (R) group with TTR $\leq$ 12 months (n = 11), and the frankly Sensitive (fS) groups with TTR $\geq$ 24 months (n = 16). These 27 patients (5.9% of the entire TCGA-OV cohort) constitute the TCGA-OV27 cohort, analyzed in the present study. All analyses described in the following sections were performed in the R environment version 3.5.2.

2.2. RNA-Seq Data Analysis

RNA-Seq data were available for 23 patients (9 R and 14 fS) of the TCGA-OV27 dataset. Raw read counts were normalized using the Trimmed Mean of M-values (TMM) method [6], implemented in the edgeR Bioconductor package [7]. TMM estimates a scaling factor used to reduce technical bias between samples due to differences in library size. Normalized data were then filtered removing genes with at least 1 count per million reads in less than 5% of samples. The final dataset included

23391 unique genes. Differential expression between R and fS was performed using the limma/voom pipeline [8]. *p*-values were corrected for multiple testing using the Benjamini–Hochberg false discovery rate (FDR) method. Ensembl gene IDs were associated to HUGO gene symbols using the GENCODE v22 annotation. Gene Set Enrichment Analysis [9] between R and fS was performed using the Fast Gene Set Enrichment Analysis (fgsea) package ranking genes according to the t-statistic obtained with limma. Gene sets of the "Hallmark" collection from the Molecular Signatures Database (MSigDB, http://software.broadinstitute.org/gsea/msigdb/) were tested. Gene sets with an FDR < 0.05 were considered significant.

2.3. Mutational Data Analysis

Mutation Annotation Format (MAF) files used to store somatic variants detected were summarized, analyzed, annotated, and visualized using the maftools Bioconductor package [10]. Only variants assumed to have high or moderate (disruptive) impact in the protein, probably causing protein truncation, loss of function or triggering nonsense mediated decay were included in the analysis of most frequently mutated genes. For the calculation of tumor mutational load we considered both high/moderate impact mutation and all somatic mutations.

The DeconstructSigs package [11] was used to perform the mutational signature analysis. This tool evaluates the contribution of 30 signatures reported in COSMIC (https://cancer.sanger.ac.uk/cosmic/signatures) [12] to the mutational profile of each sample. Mutational signatures were calculated considering all somatic mutations in a given sample. The obtained signature scores were then analyzed in association with sensitivity class using Wilcoxon rank-sum test. Samples were grouped according to the top-5 most contributing mutational signatures using unsupervised hierarchical clustering performed with Euclidean distance and Ward linkage.

To identify mutations associated to sensitivity class we used the clinicalEnrichment function of *maftools* package [10] that performs Fisher's exact tests to identify mutated genes associated with the class of interest. Analysis at the level of oncogenic pathways described in Sanchez-Vega et al. [13] was performed using the *OncogenicPathways* function of *maftools*. For each sample we classified each pathway as mutated if at least one of its genes carried a mutation. We then associated mutated pathways to sensitivity class using Fisher's exact test. The same analysis was repeated using the "Hallmark" gene sets from MSigDB.

2.4. sCNA Data Analysis

Genomic Identification of Significant Targets in Cancer (GISTIC) [14] algorithm was used to analyze sCNA data.

Segmented copy number data were analyzed using GISTIC [14] to identify significantly recurrent sCNA in the whole TCGA-OV27 cohort, independently of sensitivity class. GISTIC output was parsed using the maftools package [10]. In addition to the regions recurrently affected by sCNA, GISTIC provides a gene-level copy number status for all genes of the genome in each sample (all_thresholded.by_genes.txt output file). Thus, we tested the association with sensitivity class both for recurrently amplified or deleted regions (GISTIC FDR < 0.1) and for each single gene. For these analyses amplifications and deletions were analyzed separately. For amplifications, a region was assigned a value of 1 if amplified or 0 if the region was not altered or deleted. The same criterion was applied to deletions. The binary amplification and deletion data were then analyzed in relation to sensitivity class using Fisher's exact test. *p*-values were corrected for multiple testing using the Benjamini-Hochberg FDR method.

Per sample genomic instability was calculated according to: (i) The number of segments in the segmented copy number data; (ii) the total number of genes with a copy number alteration; (iii) the sum of deleted or amplified genes. Association between genomic instability and sensitivity class was assessed by Wilcoxon rank-sum test.

2.5. Statistical Power and Sample Size Calculation

The statistical power for Fisher's exact test applied to the TCGA-OV27 cohort for mutational and sCNA data analyses was calculated using the power2x2 function of the exact2x2 R package. From TCGA-OV27 data we observed that the genes mostly associated to the phenotype of interest were altered (mutated, amplified or deleted) in 27% and 94% of R and fS patients, respectively. Considering these proportions and hypothesizing to test 20,000 genes, the present study has a statistical power of 2.4% of detecting at least one significant finding at an FDR threshold of 5%. To achieve a power of 80% at the same FDR threshold at least 31 patients per group are required. This sample size was calculated using the ss2x2 function of the R-package.

2.6. Integrated sCNA and RNA-Seq Functional Analysis

Functional analysis was carried out on a subset of genes that showed coherent copy number status and differential expression in R compared to fS patients. Over-representation of molecular and cellular functions in the list of selected genes was carried out using: (i) Reactome canonical pathways gene sets from the C2 collection of MSigDB (http://software.broadinstitute.org/gsea/msigdb/annotate.jsp) to map the genes in known functional pathways; (ii) Ingenuity® Pathway Analysis (IPA®, Qiagen; Bioinformatics, Redwood City, CA, USA; http://www.qiagen.com/ingenuity) to derive predictions about the activation status. Enrichments with an FDR < 0.05 were considered statistically significant.

3. Results

From TCGA-OV dataset we selected patients with no residual disease (R0) after PDS with WES and sCNA data available and with a follow-up time ≥ 12 months.

Then, considering that the subgroup of R0 patients is expected to have a good prognosis, for the pilot analysis we further refined the cohort selecting Resistant (R, n = 11) with an unfavorable outcome and frankly Sensitive (fS, n = 16) patients. Overall 27 patients, the TCGA-OV27 cohort, were included in the study and their associated clinical data are summarized in Table 1.

Table 1. Clinical characteristics of The Cancer Genome Atlas (TCGA) ovarian serous cystadenocarcinoma (TCGA-OV) 27 cohort.

	Total (n = 27)	R (n = 11)	Fs (n = 16)
	Stage		
III	23	9	14
IV	4	2	2
	Grading		
G2	3	0	3
G3	23	10	13
NA	1	1	0
	Relapse		
yes	18	11	7
no	9	0	9

R = Resistant; fS = frankly Sensitive.

Transcriptomic analysis of TCGA-OV27 cohort did not reveal differentially expressed genes between R and fS patients at an FDR < 0.05. However, when we considered a nominal p-value < 0.05 and a fold-change of 2, 210 and 214 genes were down- and up-regulated respectively, in R patients. Comparison of the two groups using GSEA highlighted 29 hallmark gene sets significantly enriched in one of the two groups at an FDR < 0.05. (Figure S1). In particular, 1 gene set related to oxidative phosphorylation was positively enriched in fS patients while the remaining 28 gene sets were positively enriched in the R group. Overall, gene sets positively enriched in R patients are supporting of a more aggressive phenotype for this subset of tumors but did not highlighted specific mechanisms possibly associated with Pt-resistance.

3.1. Mutational Landscape of TCGA-OV27 Cohort

To identify genomic features associated with early relapse we then analyzed mutational data of the selected cohort. Consistent with genome landscape studies of the whole TCGA-OV cohort and most recent studies on ovarian cancer [15,16], p53 is mutated in 89% of TCGA-OV27 patients (Figure 1). Among the prevalent mutated genes we found, as expected, *CDK12, NF1,* and *RB1,* together with *CSMD1, NOTCH4,* and *TMEM132D* genes, which seem to be a specific trait of this cohort. Considering genes mutated in at least three patients we did not observe any significantly unbalanced distribution of these predominantly mutated genes within R/fS classes (Figure 1A).

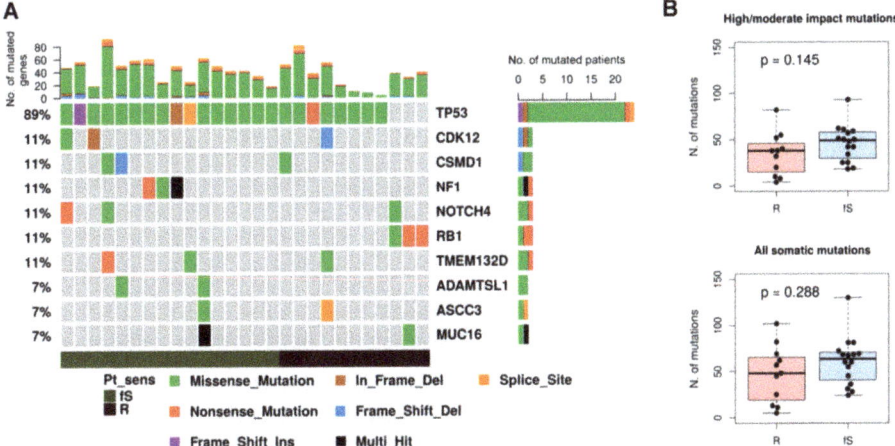

Figure 1. Mutational spectrum of TCGA-OV27 samples. (**A**) Oncoplot of the top-10 most frequently mutated genes in cytoreduction (R0) patients of the TCGA-OV27 dataset, grouped according to sensitivity class. Each column represents a sample and each row a different gene. Colored squares show mutated genes, while grey squares show no mutated genes. Different type of mutations are colored according to the variant type as indicated in the legend at the bottom. Genes annotated as "Multi_Hit" have more than one mutation in the same sample. The barplot at the top shows the number of mutated genes for each patient colored according to the mutation type. The barplot on the right reports the number of mutated patients for each gene, colored according to the mutation type. (**B**) Boxplot showing the tumor mutational load of R and fS samples, calculated both considering only mutations with high/moderate impact (upper panel) or all somatic mutations (lower panel). *P*-value was calculated by Wilcoxon rank-sum test.

We compared the tumor mutational load in the two sensitivity classes considering either only mutations with high/moderate impact (Figure 1B upper panel) or all somatic mutations (Figure 1B lower panel); even if fS patients tend to have a slightly higher number of mutations, we did not detect significant differences between the two classes.

Overall, we identified in at least one sample 1115 variants with high/moderate impact affecting 1005 unique genes. To reduce the high inter-patient heterogeneity of mutational data we grouped genes into pathways and compared pathways mutated in R or fS patients. For this analysis we considered 50 gene sets from the 'Hallmark' collection of MSigDB database that summarize well-defined biological states or processes and ten canonical oncogenic pathways [13]. We called a pathway mutated if at least one of its genes was mutated. According to our analysis, none of the pathways tested was found to be significantly associated to sensitivity class, even at a less stringent nominal p-value < 0.05 (Tables S1 and S2).

3.2. Mutational Signatures of TCGA-OV27 Cohort

Basing on the relative frequency of somatic base substitution events, 30 distinct mutational signatures, reflecting distinct mutational process associated with specific biological status and/or altered functions have been described (COSMIC; https://cancer.sanger.ac.uk/cosmic/signatures) [12]. These mutational signatures were analyzed in the TCGA-OV27 cohort considering all somatic variants independently of their functional consequences. A hierarchical clustering based on the scores of the five most represented mutational signatures identified two major clusters mainly driven by different contribution of Signature 1 (related to endogenous mutational processes) and Signature 3 (related to defective homologous repair of double-strand DNA break). Even if the association between these clusters and sensitivity was not significant (Fisher's exact test p-value = 0.054), we observed a clear trend of enrichment of R patients in the cluster driven by Signature 1 and an enrichment of fS patients in the cluster driven by Signature 3 (Figure 2). The comparison of each signature's score between the two classes is reported in Table S3 and a nominal p-value < 0.05 (Wilcoxon rank-sum test) was observed for Signature 3 only.

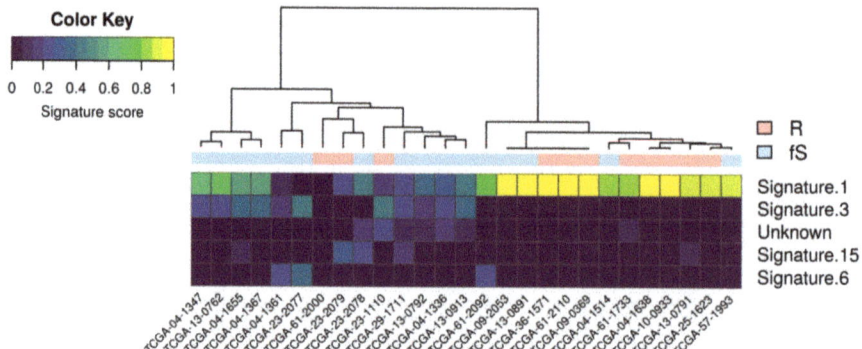

Figure 2. Mutational signatures in TCGA-OV27 cohort. Heatmap showing the contribution of the top-5 most represented COSMIC signatures in the mutational profiles of TCGA-OV27 samples.

3.3. Genomic Instability and sCNA Landscape of TCGA-OV27 Cohort

On the basis of recent studies defining sCNA as the prevalent genomic alteration affecting HGSOC [17], we assessed whether R or fS patients of our selected cohort could be distinguished by specific sCNA.

We used sCNA data to obtain a measure of genomic instability for each patient, using different approaches all based on the GISTIC algorithm. We firstly considered the number of regions with different copy number (number of segments; Figure 3A), with the assumption that a higher number of segments should describe a more fragmented (instable) genome. We next considered within each sample either the total number of genes affected by sCNA (Figure 3B) or, separately, the total number of amplified or deleted genes (Figure 3C,D). Overall, we observed a trend for higher sCNA in fS compared to R patients. This trend was significant when we considered the number of genes affected by aberrations in general (Wilcoxon rank-sum test p-value = 0.03) and this difference was mainly driven by deletions (Wilcoxon rank-sum test p-value = 0.034).

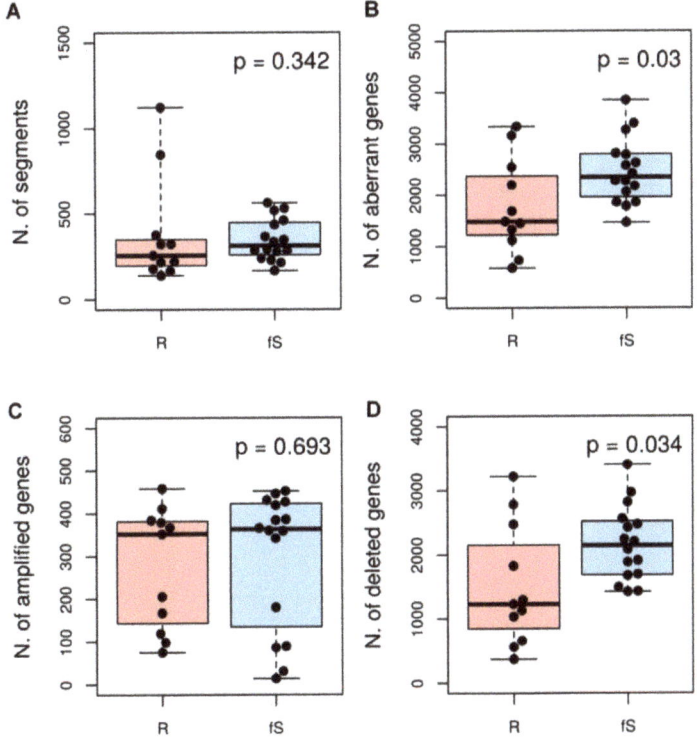

Figure 3. Association between genomic instability and sensitivity class in TCGA-OV27 dataset. As measure of genomic instability for each sample we considered: (**A**) the number of segments that represents the number of regions with different copy number levels within a genome; (**B**) the total number of amplified or deleted genes; the total number of amplified genes only (**C**) or deleted genes only (**D**). *P*-values are according to Wilcoxon rank-sum test.

To identify recurrent sCNA we applied GISTIC to copy number data of the TCGA-OV27 cohort. We identified 10 regions significantly amplified and 12 regions significantly deleted across samples (Figure 4A). All sCNA events, as well as detail in category, chromosome location genes in the region and cytobands are in Table S4.

The frequency plot distribution of sCNA detected in the TCGA-OV27 cohort (Figure 4B), shows that 3q26.2 gain, 17q11.2, 19p13.3, and 4q34.3 loss were the most frequently altered regions (>80% of patients). The frequency of samples positive for the recurrently amplified or deleted regions in the two subgroups (R and fS) of patients is showed in Figure S2. However, when we compared the frequency of the recurrent sCNA identified by GISTIC between the two sensitivity classes, no significant association to Pt-sensitivity was observed (Table S5).

We repeated the analysis of sCNA at the gene level, considering 23110 amplified or deleted genes. Due to the low number of samples available for each class, no significant findings were detected after multiple-testing correction, while we detected 1270 genes more frequently altered at a nominal p-value < 0.05 (Fisher's exact test) in R or fS patients (166 amplified and 1104 genes deleted, Table S6). Considering the explorative nature of this pilot study, we further explored the genes list being aware of the limitations associated with analysis of small group of patients and the high risk of detecting false positive hits (see Materials and Methods, Section 2.5 for power calculation of the present study). Among these genes we observed that amplifications were more frequently detected in R rather than in fS group (median percentage of patients with amplified genes: 57% in R vs 12% in fS; Range: 36–82% in

R group, 0–37% in fS group). On the other side deletions were more frequently detected in fS patients (median percentage of patients with deleted genes: 15% in R vs 62% in fS group; Range: 0–63% in R group, 19–87% in fS group).

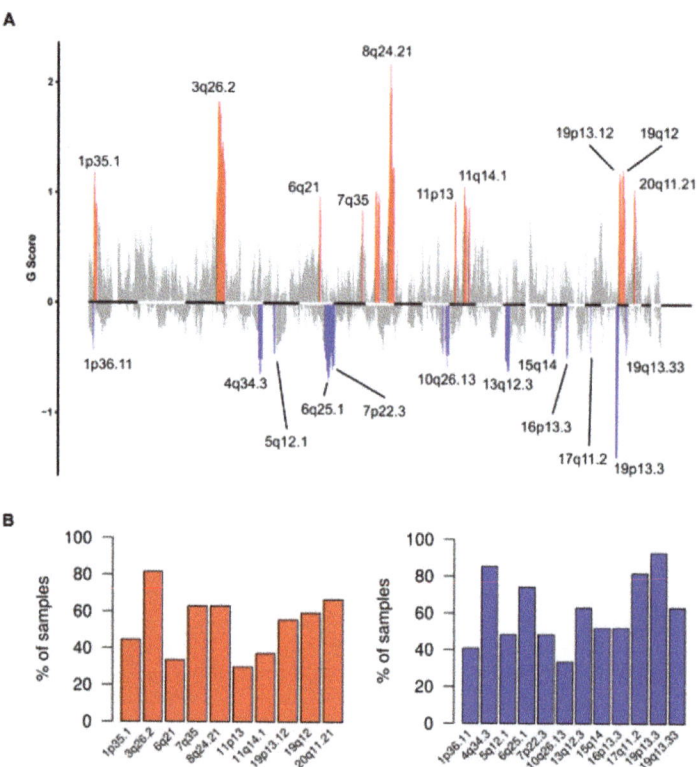

Figure 4. Recurrent somatic copy number alterations (sCNA) in R0 patients of TCGA-OV27 cohort. (**A**) Plot of G scores (defined as the amplitude of the copy number multiplied by its frequency across samples) calculated by Genomic Identification of Significant Targets in Cancer (GISTIC) for genomic regions recurrently amplified (red) or deleted (blue) in the TCGA-OV27 dataset, at an FDR < 0.1. (**B**) Barplot showing the frequency of samples positive for the recurrently amplified (left) or deleted (right) regions identified by GISTIC.

3.4. Association between sCNA and Altered Gene/Pathways Expression in Pt-Sensitivity Classes

We investigated the relationships between sCNA, alteration of genes' expression and relevant functional pathways possibly affected by these alterations.

The complete decision tree for gene selection is shown in Figure 5A. We first removed genes that were not assessed by RNA-Seq from the list of 1270 genes significantly amplified or deleted in R or fS patients. We next filtered this list according to the observed relative frequency of amplification or deletion for each sensitivity class. Finally, we removed genes whose log2 fold change (FC) was not compatible with its copy number status (e.g., a gene preferentially amplified but down-regulated in R group) and among the concordant genes we selected those with a log2 FC of at least 0.5 between R and fS patients. The final gene list included 128 genes (Table S7), consisting of 16 genes preferentially amplified and up-regulated in R group and 112 genes more frequently deleted and down-regulated in fS patients. The relative frequency of associated altered cytobands is reported in Figure 5B. Interestingly, these cytobands were not included among the significantly recurrent aberrant regions identified by GISTIC.

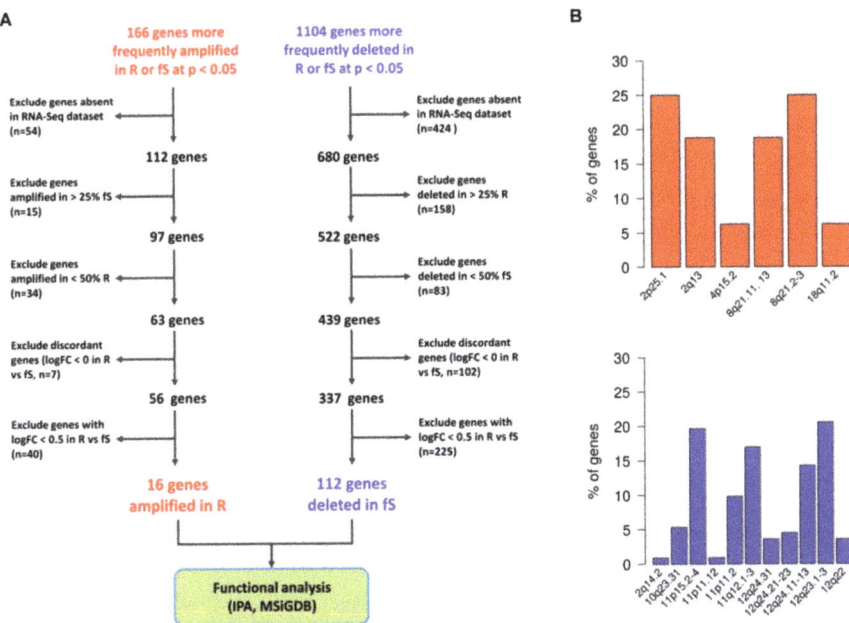

Figure 5. Association between sCNA and altered gene expression in Pt-sensitivity classes. (**A**) Selection of significant focal sCNA with concordant alteration of gene expression. Gene expression was assessed by RNA-sequencing (RNASeq) data, and for each altered gene, the logFC expression ratio of R vs fS patients was calculated. The workflow guiding selection of both amplified and deleted genes with concordant expression is shown. (**B**) Cytobands associated with significant sCNA and altered gene expression. In the plot are reported the cytobands affected by significant amplification (upper panel, red bars) and deletions (lower panel, blue bars). For each type of alteration, the relative frequency of each cytoband affected is shown.

To map the 128 altered genes into known functional pathways we firstly assessed over-representation of Reactome canonical pathways included in the C2 gene set collection of MSiGDB. Seven gene sets, related to interferon (IFN) and cytokine signaling, fatty acid and lipid metabolism, were found significantly over-represented (FDR < 0.05) and 23 out of the 128 genes overlapped with at least one of them (Figure 6).

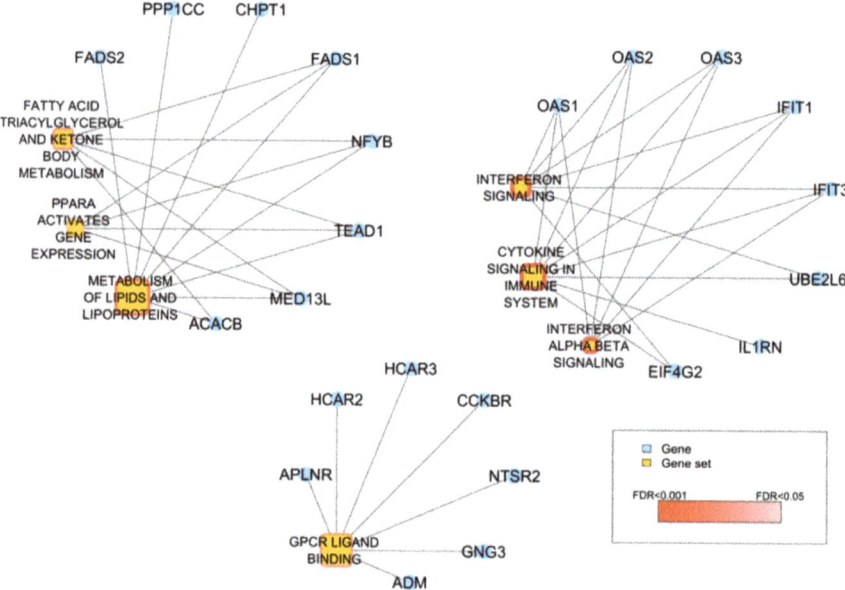

Figure 6. Over-representation analysis of the 128 genes with concordant sCNA and expression. Network showing the 7 Reactome gene sets significantly over-represented in the list of 128 genes. Yellow nodes represent gene sets and the size of the node is proportional to the number of genes catalogued in the gene set. The significance of the over-representation is represented by a dark-to-light red color scale. Blue nodes represent genes and are connected to a gene set if they are among its gene members.

Then, to examine biological relationship and investigate functional effects related to sCNA of these 128 genes, we run Ingenuity Pathway Analysis. Canonical pathways analysis confirmed a significant modulation in IFN signaling, mostly related to IFIT and OAS2 genes deletion, and fatty acid metabolism dependent on alterations in desaturase genes (FADS1 and FADS2). We also observed significant modulation of G-alpha proteins signaling pathways (Table 2). The most significant Regulatory Networks affected by the altered gene expression are listed in Table 3.

Table 2. Canonical Pathways identified by Ingenuity® Pathway Analysis (IPA).

Ingenuity Canonical Pathways	-Log(p-Value)	Genes
Interferon signaling	2.87	OAS1, IFIT1, IFIT3
Oleate biosynthesis II (animals)	2.8	FADS1, FADS2
Graft-versus-host Disease signaling	2.62	IL1RN, IL36RN, FAS
Gαs signaling	2.4	CNGB3, GNG3, HCAR3, HCAR2
γ-linolenate biosynthesis II (animals)	2.33	FADS1, FADS2
Gαi signaling	2.15	APLNR, GNG3, HCAR2, CHRM4

Table 3. Top regulatory networks identified by IPA. Genes detected in the TCGA-OV27 cohort are shown in bold.

Top Diseases and Functions	Molecules in Network	Score	Focus Molecules
Dermatological diseases and conditions, Organismal injury and abnormalities, immunological disease	ACTA2, **ADM**, **APLNR**, Akt, **CCKBR**, **CD6**, ERK, ERK1/2, **FAS**, **GLI2**, **HCAR2**, **IFIT1**, **IFIT3**, **IL1RN**, **ILK**, Interferon alpha, Jnk, **MAPK8IP1**, Mek, NFkB (complex), **OAS1**, **OAS2**, **OAS3**, P38 MAPK, PI3K (family), **PPP1CC**, Raf, SH2B3, **SLC15A3**, **SLC43A3**, TCR, **TRIM22**, **UBE2L6**, **UNG**, **WEE1**	44	24
Gastrointestinal disease, organismal injury and abnormalities, cell death and survival	**ADM**, **AHNAK**, ATG7, C3, CFTR, CLDN7, CST5, CTSS, **DENND5A**, DUSP10, **FADS1**, **FADS2**, HAS1, **HCAR3**, HLA-B, IFNGR1, IL13, IL1B, **IL36RN**, LBP, MAFF, **MS4A4A**, NFKBIE, **NRIP3**, **PQLC3**, **SEL1L3**, **SLC43A3**, SMARCA4, **STK33**, **STMN2**, **SYT7**, TNF, TP63, **TUB**, **WWP1**	27	17
Gene expression, cell cycle, cellular growth and proliferation	ACAD10, BAG1, CBS/CBSL, CCNB2, **CDK17**, **CORO1C**, CTR9, **DCHS1**, ESR1, **FGD6**, **GREB1**, HAUS8, HDAC1, HLTF, LTB, **NEDD1**, **NFYB**, NR1D1, **NR2C1**, NR3C1, NUPR1, PLK1, PRMT6, **SCUBE2**, SMARCE1, SMYD2, SMYD3, SP1, **TBX3**, **TEAD1**, TFAP2C, TNFAIP6, **TRAFD1**, YWHAG, estrogen receptor	19	13
Cellular development, cellular growth and proliferation, cell cycle	CCND1, CDCA2, CDK5, CHD7, **CMKLR1**, Ctbp, **DRAM1**, **E2F5**, ERBB2, **GCN1**, **HCAR1**, **HEY1**, JAG1, LINC-ROR, **LIPF**, MAFB, **MED13L**, NOTCH2, NOTCH4, **NUAK1**, NUMB, OIP5-AS1, PCLAF, PPARGC1A, RFC1, **RMST**, RUNX3, SLC16A1, SMTN, SOX2, SUV39H1, **TMEM119**, **TMPO**, TP53, let-7a-5p	17	12
Gene expression, cell signaling, cellular development	26s Proteasome, **ACACB**, **ACTA2**, AR, **ASCL1**, **ATP6V0D2**, BAG1, CD55, CDK5, **CDKN1C**, **CHRM4**, **CHST1**, CKAP4, DAB2, DLL4, FSH, GBP1, H2AFY, HES1, **HRK**, IER3, **LYVE1**, Lh, MED12, MTOR, NOTCH1, PGR, PRKD1, PRKD2, SMARCE1, **SMTNL1**, **SSH1**, TOP1, **TP53I11**, YWHAB	17	12
DNA replication, recombination, and repair, cell morphology, cellular function and maintenance	ACTG1, **CHPT1**, CLOCK, DDX11, DDX5, **DTX4**, **EIF4G2**, EP300, **FEN1**, GATA1, **HBB**, HNRNPC, HNRNPD, HNRNPU, HUS1, MAX, MYB, **OAS3**, OTUB1, **PARPBP**, PCLAF, PCNA, RAD51, RAD9A, RFC1, RHOA, Rnr, SATB1, **TMEM241**, TP53BP1, TRPV4, **USP44**, **UTP20**, XRN2, YBX1	15	11

The top-scoring Network (Dermatological Diseases and Conditions, Organismal Injury and Abnormalities, Immunological Disease) whose graphical representation is reported in Figure 7, shows a number of molecular relationships centered on interferon, in accordance with previously described pathway analysis. Interestingly, among the top regulatory networks we also identified a number of networks whose functions are mainly related to cell growth and proliferation and cell development. Accordingly, Cellular Development, Cell Morphology, Cellular Growth and Proliferation were the most significantly modulated Molecular Cell Function (Table S8), while Invasion, Migration and Cell Movement were the only Disease and Functions significantly predicted to be increased in R patients (Table S9).

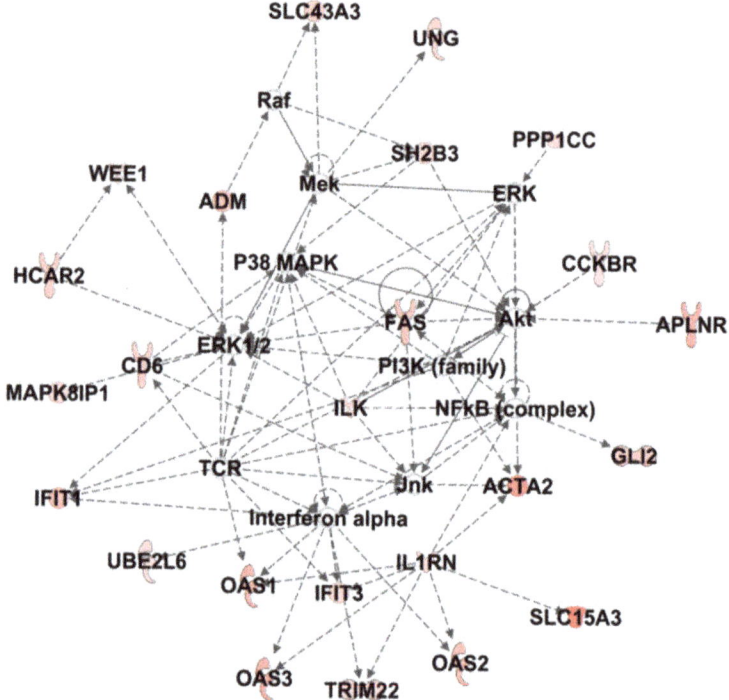

Figure 7. IPA analysis of the 128 significantly altered genes. The top-scoring regulatory network built from Core Analysis and named Dermatological Diseases and Conditions, Organismal Injury and Abnormalities, Immunological Disease is shown. Colored nodes are the genes of the dataset participating to the network.

4. Discussion

The relationship between post-operative residual tumor burden and clinical outcome is consolidated for ovarian cancer [2,18]. Consequently, the concept of optimal cytoreduction is evolving along time and, although the metric for optimal debulking is still defined as tumor nodules not greater than 1 cm, the literature and meta-data analysis clearly show that R0 patients, those with no residual tumor after primary surgery, have the best overall outcome. Nevertheless, some of those R0 patients with an expected favorable clinical outcome still experience early disease relapse, due to intrinsic molecular characteristics of their tumors. We focused our attention on this small, poorly characterized subgroup of patients with an unexpectedly unfavorable prognosis (R patients; PFS < 12 months from surgery). To possibly identify molecular traits associated with Pt-resistant disease in R0 patients we analyzed their genomic portrait in comparison to those of R0 patients with good prognosis (fS patients; PFS > 24 months from surgery).

The approach to compare the gene expression of two series of patients with marked opposite outcomes, with the assumption that this selection may enhance discovering relevant molecular pathways associated to sensitivity to pt- or cetuximab/pt-based treatment was previously applied with some success to small cohorts of gastric [19] and head and neck cancers [20]. Comparison of transcriptomes in the two R0 HGSOC Pt-sensitivity classes, showed in R patients modifications that could be commonly referred to an increased aggressiveness of tumors but were not directly suggestive of specific actionable alterations. Similarly, the mutational profile of the R0 cohort did not substantially differ from the overall TCGA study population, where, apart the prevalent p53 mutation, few other genes were commonly mutated and in a small fraction of patients, thus confirming the high mutational heterogeneity of this tumor type. Also, none of these prevalently mutated genes was significantly associated with Pt-sensitivity classes. Interestingly, from the overall analysis of the somatic mutational status we did not observe any enrichment for BRCA1/2 mutations in the fS group and not all fS patients were characterized by mutational Signature 3 related to defective Homologous Repair of double-strand DNA breaks. These findings are substantially in agreement with recent data obtained on long term survivor ovarian cancer patients [15] where the authors propose that the BRCA-associated signature alone could not be prognostic of Pt-sensitivity in HGSOC. Nevertheless, the analysis of genomic instability in our R0 cohort disclosed a higher number of sCNA in fS patients as compared to R ones. Since genomic instability can be attributed to defects in HR pathway [21] these data are in accordance with the observed enrichment of fS patient in the cluster characterized by mutational Signature 3 and overall support their Pt-sensitivity. This trend appeared to be mainly driven by deletions rather than amplification, in accordance with data obtained from focal (gene-level) sCNA analysis, which described deletions as the prominent event distinctive of the fS group. At the same time these observations confirm that the maintenance of potential oncogenic pro-survival functions is a requirement for Pt-resistance and, concordantly, their inactivation might be an opportunity to overcome Pt-resistance. Noteworthy, the sCNA profile of the R0, fS patients of the TCGA-OV27 cohort appeared to be different from the HR-deficient TCGA-OV cohort [5], possibly because of the specific molecular setting of R0 tumors, which have been shown to be intrinsically different from those ovarian tumors more massively diffused in the peritoneal cavity and less-likely to be completely removed at primary surgery [22].

sCNA are known drivers of HGSOC development and progression [17]. Interestingly, in a recent paper studying the spatial and temporal heterogeneity of HGSOC [23], the authors suggest that in this tumor type the relapsed disease is mostly related to the emergence of pre-existing rather than de-novo clones and observe that sCNA maintain a low level of intra-patient heterogeneity. Therefore, sCNA analysis promises to be an effective strategy to identify cancer-causing genes, which could be used for treatment decisions. Accordingly, Cyclin E (CCNE1) amplification is a known trait in ovarian cancers with intact HR. It occurs in around 20% of all HGSOC and since it is mutually exclusive with BRCA1/2 mutation [24], patients harboring CCNE1 amplification will not benefit from PARPi treatment and will likely be less responsive to Pt treatment [5,17]. Nevertheless, these finding provided the rationale for the development of therapeutic approach that specifically exploit the tumor dependence upon CCNE1 amplification, for instance by targeting CDK2 and AKT activities [25].

CCNE1 locates on chr19q12 cytoband, which we identified to be amplified in the whole TCGA-OV27 cohort. However, possibly due to the small number of samples analyzed, we did not identify any significant enrichment of 19q12 amplification in the R subgroup of patients and, concordantly, we did not have any evidence about significant enrichment of CCNE1 amplification in the same subgroup when we performed the analysis at gene-level. Of note, none of the cytobands identified as significantly altered in both R and fS class of R0 patients at gene level is comprised in the recurrent chromosomal aberrations identified and only 5 genes (FAS, HEY1, SH2B3, TBX3, USP44) were included in the COSMIC (Catalogue of Somatic Mutations in Cancer) Cancer Gene Census list, suggesting that new information can be acquired with this approach.

Among these newly identified genes, we found HEY1, to be amplified in the R group. Interestingly, HEY1 is a downstream mediator of Notch-dependent signals [26], it has a putative role as oncogene (COSMIC) and its expression was recently associated with an EMT phenotype, increased invasion and cell migration as well as Pt resistance in head and neck cancers [27]. These observations are in agreement with IPA describing a predicted increase in functions (cell growth and proliferation and cell development) overall suggestive of a stemness program. Also, Notch1 signaling pathway has been described to contribute to chemoresistance in ovarian cancer [28], it is a key for maintenance of cancer stem cell in ovarian cancer [29] and the development of new treatment strategies targeting these pathways to control stem-cell replication is a current active field of research.

Pt-resistance is recognized to be a multifactorial event and the search for determinants (genes) guiding response to Pt treatments still continues to be a key issue in ovarian cancer translational research. In this context, it has been proven the involvement of aberrant DNA methylation and modification of histone marks [17,30] in the development of Pt-resistance and a number of synthetically lethal approaches are under investigation, with cell cycle check points (CHK1, Wee1, DNA-PK) and related cyclins inhibitors being among the most promising (see [31,32] for an overview).

To our knowledge, this is the first study of R0 HGSOC that specifically investigates sensitivity to Pt-based therapy by transcriptomics and genomics analyses and biology behind. We are aware that our study has to be considered explorative. The major limit rests in the small number of samples included in the TCGA-OV27 cohort, which account for about 6% of the entire TCGA-OV cohort. This limitation is inherently related to the reduced number of ovarian cancer patients having these clinical characteristics and with full molecular data available. The statistical power of our analyses is constrained to 2.4% by the sample size of the TCGA-OV27 cohort, which should triplicate to endow a statistical significance. Our results should be interpreted with caution. Nevertheless, the overall data presented here, based on tumors with marked opposite treatment outcomes, are suggestive of a specific Pt-resistance molecular trait driven by sCNA, and these observations deserve to be further explored in wider cohort of patients with selected clinical characteristics. If verified and upon appropriate independent validation, it could possibly drive toward the development of a new tool based on the sCNA pattern, which may help clinicians in defining sensitivity to Pt treatment.

Supplementary Materials: The following are available online at http://www.mdpi.com/2073-4425/10/9/678/s1, Figure S1: Enrichment plots of hallmark gene sets significantly enriched at an FDR < 0.01. Gene sets were tested against the list of genes ranked according to their differential expression significance and fold change, from the most up-regulated to the most down-regulated in R versus fS. The Gene Ranks column shows the location of the genes of each gene set along the pre-ranked gene list. NES: normalized enrichment score; padj: adjusted p-value (FDR). Figure S2: Barplot showing for each sensitivity class the frequency of samples positive for the recurrently amplified (left panel) or deleted (right panel) regions identified by GISTIC. Table S1. Association between mutated hallmark gene sets and sensitivity class. P-value by Fisher's exact test. FDR: false discovery rate. Table S2. Association between mutated oncogenic pathways and sensitivity class. P-value by Fisher's exact test. FDR: false discovery rate. Table S3. Association between mutational signatures scores of the top-5 most represented COSMIC signatures and sensitivity class. P-value by Wilcoxon rank-sum test. FDR: false discovery rate. Table S4. Recurrently amplified or deleted regions in the TCGA-OV27 dataset identified by GISTIC. Table S5. Association of recurrently amplified or deleted regions identified by GISTIC and sensitivity class. P-value by Fisher's exact test. FDR: false discovery rate. Table S6. Association of copy number status at the gene level and sensitivity class. P-value by Fisher's exact test. Table S7. List of the 128 genes selected after integration of sCNA and RNA-Seq data. Table S8. IPA on 128 genes list. Molecular cell functions significantly modulated Table S9. Prediction of Disease and Function activation state by IPA on 128 genes list.

Author Contributions: Conceptualization: M.D.; M.S. and M.B.; Formal Analysis: M.D., A.D. and M.B.; Data Curation, M.D., A.D. and L.D.C.; Writing—Original Draft Preparation, M.B, M.D., A.D.; Writing—Review and Editing. M.S., D.M., E.C., M.D. and M.B.; Supervision: D.M., M.S. All authors read and approved the final manuscript.

Funding: This research was funded by Italian Ministry of Health 5 x 1000 Funds—2010 program; epithelial ovarian cancer subproject to MB and Italian Ministry of Health (5 x 1000 Funds—2013) to MB.

Acknowledgments: We thank Silvana Canevari (Fondazione IRCCS Istituto Nazionale dei Tumori Milano, Italy) for fruitful discussion and critical reading of the manuscript.

Conflicts of Interest: The authors declare no conflict of interest. The funders had no role in the design of the study; in the collection, analyses, or interpretation of data; in the writing of the manuscript, or in the decision to publish the results.

References

1. Siegel, R.L.; Miller, K.D.; Jemal, A. Cancer statistics, 2019. *CA Cancer J. Clin.* **2019**, *69*, 7–34. [CrossRef] [PubMed]
2. Jayson, G.C.; Kohn, E.C.; Kitchener, H.C.; Ledermann, J.A. Ovarian cancer. *Lancet* **2014**, *384*, 1376–1388. [CrossRef]

3. Lheureux, S.; Gourley, C.; Vergote, I.; Oza, A.M. Epithelial ovarian cancer. *Lancet* **2019**, *393*, 1240–1253. [CrossRef]
4. Ciriello, G.; Miller, M.L.; Aksoy, B.A.; Senbabaoglu, Y.; Schultz, N.; Sander, C. Emerging landscape of oncogenic signatures across human cancers. *Nat. Genet.* **2013**, *45*, 1127–1133. [CrossRef] [PubMed]
5. Cancer Genome Atlas Research Network. Integrated genomic analyses of ovarian carcinoma. *Nature* **2011**, *474*, 609–615. [CrossRef]
6. Robinson, M.D.; Oshlack, A. A scaling normalization method for differential expression analysis of RNA-seq data. *Genome Biol.* **2010**, *11*, R25. [CrossRef] [PubMed]
7. Robinson, M.D.; McCarthy, D.J.; Smyth, G.K. edgeR: A Bioconductor package for differential expression analysis of digital gene expression data. *Bioinformatics* **2010**, *26*, 139–140. [CrossRef]
8. Law, C.W.; Chen, Y.; Shi, W.; Smyth, G.K. voom: Precision weights unlock linear model analysis tools for RNA-seq read counts. *Genome Biol.* **2014**, *15*, R29. [CrossRef]
9. Subramanian, A.; Tamayo, P.; Mootha, V.K.; Mukherjee, S.; Ebert, B.L.; Gillette, M.A.; Paulovich, A.; Pomeroy, S.L.; Golub, T.R.; Lander, E.S.; et al. Gene set enrichment analysis: A knowledge-based approach for interpreting genome-wide expression profiles. *Proc. Natl. Acad. Sci. USA* **2005**, *102*, 17745–17750. [CrossRef]
10. Mayakonda, A.; Lin, D.C.; Assenov, Y.; Plass, C.; Koeffler, H.P. Maftools: Efficient and comprehensive analysis of somatic variants in cancer. *Genome Res.* **2018**, *28*, 1747–1756. [CrossRef]
11. Rosenthal, R.; McGranahan, N.; Herrero, J.; Taylor, B.S.; Swanton, C. DeconstructSigs: Delineating mutational processes in single tumors distinguishes DNA repair deficiencies and patterns of carcinoma evolution. *Genome Biol.* **2016**, *17*, 31. [CrossRef] [PubMed]
12. Alexandrov, L.B.; Nik-Zainal, S.; Wedge, D.C.; Aparicio, S.A.; Behjati, S.; Biankin, A.V.; Bignell, G.R.; Bolli, N.; Borg, A.; Borresen-Dale, A.L.; et al. Signatures of mutational processes in human cancer. *Nature* **2013**, *500*, 415–421. [CrossRef] [PubMed]
13. Sanchez-Vega, F.; Mina, M.; Armenia, J.; Chatila, W.K.; Luna, A.; La, K.C.; Dimitriadoy, S.; Liu, D.L.; Kantheti, H.S.; Saghafinia, S.; et al. Oncogenic signaling pathways in The Cancer Genome Atlas. *Cell* **2018**, *173*, 321–337. [CrossRef] [PubMed]
14. Mermel, C.H.; Schumacher, S.E.; Hill, B.; Meyerson, M.L.; Beroukhim, R.; Getz, G. GISTIC2.0 facilitates sensitive and confident localization of the targets of focal somatic copy-number alteration in human cancers. *Genome Biol.* **2011**, *12*, R41. [CrossRef] [PubMed]
15. Yang, S.Y.C.; Lheureux, S.; Karakasis, K.; Burnier, J.V.; Bruce, J.P.; Clouthier, D.L.; Danesh, A.; Quevedo, R.; Dowar, M.; Hanna, Y.; et al. Landscape of genomic alterations in high-grade serous ovarian cancer from exceptional long- and short-term survivors. *Genome Med.* **2018**, *10*, 81. [CrossRef] [PubMed]
16. Macintyre, G.; Goranova, T.E.; De, S.D.; Ennis, D.; Piskorz, A.M.; Eldridge, M.; Sie, D.; Lewsley, L.A.; Hanif, A.; Wilson, C.; et al. Copy number signatures and mutational processes in ovarian carcinoma. *Nat. Genet.* **2018**, *50*, 1262–1270. [CrossRef]
17. Patch, A.M.; Christie, E.L.; Etemadmoghadam, D.; Garsed, D.W.; George, J.; Fereday, S.; Nones, K.; Cowin, P.; Alsop, K.; Bailey, P.J.; et al. Whole-genome characterization of chemoresistant ovarian cancer. *Nature* **2015**, *521*, 489–494. [CrossRef]
18. Nick, A.M.; Coleman, R.L.; Ramirez, P.T.; Sood, A.K. A framework for a personalized surgical approach to ovarian cancer. *Nat. Rev. Clin. Oncol.* **2015**, *12*, 239–245. [CrossRef] [PubMed]
19. Lo, N.C.; Monteverde, M.; Riba, M.; Lattanzio, L.; Tonissi, F.; Garrone, O.; Heouaine, A.; Gallo, F.; Ceppi, M.; Borghi, F.; et al. Expression profiling and long lasting responses to chemotherapy in metastatic gastric cancer. *Int. J. Oncol.* **2010**, *37*, 1219–1228.
20. Bossi, P.; Bergamini, C.; Siano, M.; Cossu, R.M.; Sponghini, A.P.; Favales, F.; Giannoccaro, M.; Marchesi, E.; Cortelazzi, B.; Perrone, F.; et al. Functional genomics uncover the biology behind the responsiveness of head and neck squamous cell cancer patients to cetuximab. *Clin. Cancer Res.* **2016**, *22*, 3961–3970. [CrossRef]
21. Negrini, S.; Gorgoulis, V.G.; Halazonetis, T.D. Genomic instability—An evolving hallmark of cancer. *Nat. Rev. Mol. Cell Biol.* **2010**, *11*, 220–228. [CrossRef] [PubMed]
22. Riester, M.; Wei, W.; Waldron, L.; Culhane, A.C.; Trippa, L.; Oliva, E.; Kim, S.H.; Michor, F.; Huttenhower, C.; Parmigiani, G.; et al. Risk prediction for late-stage ovarian cancer by meta-analysis of 1525 patient samples. *J. Natl. Cancer Inst.* **2014**, *106*. [CrossRef] [PubMed]

23. Ballabio, S.; Craparotta, I.; Paracchini, L.; Mannarino, L.; Corso, S.; Pezzotta, M.G.; Vescio, M.; Fruscio, R.; Romualdi, C.; Dainese, E.; et al. Multisite analysis of high-grade serous epithelial ovarian cancers identifies genomic regions of focal and recurrent copy number alteration in 3q26.2 and 8q24.3. *Int. J. Cancer* **2019**. [CrossRef] [PubMed]
24. Etemadmoghadam, D.; Weir, B.A.; Au-Yeung, G.; Alsop, K.; Mitchell, G.; George, J.; Davis, S.; D'Andrea, A.D.; Simpson, K.; Hahn, W.C.; et al. Synthetic lethality between *CCNE1* amplification and loss of *BRCA1*. *Proc. Natl. Acad. Sci. USA* **2013**, *110*, 19489–19494. [CrossRef] [PubMed]
25. Au-Yeung, G.; Lang, F.; Azar, W.J.; Mitchell, C.; Jarman, K.E.; Lackovic, K.; Aziz, D.; Cullinane, C.; Pearson, R.B.; Mileshkin, L.; et al. Selective targeting of Cyclin E1-amplified high-grade serous ovarian cancer by cyclin-dependent kinase 2 and AKT inhibition. *Clin. Cancer Res.* **2017**, *23*, 1862–1874. [CrossRef]
26. Belandia, B.; Powell, S.M.; Garcia-Pedrero, J.M.; Walker, M.M.; Bevan, C.L.; Parker, M.G. Hey1, a mediator of notch signaling, is an androgen receptor corepressor. *Mol. Cell Biol.* **2005**, *25*, 1425–1436. [CrossRef]
27. Fukusumi, T.; Guo, T.W.; Sakai, A.; Ando, M.; Ren, S.; Haft, S.; Liu, C.; Amornphimoltham, P.; Gutkind, J.S.; Califano, J.A. The NOTCH4-HEY1 pathway induces epithelial-mesenchymal transition in head and neck squamous cell carcinoma. *Clin. Cancer Res.* **2018**, *24*, 619–633. [CrossRef]
28. Chen, C.; Wang, X.; Huang, S.; Wang, L.; Han, L.; Yu, S. Prognostic roles of Notch receptor mRNA expression in human ovarian cancer. *Oncotarget* **2017**, *8*, 32731–32740. [CrossRef]
29. Venkatesh, V.; Nataraj, R.; Thangaraj, G.S.; Karthikeyan, M.; Gnanasekaran, A.; Kaginelli, S.B.; Kuppanna, G.; Kallappa, C.G.; Basalingappa, K.M. Targeting Notch signalling pathway of cancer stem cells. *Stem Cell Investig.* **2018**, *5*, 5. [CrossRef]
30. Fang, F.; Cardenas, H.; Huang, H.; Jiang, G.; Perkins, S.M.; Zhang, C.; Keer, H.N.; Liu, Y.; Nephew, K.P.; Matei, D. Genomic and epigenomic signatures in ovarian cancer associated with resensitization to platinum drugs. *Cancer Res.* **2018**, *78*, 631–644. [CrossRef]
31. Brown, J.S.; O'Carrigan, B.; Jackson, S.P.; Yap, T.A. Targeting DNA repair in cancer: Beyond PARP inhibitors. *Cancer Discov.* **2017**, *7*, 20–37. [CrossRef] [PubMed]
32. Gourley, C.; Balmana, J.; Ledermann, J.A.; Serra, V.; Dent, R.; Loibl, S.; Pujade-Lauraine, E.; Boulton, S.J. Moving from poly (ADP-Ribose) polymerase inhibition to targeting DNA repair and DNA damage response in cancer therapy. *J. Clin. Oncol.* **2019**. [CrossRef] [PubMed]

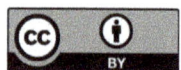

© 2019 by the authors. Licensee MDPI, Basel, Switzerland. This article is an open access article distributed under the terms and conditions of the Creative Commons Attribution (CC BY) license (http://creativecommons.org/licenses/by/4.0/).

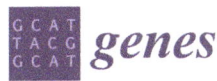

Article

Outcome Definition Influences the Relationship between Genetic Polymorphisms of *ERCC1*, *ERCC2*, *SLC22A2* and Cisplatin Nephrotoxicity in Adult Testicular Cancer Patients

Zulfan Zazuli [1,2,3], Leila S. Otten [3], Britt I. Drögemöller [4,5], Mara Medeiros [6,7], Jose G. Monzon [8], Galen E. B. Wright [4,9], Christian K. Kollmannsberger [10], Philippe L. Bedard [11], Zhuo Chen [12], Karen A. Gelmon [10], Nicole McGoldrick [13], Abhijat Kitchlu [14], Susanne J. H. Vijverberg [1], Rosalinde Masereeuw [3], Colin J. D. Ross [4,5], Geoffrey Liu [12], Bruce C. Carleton [13,15,†] and Anke H. Maitland-van der Zee [1,†,*]

1. Department of Respiratory Medicine, Amsterdam University Medical Centers, University of Amsterdam, 1105 AZ Amsterdam, The Netherlands; z.zazuli@amc.uva.nl (Z.Z.); s.j.vijverberg@amsterdamumc.nl (S.J.H.V.)
2. Department of Pharmacology-Clinical Pharmacy, School of Pharmacy, Bandung Institute of Technology, Bandung 40132, Indonesia
3. Division of Pharmacology, Utrecht Institute for Pharmaceutical Sciences, Utrecht University, 3512 JE Utrecht, The Netherlands; l.s.otten@students.uu.nl (L.S.O.); R.Masereeuw@uu.nl (R.M.)
4. British Columbia Children's Hospital Research Institute, Vancouver, BC V5Z 4H4, Canada; bdrogemoller@cmmt.ubc.ca (B.I.D.); gwright@cmmt.ubc.ca (G.E.B.W.); colin.ross@ubc.ca (C.J.D.R.)
5. Faculty of Pharmaceutical Sciences, The University of British Columbia, Vancouver, BC V6T 1Z4, Canada
6. Nephrology Research Unit, Hospital Infantil de México Federico Gómez, Mexico City 06720, Mexico; medeiro.mara@gmail.com
7. Departamento de Farmacología, Facultad de Medicina, Universidad Nacional Autónoma de México, Mexico City 04510, Mexico
8. Department of Medical Oncology, Tom Baker Cancer Centre, Calgary, AB T2N 4N2, Canada; jgmonzon@ucalgary.ca
9. Department of Medical Genetics, University of British Columbia, Vancouver, BC V6T 1Z4, Canada
10. BC Cancer Agency and University of British Columbia, Vancouver, BC V6T 1Z4, Canada; ckollmannsberger@bccancer.bc.ca (C.K.K.); kgelmon@bccancer.bc.ca (K.A.G.)
11. Princess Margaret Cancer Centre and University of Toronto, Toronto, ON M5S, Canada; philippe.bedard@uhn.ca
12. Medical Oncology and Hematology, Department of Medicine, Princess Margaret Cancer Centre-University Health Network and University of Toronto, Toronto, ON M5S, Canada; Zhuo.Chen@uhnresearch.ca (Z.C.); Geoffrey.Liu@uhn.ca (G.L.)
13. Pharmaceutical Outcomes Programme, BC Children's Hospital, Vancouver, BC V6H 3N1, Canada; nicolemcgoldrick@hotmail.com (N.M.); bcarleton@popi.ubc.ca (B.C.C.)
14. Division of Nephrology, Department of Medicine, University Health Network and University of Toronto, Toronto, ON M5S, Canada; Abhijat.Kitchlu@uhn.ca
15. Division of Translational Therapeutics, Department of Pediatrics, Faculty of Medicine, University of British Columbia, Vancouver, BC V6T 1Z4, Canada
* Correspondence: a.h.maitland@amsterdamumc.nl; Tel.: +31-(0)20-566-8137
† These authors contributed equally to this work.

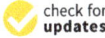

Received: 16 April 2019; Accepted: 7 May 2019; Published: 10 May 2019

Abstract: Although previous research identified candidate genetic polymorphisms associated with cisplatin nephrotoxicity, varying outcome definitions potentially contributed to the variability in the effect size and direction of this relationship. We selected genetic variants that have been significantly associated with cisplatin-induced nephrotoxicity in more than one published study (*SLC22A2* rs316019; *ERCC1* rs11615 and rs3212986; *ERCC2* rs1799793 and rs13181) and performed a replication analysis to confirm associations between these genetic polymorphisms and cisplatin nephrotoxicity using various outcome definitions. We included 282 germ cell testicular cancer patients treated with cisplatin from 2009–2014, aged >17 years recruited by the Canadian Pharmacogenomics Network for Drug Safety. Nephrotoxicity was defined using four grading tools: (1) Common Terminology Criteria for Adverse Events (CTCAE) v4.03 for acute kidney injury (AKI) or CTCAE-AKI; (2) adjusted cisplatin-induced AKI; (3) elevation of serum creatinine; and (4) reduction in the estimated glomerular filtration rate (eGFR). Significant associations were only found when using the CTCAE v4.03 definition: genotype CA of the *ERCC1* rs3212986 was associated with decreased risk of cisplatin nephrotoxicity (OR_{adj} = 0.24; 95% CI: 0.08–0.70; p = 0.009) compared to genotype CC. In contrast, addition of allele A at *SLC22A2* rs316019 was associated with increased risk (OR_{adj} = 4.41; 95% CI: 1.96–9.88; p < 0.001) while genotype AC was associated with a higher risk of cisplatin nephrotoxicity (OR_{adj} = 5.06; 95% CI: 1.69–15.16; p = 0.004) compared to genotype CC. Our study showed that different case definitions led to variability in the genetic risk ascertainment of cisplatin nephrotoxicity. Therefore, consensus on a set of clinically relevant outcome definitions that all such studies should follow is needed.

Keywords: pharmacogenetics; cisplatin; nephrotoxicity; kidney injury; genetic polymorphisms

---

1. Introduction

Cisplatin remains one of the most widely prescribed antineoplastic therapies due to its effectiveness as a component of first-line regimens against various types of cancers, including carcinomas, germ cell tumours, lymphomas and sarcomas [1,2]. In Europe, the 1- and 5-years survival rate in testicular cancer patients was 98% and 97%, respectively [3]. However, the dose-limiting toxicities of cisplatin, such as nausea and vomiting, hematotoxicity, ototoxicity and nephrotoxicity, hinder its potential antineoplastic effect. Nephrotoxicity is the most prevalent of these adverse effects caused by cisplatin, resulting in a two-fold risk of acute kidney injury and an increase in serum creatinine levels [4,5]. Approximately one third of all patients treated with cisplatin develop renal dysfunction after a single dosage of cisplatin (50–100 mg/m^2) [6]. In addition, concerns about long-term renal side effects are rising especially in cancers that occur in young patients and have a high chance of being successfully treated such as testicular cancer [7]. A previous study suggested that circulating platinum is still detectable in the plasma of testicular cancer survivors even 20 years after the last administration of cisplatin [8].

Cisplatin is mainly excreted through the kidneys. Therefore, renal tubular injury is a common clinical manifestation of cisplatin accumulation in renal tubular cells. Cisplatin levels in tubular epithelial cells may increase up to five times higher levels than blood levels [9]. After uptake via organic cation transporter 2 (OCT2) and high-affinity copper transporter 1 (CTR1) in the renal tubules, multiple mechanisms lead to cytotoxicity: complex intracellular pathways lead to DNA damage and cell death and an inflammatory response speeds up renal damage even more [10]. Cisplatin may induce vascular injury as well, which accelerates tubular cell death. These multifactorial processes lead to tubular necrosis and eventually loss of kidney function [10]. This loss of function manifests itself in multiple ways: acute kidney injury (as measured by decreased glomerular filtration rate (GFR)), decreased magnesium and potassium levels and increased serum creatinine (SCr) are paramount but cisplatin may also cause hypocalcaemia, renal salt wasting and even chronic kidney disease [10]. Various patient-related (e.g., age, gender, chronic comorbid illness, pre-existing kidney disease) and treatment-related factors (cisplatin dose per cycle, cumulative dosage, hydration) have been associated with cisplatin nephrotoxicity [11]. In addition, previous studies also suggest that variations in genes involved in cisplatin pharmacodynamics and pharmacokinetics contribute to cisplatin nephrotoxicity [12–18].

Genetic variations have been reported to play a role both as protective and as risk factors for cisplatin nephrotoxicity. In a recent systematic review we reported that variants in *ERCC1*, *ERCC2* and *SLC22A2* genes were associated with cisplatin nephrotoxicity and replicated in at least one other study [19]. *ERCC1* and *ERCC2* polymorphisms have been associated with alterations of DNA repair process in cells [20–22] including possibly the nephron following cisplatin exposure [19]. In addition, *ERCC1* polymorphisms may alter cell sensitivity to cisplatin [23]. Polymorphisms in *SLC22A2*, a gene which product is the organic cation transporter OCT2 responsible for cellular cisplatin uptake in renal proximal tubule cells [24,25], affects the severity of tubular injury process due to cisplatin accumulation. However, variability in effect size and direction of association have been reported. Consequently, this complicates the understanding of the true impact of genetic variants. Differences in clinical characteristics for example, age, type of cancer, cisplatin dose and ethnicity might be related to variability of results. We expect that differences in how cisplatin nephrotoxicity is defined contribute to the variability in results as no widely accepted single cisplatin nephrotoxicity definition exists.

Our aim is to validate the use of already associated genetic variants to predict cisplatin nephrotoxicity and to determine if different cisplatin nephrotoxicity definitions contributed to the variability in effect size and direction of already published associations between these genetic polymorphisms and cisplatin nephrotoxicity. This approach was important to highlight the need of consensus on a set of clinically relevant cisplatin nephrotoxicity definitions that future studies is able to follow.

2. Materials and Methods

This study is reported according to Strengthening the Reporting of Genetic Association Studies (STREGA) guidelines [26].

2.1. Study Design and Participants

The retrospective study included males (≥17 years old) diagnosed with germ cell testicular cancer treated with cisplatin between January 1979 and February 2013. These patients were part of a previously conducted study on cisplatin-induced adverse events and were recruited through the Canadian Pharmacogenomics Network for Drug Safety (CPNDS) in multiple Canadian centres in Ontario and British Columbia from 2009–2013 [27].

Patients were included if they had normal kidney function, were treatment-naïve and had received 100 mg/m^2 cisplatin per cycle. Patients suffering from other diseases than testicular cancer, non-genotyped patients, patients with pre-existing electrolyte disorders or patients that had received abdominal radiation were excluded from this study. All subjects gave their informed consent for inclusion prior their participation in the study. The study was conducted in accordance with the Declaration of Helsinki and the protocol was approved by the UBC C&W Research Ethics Board (ethics certificate no. H04-70358).

2.2. Clinical Data Collection

Information concerning co-medication, chemotherapy protocols, duration of the treatment, cumulative dosage of platinum, serum magnesium levels (Mg), serum potassium levels (K), serum sodium levels (Na), serum phosphate levels (PO4) and serum creatinine (SCr) levels was obtained from the medical records. The glomerular filtration rate (GFR) was not available in all patient records. Therefore, estimated glomerular filtration rate (eGFR) was calculated using the CKD-EPI equation [28] as per the KDIGO recommendation [29].

Only cisplatin-induced nephrotoxicity related variables were included as covariates in our analysis (i.e., disease-related variables were excluded). Height and body weight were not included as covariates, as the dosage was already adjusted for this (mg/m^2). Alcohol consumption, family history of cancer, prior surgery and albumin levels were not available in the medical records and were therefore not be included in the genetic association analyses. All patients in our cohort were cisplatin-naïve at the time of testicular cancer diagnosis.

Age was calculated at the start date of cisplatin treatment. Ethnicity was analysed through ancestry proportions and principal components (PCs) using EIGENSOFT v.5.0 (Harvard and Massachusetts Institute of Technology, Cambridge, MA, USA) and ADMIXTURE. Cardiovascular disease and diabetes data were not available in the database and were for that reason determined based on co-medications [30–34]. Potentially nephrotoxic co-medications were identified from the start until the end date of cisplatin treatment and grouped according to their mechanism of action [35]. The amount of hydration depended on standardized chemotherapy regimen and was derived from Canadian protocols for testicular cancer [36,37]. Cumulative dose was assessed and where carboplatin had been substituted for cisplatin, a conversion factor of 1:4 for cisplatin: carboplatin was used [1,38]. For the baseline SCr and electrolyte measurement, the measurement closest to the start date within 30 days prior to start was taken.

2.3. Outcome Definition

To assess the relationship between cisplatin-induced nephrotoxicity and genetic variants, multiple outcomes were studied. Multiple outcomes were used to determine if different cisplatin nephrotoxicity definitions contributed to the variability in effect size and direction of already published associations between these genetic polymorphisms and cisplatin nephrotoxicity. A new tailored definition for cisplatin-induced nephrotoxicity was formulated based on expert opinions to optimize clinical relevance (see below "Adjusted Acute Kidney Injury" Outcome Definition). Since the results for this definition were not comparable with previously published studies, CTCAE-AKI grading and the differences in SCr and eGFR before and after cisplatin-treatment (ΔSCr and ΔeGFR) were assessed as well.

2.3.1. "Adjusted Acute Kidney Injury" (Adjusted-AKI) Outcome Definition

The definition of cisplatin-induced nephrotoxicity combines SCr-based staging and electrolyte disturbances (i.e., National Cancer Institute Common Terminology Criteria for Adverse Events (NCI-CTCAE) v.4.03 definitions for electrolyte disturbances) [39] (Table 1). Measurements from start date up to 90 days after the end of cisplatin treatment were collected. The measurement closest to the start date with a cut-off of 30 days was taken as the baseline value when calculating the increase in SCr.

Hyperhydration during administration may cause a hypervolemic state which may provoke hyponatremia [40]. To increase sensitivity and decrease false-positive or overestimated results, hyponatremia must have persisted for longer than two consecutive months. For further statistical analyses, these categories were divided into case, control and ambiguous groups (Table 2). Two separate investigators designated the patients in one of three categories and discrepancies were resolved through discussion between a clinical pharmacologist and nephrologist.

Table 1. Adjusted Acute Kidney Injury (Adjusted-AKI) grading.

Grade	Definition	Characteristic(s)
0	An increase in serum creatinine, up to 1.5 times baseline value AND Electrolyte disorders grade 0 CTCAE: • Hypomagnesemia: ≥LLN–1.2 mg/dL; <LLN–0.5 mmol/L, OR • Hypokalaemia: ≥LLN–3.0 mmol/L, OR • Hypophosphatemia: ≥LLN–2.5 mg/dL; <LLN–0.8 mmol/L, OR • Hyponatremia: ≥LLN–130 mmol/L (>2 months)	Asymptomatic
1	Between 1.5–1.9 times baseline SCr OR ≥0.3 mg/dL (≥26.5 µmol/L) increase in SCr OR Electrolyte disorders grade 1 CTCAE: • Hypomagnesemia: <LLN–1.2 mg/dL; <LLN–0.5 mmol/L, OR • Hypokalaemia: <LLN–3.0 mmol/L, OR • Hypophosphatemia: <LLN–2.5 mg/dL; <LLN–0.8 mmol/L, OR • Hyponatremia: <LLN–130 mmol/L (>2 months)	Possible Symptomatic
2	An increase in serum creatinine between 2.0–2.9 times baseline SCr ORElectrolyte disorders grade 2 CTCAE: • Hypomagnesemia: <1.2–0.9 mg/dL; <0.5–0.4 mmol/L, OR • Hypokalaemia: <LLN–3.0 mmol/L, OR • Hypophosphatemia: <2.5–2.0 mg/dL; <0.8–0.6 mmol/L, OR • Hyponatremia: <LLN–130–120 mmol/L (>2 months)	Clinically relevant, required intervention
3	An increase in serum creatinine at least 3.0 times baseline OR Increase in serum creatinine to ≥4.0 mg/dL (≥353.6 µmol/L) OR Initiation of renal replacement therapy, OR Electrolyte disorders ≥grade 3 CTCAE: • Hypomagnesemia: <0.9 mg/dL; <0.4 mmol/L, OR • Hypokalaemia: <3.0 mmol/L; hospitalization indicated, OR • Hypophosphatemia: <2.0 mg/dL; <0.6 mmol/L, OR • Hyponatremia: <LLN–120 mmol/L (>2 months)	Required close monitoring

Table 2. Case-control designation according to Adjusted-AKI outcome definition.

Case	Control	Ambiguous
Acute nephrotoxicity ≥ grade 1 OR Received electrolyte supplementation	Acute nephrotoxicity < grade 1 AND No supplementation	No lab values available during the time frame (3 months before initiation and 3 months after the last administration of cisplatin) OR Incomplete data e.g., initiation and end date of cisplatin therapy OR Pre-existing renal disease (electrolyte disturbances, not SCr or eGFR)

SCr: serum creatinine; eGFR: estimated glomerular filtration rate.

2.3.2. CTCAE-AKI Outcome Definition

The SCr-based CTCAE v.4.03 definition of "Acute Kidney Injury" was also used to define cisplatin-induced nephrotoxicity [39]. Patients were divided into cases (≥grade 1) and controls (<grade 1) (Table 3). The lowest SCr measurement up to 30 days before start of cisplatin treatment was taken as baseline. The follow up value used was the highest SCr value within 90 days after the end of cisplatin treatment.

Table 3. Case-control designation according to Common Terminology Criteria for Adverse Events (CTCAE)-AKI Outcome Definition.

Case	Control	Ambiguous
Acute kidney injury ≥ grade 1	Acute kidney injury < grade 1	No lab values available during the time frame (3 months before initiation and 3 months after the last administration of cisplatin) OR Incomplete data e.g., initiation and end date of cisplatin therapy

2.3.3. "ΔSCr and ΔeGFR" Outcome Definition

To calculate the differences between baseline and follow up SCr and eGFR (ΔSCr and ΔeGFR), the same procedure of creatinine serum measurements was applied as with the CTCAE outcome definition.

2.4. Genotype Data

2.4.1. Candidate Genes

The list of candidate genes and related variants was selected from a systematic review [19]. Candidate genes were included if they were found to be significantly associated with nephrotoxicity (any outcome definition) in a published study and the relationship had been replicated at least once. The following five single nucleotide polymorphisms (SNPs) meeting these criteria were included in this study: *ERCC1* rs11615 (chr19:45420395; A>G; a synonymous variant) and rs3212986 (chr19:45409478; C>A/C>G/C>T; non-coding transcript variant), *ERCC2* rs13181 (chr19:45351661; T>A/T>G; stop gained) and rs1799793 (chr19:45364001; C>A/C>T; a missense variant)) and *SLC22A2* rs316019 (chr6:160249250; A>C; a missense variant).

2.4.2. Genotyping

DNA was collected from saliva using Oragene collection kits (DNK Genotek Inc., Ottawa, ON, Canada) and was extracted according to the manufacturer's protocol. Genomic DNA samples for all patients were genotyped for 7907 variants located within absorption, distribution, metabolism, excretion (ADME) gene regions using the Illumina Infinium Panel (Illumina, San Diego, CA, USA), according to the manufacturer's instructions at the Canadian Pharmacogenomics Network for Drug Safety at the University of British Columbia. The genotyping details and the ADME custom panel used have been described in previously [27].

2.4.3. Quality Control of Genotype Data

Variants are filtered on SNP call rate (>95%), sample call rate (samples missing ≥2 SNPs excluded), Hardy-Weinberg equilibrium (HWE, p-value > 0.05, in controls) and minor allele frequency (MAF, >0.05, in patients with a European proportion ancestry ≥80%). HWE was calculated using Fisher's exact test.

2.5. Statistical Analyses

The genetic association between SNPs and the categorical clinical outcomes reflecting nephrotoxicity (i.e., adjusted-AKI and CTCAE-AKI) were examined using logistic regression assuming an additive model. MAFs for the whole cohort in both designations were calculated for each SNP. An allele frequency lower than 0.5 indicated the minor allele and was also classified as the risk allele. Power analyses were performed assuming a 0.05 significance level, assuming 5% MAF and with an OR > 3 as effect size with the goal of achieving a power of at least 80%. To assess differences between cases and controls (adjusted AKI and CTCAE-AKI designation) for continuous clinical variables, a Mann-Whitney U test was used. The differences between categorical clinical variables and cases and controls (adjusted AKI and CTCAE-AKI designation) were evaluated using a Chi-squared tests. A logistic regression model analysis that included potential confounders (counting subject ancestry) was used to calculate adjusted odds ratios (OR) and the 95% confidence intervals (95% CI) separately for outcomes defined using an adjusted-AKI and CTCAE-AKI designation. Cochran-Armitage trend test was conducted to test the assumption of an additive genetic model. Multiple linear regression was performed to assess the association between genetic variants and the continuous variables ΔeGFR and ΔSCr, adjusting for potential confounders. Key assumptions for multiple linear regression analysis—for example, multivariate normality, no multicollinearity and homoscedasticity—were fulfilled. Clinical variables which caused changes of the crude regression coefficient by 10% or more is considered a confounder and is added to the model. Multiple testing was accounted for using Bonferroni adjustments ($p = 0.05/5 = 0.01$). Statistical analyses were performed using SPSS v.25 (IBM Corporation, Armonk, NY, USA).

3. Results

3.1. Study Population

The study included 282 testicular-cancer patients from five adult oncology centres in British Columbia and Ontario through active surveillance of the Canadian Pharmacogenomics Network for Drug Safety (CPNDS) [41]. Ambiguous patients (Tables 2 and 3) or patients with missing SCr or eGFR data were excluded from further analyses. From the primary cohort, 72 patients were excluded because they were not genotyped (N = 61), had received abdominal radiation (N = 4) or because they were not diagnosed with testicular cancer (N = 7). From the secondary cohort (N = 210), 47 patients were excluded for the adjusted-AKI analyses due to pre-existing renal disease, incomplete data regarding the start- and/or end date of cisplatin therapy or absence of laboratory values. For the CTCAE-AKI outcome and ΔSCr analyses, 51 patients were excluded due to lack of SCr data. For the ΔeGFR analyses, 52 patients were excluded due to lack of eGFR data.

For genetic association analyses 167, 159, 158 and 159, patients were eligible for the adjusted AKI designation, the CTCAE-AKI designation and ΔeGFR and ΔSCr analyses, respectively (Figure 1). These patient cohorts were similar with respect to baseline characteristics. The mean age (± standard deviation) of the testicular-cancer patients was 31.8 ± 10.2 (Table 4). European has the highest ancestry proportion in our dataset (0.72 ± 0.26) followed by South Asian, East Asian, American and African. The detailed of ancestry analysis has been published elsewhere [27]. Patients had a low number of comorbidities: 1.0% (N = 2) suffered from diabetes and 3.3% (N = 7) from a cardiovascular disease. Only 2.9% (N = 6) of the patients received carboplatin within 90 days after cisplatin treatment ended (these dosages were included in the calculation of total platinum exposure). A majority of patients received the regimen of cisplatin with bleomycin and etoposide (BEP; 65%, N = 136). Because data on phosphate levels were missing for 207 patients, this electrolyte was excluded from further analyses.

3.2. Genotyping Results

The lowest SNP call rate was 97.5% for *SLC22A2* rs316019 (Table S2). HWE was fulfilled in the control group of all evaluated SNPs for adjusted-AKI outcome ($p > 0.05$) but not in the control group of *ERCC1* rs1799793 for the CTCAE-AKI outcome ($p = 0.013$) (Tables S1 and S2).

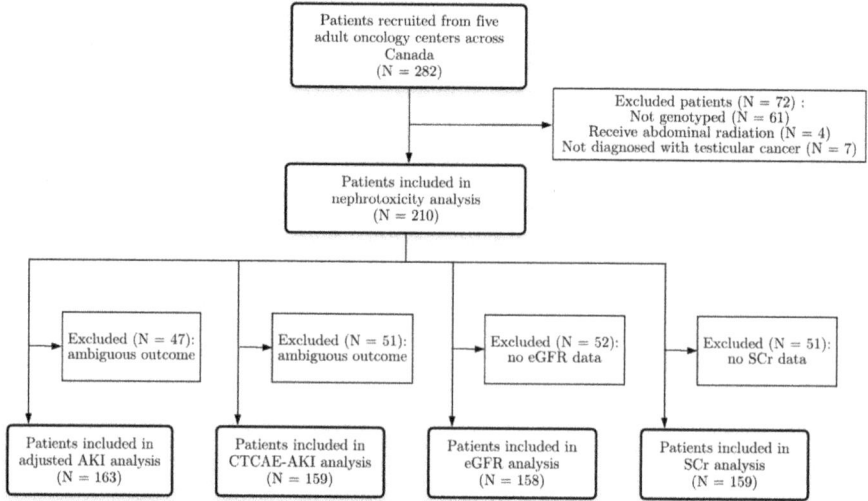

Figure 1. Flowchart of patient inclusion in statistical analyses.

Table 4. Clinical characteristics testicular cancer patients included in nephrotoxicity analyses (N = 210).

Characteristics		
Age at start treatment, mean ± SD, years		31.8 ± 10.2
Ancestry, mean ± SD, proportion	European	0.72 ± 0.26
	East-Asian	0.09 ± 0.23
	American	0.05 ± 0.10
	African	0.03 ± 0.03
	South-Asian	0.11 ± 0.15
Cardiovascular disease, no. (%)		7 (3.3)
Diabetes, no. (%)		2 (1.0)
Potentially nephrotoxic co-medications, mean ± SD, total number per patient		2 ± 2
Potentially nephrotoxic co-medications, no. (%)	ACEIs [a]	3 (1.4)
	Aminoglycosides	4 (1.9)
	ARBs [b]	1 (0.5)
	Benzodiazepines	30 (14)
	NSAIDs [c]	6 (2.9)
	Betalactams	26 (12)
	PPIs [d]	25 (12)
	Quinolones	29 (14)
	Statins	2 (1.0)
	Acetaminophen	29 (14)
	Other	104 (50)
Baseline [SCr], mean ± SD, umol/L		84 ± 16
Baseline [K$^+$], mean ± SD, mmol/L		4.1 ± 0.4
Baseline [Mg^{2+}], mean ± SD, mmol/L		0.85 ± 0.10
Baseline [Na$^+$], mean ± SD, mmol/L		138 ± 2.49
Baseline [PO4$^-$], mean ± SD, mmol/L		1.09 ± 0.23
Cumulative platinum dose, mean ± SD, mg/m^2		380 ± 123
Duration cisplatin treatment, mean ± SD	Weeks	8.7 ± 3.3
	Cycles	3.8 ± 1.1
Chemotherapy protocol, no. (%), BEP		136 (65)
Chemotherapy hydration, mean ± SD, L/cycle		10.7 ± 0.5

[a] ACEIs: Angiotensin-converting enzyme inhibitors, [b] ARBs: Angiotensin-II-Receptor Blockers, [c] NSAIDs: non-steroidal anti-inflammatory drugs, [d] PPIs: proton-pump inhibitors, BEP: bleomycin, etoposide, and cisplatin.

3.3. Adjusted AKI Analysis

For this outcome, 75 cases and 88 controls were identified (Table S3). Cases had significantly lower baseline magnesium compared to controls (0.83 vs. 0.88 mmol/L, $p = 0.008$). Quinolone usage was significantly higher in cases versus controls (24% vs. 5.7%, $p = 0.001$). Cases received significantly more platinum (400 vs. 300 mg/m^2, $p = 0.001$) and were treated longer with platinum (4 vs. 3 cycles, $p = 0.001$) compared to controls.

Genetic association analyses on the adjusted AKI designation were corrected for quinolone usage, cumulative dose, baseline magnesium and ancestry using principal components (PC's) to account for population structure. None of the genetic variants were found to be significantly associated with the risk of nephrotoxicity using this definition (Tables 5 and 6). In addition, Cochran-Armitage trend test also showed no significant trend to confirm the additive effect of minor allele (Table 6).

Table 5. Strength of genotypic association between genetic polymorphisms and cisplatin nephrotoxicity in adjusted-AKI outcome (N = 163).

Gene–SNP	OR	95% CI	p-Value	OR$_{adj}$	95% CI$_{adj}$	p-Value$_{adj}$
ERCC1 rs11615						
GG	1 #			1 #		
GA	1.30	0.63–2.67	0.48	1.45	0.64–3.27	0.38
AA	1.24	0.51–3.02	0.63	1.47	0.50–4.28	0.48
ERCC1 rs3212986						
CC	1 #			1 #		
CA	0.71	0.37–1.36	0.31	0.63	0.30–1.34	0.23
AA	1.00	0.30–3.37	1.00	1.44	0.32–6.43	0.63
ERCC2 rs13181						
AA	1 #			1 #		
CA	0.84	0.42–1.66	0.61	0.59	0.26–1.33	0.20
CC	1.60	0.65–3.93	0.31	1.43	0.50–4.07	0.51
ERCC2 rs1799793						
AA	1 #			1 #		
CA	1.00	0.49–2.03	1.00	0.92	0.40–2.15	0.85
CC	0.50	0.21–1.17	0.11	0.55	0.21–1.43	0.22
SLC22A2 rs316019						
CC	1 #			1 #		
AC	1.15	0.51–2.57	0.71	1.10	0.43–2.79	0.85
AA	2.46	0.22–27.78	0.47	1.70	0.11–25.57	0.70

$_{adj}$ Adjusted for: cumulative dose, quinolone usage, all ancestries (from four PCs) and baseline magnesium. # Reference category.

Table 6. Odds ratio of minor allele addition in adjusted-AKI outcome (N = 163) and Cochran-Armitage trend test result for additive model assumption.

Gene–SNP	OR	95% CI	p-Value	OR$_{adj}$	95% CI$_{adj}$	p-Value$_{adj}$	Cochran-Armitage Trend Test p-Value
ERCC1 rs11615 GG vs. GA vs. AA	1.13	0.73–1.75	0.586	1.23	0.73–2.05	0.436	0.586
ERCC1 rs3212986 AA vs. CA vs. CC	0.86	0.54–1.40	0.551	0.89	0.51–1.54	0.669	0.537
ERCC2 rs13181 CC vs. CA vs. AA	1.19	0.75–1.88	0.461	1.04	0.61–1.78	0.875	0.497
ERCC2 rs1799793 CC vs. CA vs. AA	0.70	0.45–1.09	0.114	0.73	0.44–1.19	0.206	0.280
SLC22A2 rs316019 AA vs. CA vs. CC	1.28	0.64–2.59	0.488	1.17	0.53–2.60	0.702	0.502

$_{adj}$ Adjusted for: cumulative dose, quinolone usage, all ancestries (as PC's) and baseline magnesium.

3.4. CTCAE-AKI Analysis

For this outcome, 36 cases and 123 controls were identified (Table S4). Cases were significantly older compared to controls (35 vs. 29 years old, $p = 0.002$) and differed from controls in ancestry: cases had a lower proportion who were of East-Asian ancestry (0 vs. 0.023, $p = 0.041$) and higher proportion who were of European ancestry (0.853 vs. 0.811, $p = 0.017$). Cases used proton-pump inhibitors (PPIs) significantly more often compared to controls (25% vs. 8%, $p = 0.015$). Cases received significantly more platinum (400 vs. 300 mg/m^2, $p = 0.005$) and were treated longer with platinum (4 vs. 3 cycles, $p = 0.007$) compared to controls. Furthermore, therapy regimens varied between cases and controls: cases were less often treated with a bleomycin-etoposide-platinum (BEP) protocol (53% vs. 72%, $p = 0.041$) and cases received chemotherapy hydration less often (10.75 (IQR = 10.50–10.75) vs. 10.75 (IQR = 0) L/cycle, $p = 0.004$).

The results of genotypic logistic regression are provided in Table 7. When corrected for age, ancestry from four PCs, chemotherapy protocol, cumulative dosage, hydration and PPI usage, patients carrying *ERCC1* rs3212986 heterozygous genotypes were found to have fewer nephrotoxicity events when compared with patients carrying the homozygous wildtype (OR$_{adj}$ = 0.24, CI = 0.08–0.70, $p = 0.009$). Patients carrying *SLC22A2* rs316019 heterozygous genotypes were found to have a greater number of nephrotoxicity events than patients who carrying the wildtype (normal) genotype before and after adjusting for the same covariates (OR$_{adj}$ = 5.06, CI = 1.69–15.16, $p = 0.004$). Besides this, the *SLC22A2* rs316109 homozygous variant carriers had more nephrotoxicity events than patients carrying the wildtype genotype, however after Bonferroni correction this was no longer statistically significant (OR$_{adj}$ = 38.12, CI = 1.89–767.51, $p = 0.017$).

Table 7. Strength of genotypic association between genetic polymorphisms and cisplatin nephrotoxicity in CTCAE-AKI designation (N = 159).

Gene–SNP	OR	95% CI	*p*-Value	OR$_{adj}$	95% CI$_{adj}$	*p*-Value$_{adj}$
ERCC1 rs11615						
GG	1 #			1 #		
GA	1.30	0.57–2.99	0.55	1.23	0.45–3.39	0.68
AA	0.48	0.14–1.65	0.24	0.53	0.12–2.37	0.41
ERCC1 rs3212986						
CC	1 #			1 #		
CA	0.45	0.20–1.02	0.06	0.24	0.08–0.70	0.009 *
AA	0.48	0.10–2.36	0.37	0.43	0.07–2.47	0.34
ERCC2 rs13181						
AA	1 #			1 #		
CA	1.16	0.49–2.73	0.74	0.59	0.20–1.76	0.37
CC	3.16	1.17–8.58	0.02	1.72	0.53–5.65	0.35
ERCC2 rs1799793						
AA	1 #			1 #		
CA	1.52	0.65–3.54	0.33	2.39	0.84–6.77	0.10
CC	0.57	0.18–1.79	0.33	0.66	0.16–2.64	0.56
SLC22A2 rs316019						
CC	1 #			1 #		
AC	3.24	1.36–7.74	0.008 *	5.06	1.69–15.16	0.004 *
AA	9.18	0.80–105.80	0.08	38.12	1.89–767.51	0.02

$_{adj}$ Adjusted for: age, all ancestries (as PC's), chemotherapy protocol, cumulative dosage, hydration and PPI usage, # Reference category, * significant ($p < 0.01$).

Additive effect of risk allele was found significant only on *SLC22A2* rs316109. The OR was even higher after adjustment (OR$_{adj}$ = 4.41, CI = 1.96–9.88, $p < 0.001$). In contrast, addition of minor allele on *ERCC1* rs3212986 produce protective effect although the result was not significant (OR$_{adj}$ = 0.52,

CI = 0.26–1.07, p = 0.076). The additive effect of minor allele was confirmed by Cochran-Armitage trend test but only for *SLC22A2* rs316019 and *ERCC2* rs13181 (Table 8).

Table 8. Odds ratio of minor allele addition in CTCAE-AKI designation (N = 159) and Cohcran-Armitage trend test result for additive model assumption.

Gene–SNP	OR	95% CI	p-Value	OR$_{adj}$	95% CI$_{adj}$	p-Value$_{adj}$	Cohcran-Armitage Trend Test p-Value
ERCC1 rs11615 GG vs. GA vs. AA	0.78	0.46–1.33	0.364	0.92	0.50–1.68	0.777	0.368
ERCC1 rs3212986 AA vs. CA vs. CC	0.57	0.30–1.06	0.077	0.52	0.26–1.07	0.076	0.067
ERCC2 rs13181 CC vs. CA vs. AA	1.84	1.07–3.15	0.027	1.39	0.75–2.58	0.293	0.039 *
ERCC2 rs1799793 CC vs. CA vs. AA	0.81	0.48–1.38	0.447	0.85	0.47–1.53	0.578	0.473
SLC22A2 rs316019 AA vs. CA vs. CC	3.29	1.60–6.81	0.001 **	4.41	1.96–9.88	<0.001 **	0.001 **

$_{adj}$ Adjusted for: age, all ancestries (as PC's), chemotherapy protocol, cumulative dosage, hydration and PPI usage, * significant (p < 0.05); proof of trend, ** significant (p < 0.01).

3.5. ΔSCr and ΔeGFR Analysis

Multiple linear regression was used to predict ΔSCr and ΔeGFR based on genotype for each SNP before and after adjustment for confounding variables. The analysis did not reveal any statistically significant results (Table 9). However, there was a very slight trend for the *ERCC1* rs3212986 variant to be protective and the *SLC22A2* rs316019 homozygous variant to be a risk factor, based on box-plots (Figures S1 and S2).

Table 9. Multiple linear regression analysis results between genetic polymorphisms and ΔSCr and ΔeGFR.

Gene–SNP	ΔSCr [a]				ΔeGFR [b]			
	R^2	p-Value	R^2_{adj}	p-Value $_{adj}$	R^2	p-Value	R^2_{adj}	p-Value $_{adj}$
ERCC1 rs11615 GG vs. GA vs. AA	0.01	0.218	0.055	0.17	0.006	0.347	0.042	0.20
ERCC1 rs3212986 AA vs. CA vs. CC	0.008	0.268	0.058	0.16	0.013	0.167	0.052	0.12
ERCC2 rs13181 CC vs. CA vs. AA	0.001	0.652	0.046	0.28	0	0.796	0.035	0.29
ERCC2 rs1799793 CC vs. CA vs. AA	0.001	0.77	0.046	0.27	0.001	0.668	0.036	0.29
SLC22A2 rs316019 AA vs. CA vs. CC	0.002	0.599	0.047	0.27	0.006	0.343	0.039	0.25

[a] adjusted for cardiovascular disease, duration (weeks), aminoglycoside users and baseline magnesium, [b] adjusted for duration (weeks), baseline potassium and beta-lactams use.

4. Discussion

4.1. Main Findings

Previous studies assessing the associations between *ERCC1* rs3212986 and *SLC22A2* rs316019 genotypes and cisplatin-induced nephrotoxicity have reported conflicting results. In this study, associations between genetic variants and multiple definitions of cisplatin-induced nephrotoxicity were analysed in the same dataset and demonstrated that different definitions of cisplatin nephrotoxicity contributed to variability of results. We could not reproduce the same genetic associations that were previously reported, when using the adjusted-AKI or continuous outcomes [13,16,18,42]. In contrast, when using the CTCAE-AKI outcome in the same patient sample, the *ERCC1* rs3212986 heterozygous genotype was reno-protective whilst the *SLC22A2* rs316019 homozygous genotype was a risk factor for cisplatin-induced nephrotoxicity. We also found that additive effect of risk allele was found significant only on *SLC22A2* rs316109.

Several published studies could not detect any significant associations between the CTCAE-AKI outcome definition of cisplatin-induced nephrotoxicity and *ERCC1* rs3212986 [14,43–45]; the reasons for this lack of association include lack of study power, population stratification or phenotypic heterogeneity. However, studies carried out by Tzvetkov et al. and Khrunin et al. did reveal associations between *ERCC1* rs3212986 genotypes and cisplatin-induced nephrotoxicity. Tzvetkov et al. found that homozygous variants were not associated with a decrease of eGFR, while the C allele carriers (major allele) had mean decrease of 11.5 ± 1.8% of eGFR ($p = 0.004$) [13]. By applying the same genetic model, we also found that the C allele carriers of this SNP have higher mean eGFR reduction than the homozygous variant subjects although the result was not statistically significant (18.9 ± 22.6 vs. 13.5 ± 23.0 mL/min/1.73 m^2; $p = 0.412$). This finding suggested protective effect of the variant genotype of rs3212986. Furthermore, we found that variant genotypes were protective against cisplatin nephrotoxicity when applying the CTCAE-AKI definition of nephrotoxicity: heterozygous carriers of the *ERCC1* rs3212986 had an OR$_{adj}$ of 0.24 (95% CI: 0.08–0.70) while the homozygous variant had an OR$_{adj}$ of 0.43 (95% CI: 0.07–2.47; $p = 0.341$). Addition of minor allele on this SNP produce protective effect although the result was not significant (ORadj = 0.52, CI = 0.26–1.07, $p = 0.076$). In contrast to these findings, Khrunin et al. reported a higher prevalence of cisplatin-induced nephrotoxicity among heterozygous genotypes compared with homozygous wildtype (OR = 3.29, 95% CI = 1.40–7.73, $p = 0.009$) [12].

The relationship between *SLC22A2* rs316019 genotypes and cisplatin-induced nephrotoxicity has been assessed in multiple studies. Filipski et al. reported a significant increase in SCr compared to baseline in homozygous wildtype patients after the first cycle ($p = 0.0009$) but found no significant increase in heterozygous patients ($p = 0.12$) [18]. Iwata et al. reported a significant higher increase in SCr in homozygous wildtype patients compared to heterozygous patients (0.34 ± 0.33 vs. 0.14 ± 0.12 mg/dL, $p = 0.04$, respectively) [16]. In addition, Zhang et al. observed a higher increase of cystatin C in homozygous wildtype patients compared to heterozygous and homozygous variant patients (0.043 ± 0.107 vs. −0.013 ± 0.120 mmol/L, $p = 0.009$, respectively) [46]. These results indicate that the homozygous wildtype genotype may be a risk factor for developing cisplatin-induced nephrotoxicity. In contrast, our results suggest that both homozygous and heterozygous variant carriers have an increased risk of cisplatin-induced nephrotoxicity when using the CTCAE-AKI definition. This finding also supported by significant additive effect of risk allele on *SLC22A2* rs316109 when applying additive genetic model. However, our study identified a possible greater risk of nephrotoxicity as defined by ΔSCr in patients carrying the homozygous variant (Figure S1); these data are consistent with Zhang et al. and Hinai et al., who reported a higher increase of SCr in heterozygous and homozygous variant than in homozygous wildtype subjects, although the result is not statistically significant (0.83 ± 7.39 vs. 2.09 ± 6.30 mmol/L, $p = 0.35$ and 0.30 ± 0.30 vs. 0.40 ± 0.53 mg/dL, $p = 0.25$, respectively) [46].

Other factors could also contribute to the discrepancy in results between our study and previous studies. Our results suggest that cisplatin-induced nephrotoxicity is confounded by ethnic origin. The CTCAE-AKI outcome was related to East-Asian and European ancestry. Our results suggest that East-Asian ancestry may be a protective factor and European ancestry may be a risk factor for cisplatin-induced nephrotoxicity. This may also explain the differences of results between our study and the studies of Iwata et al. and Hinai et al. that included subjects of East Asian ancestry. Discrepancies regarding the ΔSCr—and hence, ΔeGFR—among those studies could also be explained by the age of the population. Hinai et al. and Iwata et al. both studied an older population: 68.0 ± 9.7 and 65.8 ± 7.7 years old (mean ± SD) [16,42]. As highlighted before, older age could attribute to a higher increase in SCr [47]. This may explain the elevated SCr levels in the wildtype homozygous group of *SLC22A2* rs316019 found by Iwata et al. and Hinai et al. compared to our study. Furthermore, our population received a high dose cisplatin (100 mg/m^2 per cycle) compared to dosages used in other indications and compared to the other studies [16,42]: patients analysed by Hinai et al. received 80 mg/m² per cycle and Iwata et al. treated their patients with 60–80 mg/m² cisplatin per cycle. The higher cisplatin-dose in our study could have attributed to a possible higher incidence of cisplatin-induced nephrotoxicity.

This study further shows that different outcome definitions produce different results. The main difference in the outcomes definitions is the inclusion of electrolyte disturbances in the adjusted AKI outcome definition (Table 10). Our results suggest that the genetic associations were found when the SCr based definition was used but not when using an electrolyte-based definition that forms the adjusted AKI outcome definition. Acute kidney injury caused by cisplatin mainly manifests itself as renal tubular injury and is therefore characterized earlier by electrolyte abnormalities (phosphate, magnesium, potassium and sodium) [48]. However, incorporating serum abnormalities with creatinine serum levels in one single definition of cisplatin nephrotoxicity should be further validated.

Table 10. Multiple outcome definitions of cisplatin-induced nephrotoxicity used in this study.

	Adjusted-AKI	CTCAE-AKI	ΔeGFR	ΔSCr
Basis of Determination	SCr + Mg/K/PO₄/Na	SCr	CKD-EPI equation (SCr+age+sex+ethnicity)	SCr
Data Characteristics	Categorical	Categorical	Continuous	Continuous
Advantage	Tailored on cisplatin-induced nephrotoxicity	• Mostly used in clinics and studies in cancer subjects • Easily calculated	• Easily calculated • CKD-EPI is the equation recommended by KDIGO	• Routinely measured in patients
Disadvantage	• Not comparable with other studies • Not validated yet	• Is ≥ grade 1 cut-off clinically relevant? • SCr often increase late resulting in failing to detect early stage nephrotoxicity	• Could not correct for cystatin-C due to unavailable data in routine practice • Disregarding the clinical value of baseline eGFR	• Highly influenced by various individual factors (e.g., age, gender, body weight, diet etc.) • SCr often increase late resulting in failing to detect early stage nephrotoxicity • Disregarding the clinical value of baseline SCr

4.2. Gene Expression and Regulation

ERCC1 rs3212986, located at the 3' UTR (non-coding region) was not associated with changes in protein and mRNA expression [49,50]. However, the tissue expression quantitative trait loci (eQTL) analysis from the Genotype-Tissue Expression (GTEx) Project reported a significant association between rs3212986 and gene expression in various tissues [51]. Unfortunately, no association has been found between rs3212986 and ERCC1 expression in kidney cortex tissue. SLC22A2 rs316019, a nonsynonymous missense mutation (p.270Ala>Ser), is the only common coding polymorphism of SLCC2A2 with an allele frequency ranging from 9–16% and is reported to cause changes in transporter function [52]. No significant eQTLs were found for rs316019 in the eQTL tissues database [51]. Specific functional validation of ERCC1 rs3212986 and SLC22A2 rs316019 in kidney tubular tissue is needed to elucidate their role in cisplatin nephrotoxicity and how they affect protein expression involved in cisplatin nephrotoxicity pathway (e.g., OCT2).

4.3. Strength and Limitations of the Study

Compared to the previously published studies, our study was conducted in an appropriate population of relatively young adult male patients, who had a low number of comorbidities. By studying a dataset of testicular cancer patients, we minimized the influence of gender, older age, comorbidities and long-term use of medications that could have affected the renin-angiotensin systems (e.g., angiotensin converting enzyme inhibitors and angiotensin receptor blockers) and nephrotoxic compounds (e.g., non-steroidal anti-inflammatory drugs).

Our study had several limitations. The retrospective design led to several potential but unavoidable bias. Since laboratory measurements that were available were mostly measured in patients who were monitored more intensively, any missing data was non-random. Hence, the measurements that were available more likely to found individuals who were prone to cisplatin-induced nephrotoxicity. This resulted in selection bias and a possible overestimation of the amount of cases. The relatively small sample size was also a possible cause of failing to detect an association in this candidate gene study. A large prospective cohort study with a genome-wide approach is recommended to explore additional genetic variants that might be of importance. Furthermore, slightly different number of cohorts were used for each outcome. This may also have influenced the associations observed with each outcome.

5. Conclusions

In conclusion, the results of this study imply that the use of different outcome definitions lead to altered results. Consensus on a set of clinically relevant outcome definitions that future studies can follow are needed. The adjusted acute kidney injury definition that includes electrolyte imbalances seems more appropriate for cisplatin-induced nephrotoxicity. However, further validation of the definition and staging is necessary before it can be applied in further research or clinical settings. Furthermore, this study provides more evidence for associations between genetic variants and cisplatin-induced nephrotoxicity by using serum creatinine-based grading. These findings imply that genetic variations are involved in the inter-individual susceptibility to cisplatin-induced nephrotoxicity. Thus, in the future genotyping will make it possible to optimize therapy with cisplatin for the individual patients by improving cisplatin dosage selection–lower doses for patients prone to renal toxicity and higher doses for patient not susceptible to developing renal toxicity.

Supplementary Materials: The following are available online at http://www.mdpi.com/2073-4425/10/5/364/s1, Table S1: Genotyping details for adjusted-AKI outcome in patients with European proportion ancestry ≥80% (N = 93), Table S2: Genotyping details for AKI-CTCAE outcome in patients with European proportion ancestry ≥80% (N = 88), Table S3: Clinical characteristics of cases and controls in adjusted-AKI outcome (N = 163), Table S4: Clinical characteristics of cases and controls in AKI-CTCAE outcome (N = 159), Figure S1: Boxplot chart of SCr elevation (ΔSCr) by genotype of studied SNPs, Figure S2: Boxplot chart of eGFR reduction (ΔeGFR) by genotype of studied SNPs.

Author Contributions: Conceptualization, Z.Z., B.I.D., S.J.H.V., R.M., G.L., B.C.C. and A.H.M.-v.d.Z.; Data curation, G.E.B.W., N.M., C.J.D.R. and B.C.C.; Formal analysis, Z.Z., L.S.O., B.I.D. and B.C.C.; Funding acquisition, B.C.C. and Z.Z.; Investigation, Z.Z., L.S.O., B.I.D., M.M., J.G.M., G.E.B.W., C.K.K., P.L.B., Z.C., K.A.G., N.M., C.J.D.R., G.L., B.C.C. and A.H.M.-v.d.Z.; Methodology, Z.Z., B.I.D., M.M., A.K., S.J.H.V., C.J.D.R., B.C.C. and A.H.M.-v.d.Z.; Project administration, B.C.C. and A.H.M.-v.d.Z.; Resources, J.G.M., G.E.B.W., C.K.K., P.L.B., Z.C., K.A.G., C.J.D.R, G.L. and B.C.C.; Supervision, B.I.D., S.J.H.V., R.M., B.C.C. and A.H.M.-v.d.Z.; Visualization, Z.Z. and L.S.O.; Writing—original draft, Z.Z. and L.S.O.; Writing—review & editing, Z.Z., L.S.O., B.I.D., M.M., J.G.M., G.E.B.W., C.K.K., P.L.B., Z.C., K.A.G., N.M., A.K., S.J.H.V., R.M., C.J.D.R., G.L., B.C.C. and A.H.M.-v.d.Z.

Funding: This research was funded by the Canadian Foundation for Innovation/Canadian Institutes of Health Research (CIHR) (grant number CIHR CRI-88362), the CIHR-Drug Safety and Effectiveness Network (grants number CIHR TD1 137714 and CIHR TD2 117588), Genome BC and Genome Canada (grant number 272PGX), the BC Children's Hospital Research Institute Bertram Hoffmeister Postdoctoral Fellowship Award (B.I.D), Michael Smith Foundation for Health Research Scholar Program (C.J.D.R) and Indonesia Endowment Fund for Education (LPDP) Ministry of Finance, the Republic of Indonesia (as a part of ZZ's Ph.D. project, grant no. 20161022049506). The APC was funded by Indonesia Endowment Fund for Education (LPDP).

Acknowledgments: We gratefully acknowledge the participation of all patients and families who took part in this study. We also acknowledge the contributions of the Canadian Pharmacogenomics Network for Drug Safety (CPNDS) Consortium.

Conflicts of Interest: The authors declare no conflict of interest. The funders had no role in the design of the study; in the collection, analyses or interpretation of data; in the writing of the manuscript or in the decision to publish the results.

References

1. Dasari, S.; Tchounwou, P.B. Cisplatin in cancer therapy: Molecular mechanisms of action. *Eur. J. Pharmacol.* **2014**, *740*, 364–378. [CrossRef]
2. Rancoule, C.; Guy, J.B.; Vallard, A.; Ben Mrad, M.; Rehailia, A.; Magne, N. 50th anniversary of cisplatin. *Bull. Cancer* **2017**, *104*, 167–176. [CrossRef]

3. Hoffmann, R.; Plug, I.; McKee, M.; Khoshaba, B.; Westerling, R.; Looman, C.; Rey, G.; Jougla, E.; Lang, K.; Parna, K.; et al. Innovations in health care and mortality trends from five cancers in seven European countries between 1970 and 2005. *Int. J. Public. Health* **2014**, *59*, 341–350. [CrossRef]
4. Sakaeda, T.; Kadoyama, K.; Okuno, Y. Adverse event profiles of platinum agents: Data mining of the public version of the FDA adverse event reporting system, AERS and reproducibility of clinical observations. *Int. J. Med. Sci.* **2011**, *8*, 487–491. [CrossRef]
5. Arany, I.; Safirstein, R.L. Cisplatin nephrotoxicity. *Semin. Nephrol.* **2003**, *23*, 460–464. [CrossRef]
6. Sahni, V.; Choudhury, D.; Ahmed, Z. Chemotherapy-associated renal dysfunction. *Nat. Rev. Nephrol.* **2009**, *5*, 450–462. [CrossRef]
7. Chovanec, M.; Abu Zaid, M.; Hanna, N.; El-Kouri, N.; Einhorn, L.H.; Albany, C. Long-term toxicity of cisplatin in germ-cell tumor survivors. *Ann. Oncol.* **2017**, *28*, 2670–2679. [CrossRef] [PubMed]
8. Gietema, J.A.; Meinardi, M.T.; Messerschmidt, J.; Gelevert, T.; Alt, F.; Uges, D.R.A.; Sleijfer, D.T. Circulating plasma platinum more than 10 years after cisplatin treatment for testicular cancer. *Lancet* **2000**, *355*, 1075–1076. [CrossRef]
9. Bajorin, D.F.; Bosl, G.J.; Alcock, N.W.; Niedzwiecki, D.; Gallina, E.; Shurgot, B. Pharmacokinetics of cis-diamminedichloroplatinum(II) after administration in hypertonic saline. *Cancer Res.* **1986**, *46*, 5969–5972. [PubMed]
10. Pabla, N.; Dong, Z. Cisplatin nephrotoxicity: Mechanisms and renoprotective strategies. *Kidney Int.* **2008**, *73*, 994–1007. [CrossRef]
11. Manohar, S.; Leung, N. Cisplatin nephrotoxicity: A review of the literature. *J. Nephrol.* **2018**, *31*, 15–25. [CrossRef]
12. Khrunin, A.V.; Moisseev, A.; Gorbunova, V.; Limborska, S. Genetic polymorphisms and the efficacy and toxicity of cisplatin-based chemotherapy in ovarian cancer patients. *Pharmacogenomics J.* **2010**, *10*, 54–61. [CrossRef]
13. Tzvetkov, M.V.; Behrens, G.; O'Brien, V.P.; Hohloch, K.; Brockmoller, J.; Benohr, P. Pharmacogenetic analyses of cisplatin-induced nephrotoxicity indicate a renoprotective effect of ERCC1 polymorphisms. *Pharmacogenomics* **2011**, *12*, 1417–1427. [CrossRef]
14. Windsor, R.E.; Strauss, S.J.; Kallis, C.; Wood, N.E.; Whelan, J.S. Germline genetic polymorphisms may influence chemotherapy response and disease outcome in osteosarcoma: A pilot study. *Cancer* **2012**, *118*, 1856–1867. [CrossRef] [PubMed]
15. Powrozek, T.; Mlak, R.; Krawczyk, P.; Homa, I.; Ciesielka, M.; Koziol, P.; Prendecka, M.; Milanowski, J.; Malecka-Massalska, T. The relationship between polymorphisms of genes regulating DNA repair or cell division and the toxicity of platinum and vinorelbine chemotherapy in advanced NSCLC patients. *Clin. Transl. Oncol.* **2016**, *18*, 125–131. [CrossRef]
16. Iwata, K.; Aizawa, K.; Kamitsu, S.; Jingami, S.; Fukunaga, E.; Yoshida, M.; Yoshimura, M.; Hamada, A.; Saito, H. Effects of genetic variants in SLC22A2 organic cation transporter 2 and SLC47A1 multidrug and toxin extrusion 1 transporter on cisplatin-induced adverse events. *Clin. Exp. Nephrol.* **2012**, *16*, 843–851. [CrossRef]
17. Zhang, L.; Gao, G.; Li, X.; Ren, S.; Li, A.; Xu, J.; Zhang, J.; Zhou, C. Association between single nucleotide polymorphisms (SNPs) and toxicity of advanced non-small-cell lung cancer patients treated with chemotherapy. *PLoS ONE* **2012**, *7*, e48350. [CrossRef]
18. Filipski, K.K.; Mathijssen, R.H.; Mikkelsen, T.S.; Schinkel, A.H.; Sparreboom, A. Contribution of organic cation transporter 2 (OCT2) to cisplatin-induced nephrotoxicity. *Clin. Pharmacol. Ther.* **2009**, *86*, 396–402. [CrossRef] [PubMed]
19. Zazuli, Z.; Vijverberg, S.; Slob, E.; Liu, G.; Carleton, B.; Veltman, J.; Baas, P.; Masereeuw, R.; Maitland-van der Zee, A.H. Genetic Variations and Cisplatin Nephrotoxicity: A Systematic Review. *Front. Pharmacol.* **2018**, *9*, 1111. [CrossRef]
20. Giachino, D.F.; Ghio, P.; Regazzoni, S.; Mandrile, G.; Novello, S.; Selvaggi, G.; Gregori, D.; DeMarchi, M.; Scagliotti, G.V. Prospective assessment of XPD Lys751Gln and XRCC1 Arg399Gln single nucleotide polymorphisms in lung cancer. *Clin. Cancer Res.* **2007**, *13*, 2876–2881. [CrossRef]
21. Friboulet, L.; Olaussen, K.A.; Pignon, J.P.; Shepherd, F.A.; Tsao, M.S.; Graziano, S.; Kratzke, R.; Douillard, J.Y.; Seymour, L.; Pirker, R.; et al. ERCC1 isoform expression and DNA repair in non-small-cell lung cancer. *N. Engl. J. Med.* **2013**, *368*, 1101–1110. [CrossRef]

22. Xiong, Y.; Huang, B.Y.; Yin, J.Y. Pharmacogenomics of platinum-based chemotherapy in non-small cell lung cancer: Focusing on DNA repair systems. *Med. Oncol.* **2017**, *34*, 48. [CrossRef] [PubMed]
23. Han, Y.; Liu, J.; Sun, M.; Zhang, Z.; Liu, C.; Sun, Y. A Significant Statistical Advancement on the Predictive Values of ERCC1 Polymorphisms for Clinical Outcomes of Platinum-Based Chemotherapy in Non-Small Cell Lung Cancer: An Updated Meta-Analysis. *Dis. Markers* **2016**, *2016*, 7643981. [CrossRef]
24. Miller, R.P.; Tadagavadi, R.K.; Ramesh, G.; Reeves, W.B. Mechanisms of Cisplatin nephrotoxicity. *Toxins* **2010**, *2*, 2490–2518. [CrossRef]
25. Wensing, K.U.; Ciarimboli, G. Saving ears and kidneys from cisplatin. *Anticancer Res.* **2013**, *33*, 4183–4188. [PubMed]
26. Little, J.; Higgins, J.P.; Ioannidis, J.P.; Moher, D.; Gagnon, F.; von Elm, E.; Khoury, M.J.; Cohen, B.; Davey-Smith, G.; Grimshaw, J.; et al. Strengthening the reporting of genetic association studies (STREGA): An extension of the STROBE Statement. *Hum. Genet.* **2009**, *125*, 131–151. [CrossRef] [PubMed]
27. Drogemoller, B.I.; Monzon, J.G.; Bhavsar, A.P.; Borrie, A.E.; Brooks, B.; Wright, G.E.B.; Liu, G.; Renouf, D.J.; Kollmannsberger, C.K.; Bedard, P.L.; et al. Association Between SLC16A5 Genetic Variation and Cisplatin-Induced Ototoxic Effects in Adult Patients With Testicular Cancer. *JAMA Oncol.* **2017**, *3*, 1558–1562. [CrossRef]
28. Levey, A.S.; Stevens, L.A.; Schmid, C.H.; Zhang, Y.L.; Castro, A.F., 3rd; Feldman, H.I.; Kusek, J.W.; Eggers, P.; Van Lente, F.; Greene, T.; et al. A new equation to estimate glomerular filtration rate. *Ann. Intern. Med.* **2009**, *150*, 604–612. [CrossRef] [PubMed]
29. Group, K.D.I.G.O.K.C.W. KDIGO 2012 Clinical Practice Guideline for the Evaluation and Management of Chronic Kidney Disease. *Kidney Int. Suppl.* **2013**, *3*, 1–150.
30. Winkelmayer, W.C.; Levin, R.; Setoguchi, S. Associations of kidney function with cardiovascular medication use after myocardial infarction. *Clin. J. Am. Soc. Nephrol.* **2008**, *3*, 1415–1422. [CrossRef]
31. Becquemont, L.; Bauduceau, B.; Benattar-Zibi, L.; Berrut, G.; Bertin, P.; Bucher, S.; Corruble, E.; Danchin, N.; al-Salameh, A.; Derumeaux, G.; et al. Association between Cardiovascular Drugs and Chronic Kidney Disease in Non-Institutionalized Elderly Patients. *Basic Clin. Pharmacol. Toxicol.* **2015**, *117*, 137–143. [CrossRef]
32. Aronow, W.S.; Frishman, W.H.; Cheng-Lai, A. Cardiovascular drug therapy in the elderly. *Cardiol. Rev.* **2007**, *15*, 195–215. [CrossRef]
33. Shlipak, M.G.; Smith, G.L.; Rathore, S.S.; Massie, B.M.; Krumholz, H.M. Renal function, digoxin therapy and heart failure outcomes: Evidence from the digoxin intervention group trial. *J. Am. Soc. Nephrol.* **2004**, *15*, 2195–2203. [CrossRef]
34. Diabetes Canada Clinical Practice Guidelines Expert, C.; Lipscombe, L.; Booth, G.; Butalia, S.; Dasgupta, K.; Eurich, D.T.; Goldenberg, R.; Khan, N.; MacCallum, L.; Shah, B.R.; et al. Pharmacologic Glycemic Management of Type 2 Diabetes in Adults. *Can. J. Diabetes* **2018**, *42*, S88–S103.
35. Awdishu, L.; Mehta, R.L. The 6R's of drug induced nephrotoxicity. *BMC Nephrol.* **2017**, *18*, 124. [CrossRef]
36. BCCA Genitourinary Chemotherapy Protocols. BC Cancer, Provincial Health Services Authority. Available online: http://www.bccancer.bc.ca/health-professionals/clinical-resources/chemotherapy-protocols/genitourinary#Testicular (accessed on 21 February 2018).
37. CCA Genitourinary Cancer Guidelines and Advice. Cancer Care Ontario. Available online: https://www.cancercareontario.ca/en/guidelines-advice/types-of-cancer/genitourinary?f%5B0%5D=field_type_of_cancer%3A656&f%5B1%5D=field_type_of_cancer%3A681 (accessed on 21 February 2018).
38. Rantanen, V.; Grenman, S.; Kulmala, J.; Grenman, R. Comparative evaluation of cisplatin and carboplatin sensitivity in endometrial adenocarcinoma cell lines. *Br. J. Cancer* **1994**, *69*, 482–486. [CrossRef]
39. Common Terminology Criteria for Adverse Events (CTCAE) Version 4.0. National Cancer Institute. Available online: https://evs.nci.nih.gov/ftp1/CTCAE/About.html (accessed on 15 February 2018).
40. Castillo, J.J.; Vincent, M.; Justice, E. Diagnosis and management of hyponatremia in cancer patients. *Oncologist* **2012**, *17*, 756–765. [CrossRef]
41. CPNDS. Welcome to The Canadian Pharmacogenomics Network for Drug Safety (CPNDS). Available online: http://cpnds.ubc.ca/ (accessed on 8 January 2019).
42. Hinai, Y.; Motoyama, S.; Niioka, T.; Miura, M. Absence of effect of SLC22A2 genotype on cisplatin-induced nephrotoxicity in oesophageal cancer patients receiving cisplatin and 5-fluorouracil: Report of results discordant with those of earlier studies. *J. Clin. Pharm. Ther.* **2013**, *38*, 498–503. [CrossRef]

43. KimCurran, V.; Zhou, C.; Schmid-Bindert, G.; Shengxiang, R.; Zhou, S.; Zhang, L.; Zhang, J. Lack of correlation between ERCC1 (C8092A) single nucleotide polymorphism and efficacy/toxicity of platinum based chemotherapy in Chinese patients with advanced non-small cell lung cancer. *Adv. Med. Sci.* **2011**, *56*, 30–38. [CrossRef]
44. Goekkurt, E.; Al-Batran, S.E.; Hartmann, J.T.; Mogck, U.; Schuch, G.; Kramer, M.; Jaeger, E.; Bokemeyer, C.; Ehninger, G.; Stoehlmacher, J. Pharmacogenetic analyses of a phase III trial in metastatic gastroesophageal adenocarcinoma with fluorouracil and leucovorin plus either oxaliplatin or cisplatin: A study of the arbeitsgemeinschaft internistische onkologie. *J. Clin. Oncol.* **2009**, *27*, 2863–2873. [CrossRef] [PubMed]
45. Erculj, N.; Kovac, V.; Hmeljak, J.; Dolzan, V. The influence of platinum pathway polymorphisms on the outcome in patients with malignant mesothelioma. *Ann. Oncol.* **2012**, *23*, 961–967. [CrossRef]
46. Zhang, J.; Zhou, W. Ameliorative effects of SLC22A2 gene polymorphism 808 G/T and cimetidine on cisplatin-induced nephrotoxicity in Chinese cancer patients. *Food Chem. Toxicol.* **2012**, *50*, 2289–2293. [CrossRef] [PubMed]
47. Tiao, J.Y.; Semmens, J.B.; Masarei, J.R.; Lawrence-Brown, M.M. The effect of age on serum creatinine levels in an aging population: relevance to vascular surgery. *Cardiovasc. Surg.* **2002**, *10*, 445–451. [CrossRef]
48. McMahon, K.R.; Rod Rassekh, S.; Schultz, K.R.; Pinsk, M.; Blydt-Hansen, T.; Mammen, C.; Tsuyuki, R.T.; Devarajan, P.; Cuvelier, G.D.; Mitchell, L.G.; et al. Design and Methods of the Pan-Canadian Applying Biomarkers to Minimize Long-Term Effects of Childhood/Adolescent Cancer Treatment (ABLE) Nephrotoxicity Study: A Prospective Observational Cohort Study. *Can. J. Kidney Health Dis.* **2017**, *4*, 2054358117690338. [CrossRef] [PubMed]
49. Woelfelschneider, A.; Popanda, O.; Lilla, C.; Linseisen, J.; Mayer, C.; Celebi, O.; Debus, J.; Bartsch, H.; Chang-Claude, J.; Schmezer, P. A distinct ERCC1 haplotype is associated with mRNA expression levels in prostate cancer patients. *Carcinogenesis* **2008**, *29*, 1758–1764. [CrossRef] [PubMed]
50. Zhuo, Z.J.; Liu, W.; Zhang, J.; Zhu, J.; Zhang, R.; Tang, J.; Yang, T.; Zou, Y.; He, J.; Xia, H. Functional Polymorphisms at ERCC1/XPF Genes Confer Neuroblastoma Risk in Chinese Children. *EBioMedicine* **2018**, *30*, 113–119. [CrossRef] [PubMed]
51. Consortium, G. *The Genotype-Tissue Expression (GTEx)*, GTEx Consortium, 2017.
52. Zolk, O. Disposition of metformin: variability due to polymorphisms of organic cation transporters. *Ann. Med.* **2012**, *44*, 119–129. [CrossRef] [PubMed]

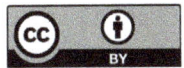

© 2019 by the authors. Licensee MDPI, Basel, Switzerland. This article is an open access article distributed under the terms and conditions of the Creative Commons Attribution (CC BY) license (http://creativecommons.org/licenses/by/4.0/).

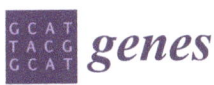

Article

Quantifying Risk Pathway Crosstalk Mediated by miRNA to Screen Precision drugs for Breast Cancer Patients

Yingqi Xu [1], Shuting Lin [1], Hongying Zhao [1], Jingwen Wang [1], Chunlong Zhang [1], Qun Dong [1], Congxue Hu [1], Desi Shang [1], Li Wang [1] and Yanjun Xu [1,*]

College of Bioinformatics Science and Technology, Harbin Medical University, Harbin 150081, China
* Correspondence: xuyanjun@hrbmu.edu.cn

Received: 19 July 2019; Accepted: 26 August 2019; Published: 28 August 2019

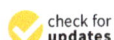

Abstract: Breast cancer has become the most common cancer that leads to women's death. Breast cancer is a complex, highly heterogeneous disease classified into various subtypes based on histological features, which determines the therapeutic options. System identification of effective drugs for each subtype remains challenging. In this work, we present a computational network biology approach to screen precision drugs for different breast cancer subtypes by considering the impact intensity of candidate drugs on the pathway crosstalk mediated by miRNAs. Firstly, we constructed and analyzed the subtype-specific risk pathway crosstalk networks mediated by miRNAs. Then, we evaluated 36 Food and Drug Administration (FDA)-approved anticancer drugs by quantifying their effects on these subtype-specific pathway crosstalk networks and combining with survival analysis. Finally, some first-line treatments of breast cancer, such as Paclitaxel and Vincristine, were optimized for each subtype. In particular, we performed precision screening of subtype-specific therapeutic drugs and also confirmed some novel drugs suitable for breast cancer treatment. For example, Sorafenib was applicable for the basal subtype treatment, Irinotecan was optimum for Her2 subtype treatment, Vemurafenib was suitable for the LumA subtype treatment, and Vorinostat could apply to LumB subtype treatment. In addition, the mechanism of these optimal therapeutic drugs in each subtype of breast cancer was further dissected. In summary, our study offers an effective way to screen precision drugs for various breast cancer subtype treatments. We also dissected the mechanism of optimal therapeutic drugs, which may provide novel insight into the precise treatment of cancer and promote researches on the mechanisms of action of drugs.

Keywords: breast cancer subtype; miRNA; pathway; crosstalk network; precision drugs

1. Introduction

Breast cancer is the most common cancer type that leads to women's death, especially in China. The high heterogeneity of breast cancer makes it a great challenge to adopt therapeutic options [1], because a heterogeneous group of diseases may exhibit distinct features in terms of histological, prognostic, and clinical outcomes [2]. At present, breast cancer can mainly be classified into four primary subtypes, including her2-enriched, luminal A, luminal B, and basal-like [3,4], distinguished by the expression of some signature genes such as the estrogen receptor (ER), progesterone receptor (PR), and HER2. Different subtypes have distinct biological behaviors and prognosis, and also exhibit various responses to drug therapy [5,6]. Thus, further research on the biological heterogeneity of each subtype of breast cancer will be an effective way to improve the therapeutic efficacy and prognosis of breast cancer [7].

The oncogenesis processes may result from the dysregulations of a series of important biological pathways [8]. Some studies have shown that the pathway crosstalk exists extensively in the processes of development and cell fate [9–11]. Cancer cells have been found to be able to establish alternative signaling pathways through crosstalk to adapt to drug treatment. In addition, crosstalk can also promote cancer therapy by inhibiting the main oncogenic pathways. The inhibition of functional redundancy and pathway crosstalk that promotes the survival of cancer cells can prevent the resistance in tumor treatment [12]. Therefore, it is essential to dissect the crosstalk of dysfunctional pathways and further capture the key molecules that mediate this functional crosstalk in breast cancer.

MicroRNAs are endogenous, non-coding RNA molecules that have been widely regarded as important post-transcriptional regulators by damping the expression level of their target genes. In recent years, studies have indicated that miRNAs are important component elements of biological pathways [13]. They regulate the function of biological pathways through target genes, and then work together with them to disrupt the pathways of diseases. According to estimates, many microRNAs play vital roles by regulating processes that are implicated with the development of cancer [14], such as proliferation, apoptosis, cell cycle, angiogenesis, etc. Some studies suggest that the crosstalk between miRNAs and the Wnt pathway may impact oncogenesis, cancer metastasis, and even drug-resistance processes [15]. Furthermore, miRNAs can also mediate the functional crosstalk of pathways related with oncogenic processes by targeting their shared or interacted genes, thus promoting the initiation and progression of tumors.

In recent years, miRNAs have shown great promise to serve as a target for drug therapy of cancer. More importantly, some studies have nominated miRNA-based therapy as a promising strategy for the treatment of breast cancer [16]. Some evidence demonstrates that drugs could modulate the expression of miRNAs in various diseases as well. For example, an experiment has validated that simvastatin could lead to cell death of breast cancer by up-regulating miR-140-5p [17]. Triiodothyronine has been demonstrated to modulate miR-204 and thus facilitate the proliferation process in breast cancer [18]. Especially, Shenoda et al. have also demonstrated that miRNA could mediate the expression of genes related with drug metabolism [19]. Furthermore, Liu et al. have established a database SM2miR [20], which provides a comprehensive resource about the influences of drugs on miRNA expression and offers unprecedented opportunities for researchers on the screening and action mechanism of drugs for disease treatment. In addition, our previous research also displays that miRNA participates in the crosstalk among pathways that play important roles in cancer development [21], indicating that it might be more effective for screening cancer treatment to evaluate the effects of drugs on the miRNA-mediated crosstalk between pathways.

In order to match the best treatment for breast cancer, in the present study, we firstly integrated the disease high-throughput molecular profiles, miRNA regulation data, and pathway and drug data to construct and analyze the miRNA-mediated pathway crosstalk network for various breast cancer subtypes. Then, we derived a novel computational method to screen precision drugs for different breast cancer subtypes by quantifying the impact intensity of candidate drugs on the pathway crosstalk mediated by miRNAs. Finally, survival analysis was combined for further screening and optimization of the drugs for breast cancer treatment (Figure 1). In summary, our study proposes an effective method to screen precision drugs for various breast cancer subtype treatments. We also dissected the mechanism of optimal therapeutic drugs, which may promote the shift from inexact medicine to precision life science.

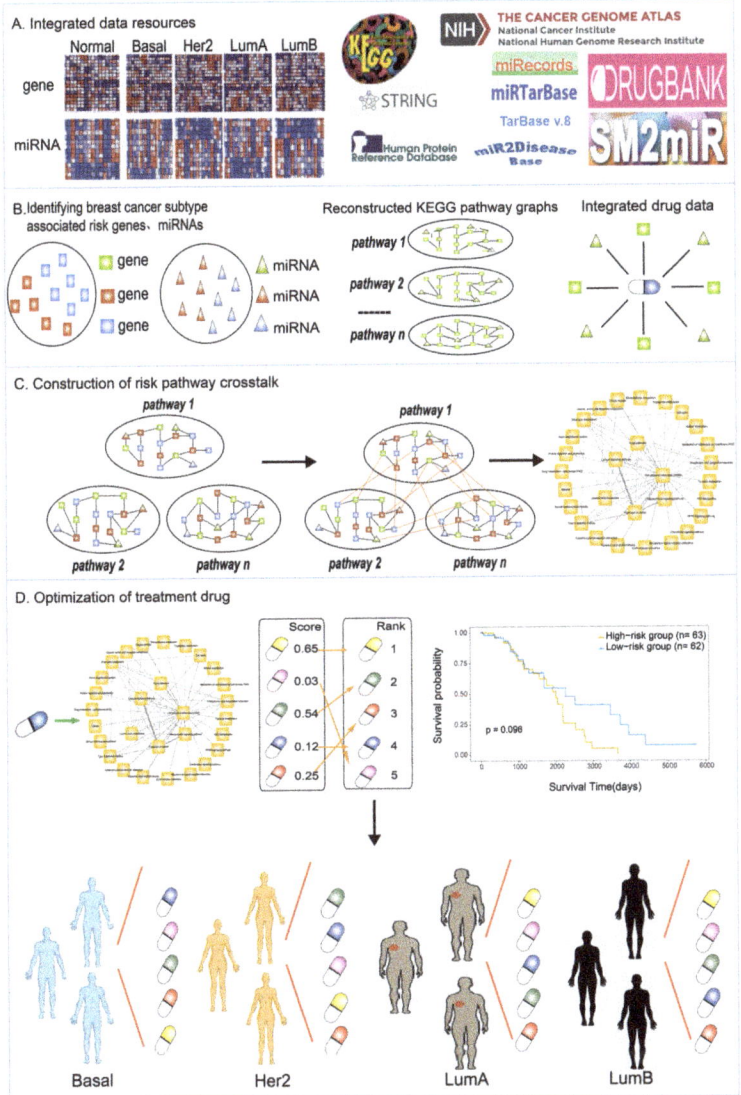

Figure 1. The workflow of optimizing drugs for different subtypes of breast cancer. (**A**) In this work, breast cancer was taken as the research model. Firstly, we integrated related data resources, including gene/miRNA expression profile of each breast cancer subtype and matching patients' survival information, miRNA-target relationship data, PPI network and pathway data, and drug and drug target data. (**B**) We identified the differential genes/miRNAs of each breast cancer subtype, and then reconstructed KEGG pathway based on miRNA-target interactions, which contained both genes and miRNAs. We also screened the target genes and target miRNAs of Food and Drug Administration (FDA)-approved anticancer drugs. (**C**) Identification of breast cancer subtype-associated risk pathways based on the differential genes/miRNAs, and calculated crosstalk for any two interrelated risk pathways. Furthermore we constructed miRNA-mediated specific pathway crosstalk networks in different subtypes of breast cancer, respectively. (**D**) The effectiveness assessment of drugs on dysfunction crosstalk network to screen candidate drugs, combined with survival analysis to optimize drugs for each breast cancer subtype. (See Methods section for details.)

2. Material and Methods

2.1. Sample Matched miRNA/Gene Expression Profiles and Clinical Data

The matched miRNA and gene expression data of breast cancer were downloaded from TCGA (The Cancer Genome Atlas) database (http://tcga-data.nci.nih.gov/), including 553 human breast cancer samples and 87 normal samples. These breast cancer samples were divided into four subtypes, including basal-like (n= 97), Her2 (n = 47), luminal A (n = 291) and luminal B (n = 118) according to the guidelines in Cirielloet et al. [22]. All selected expression datasets were log2-transformed, then standardized. Furthermore, clinical survival data of these samples in each subtype were also obtained.

2.1.1. miRNA-Target Relationship Data

In this study, we collected experimentally verified miRNA-target interactions data from four well-known data resources: miRTarBase [23], mir2Disease [24], miRecords (V4.0) [25], and TarBase (V6.0) [26]. MiRNA-target relationships in homo species were extracted and combined together to obtain a more comprehensive dataset. In total, 57,863 miRNA-target relationships involving 579 miRNAs and 14,652 target genes were collected and used for further analysis.

2.1.2. PPI Network and Pathway Data

The protein–protein interaction (PPI) network data used in this study were integrated from two databases, HPRD (Human Protein Reference Database) and STRING (Search Tool for the Retrieval of Interacting Genes/Proteins) [27,28]. The interactions stored in HPRD were mainly from experimental validation and text mining. For each recorded entry in the STRING database, a weighted score was given to measure their confidence of interaction by considering multiple factors. To collect high-quality interaction data, we only extracted interactions with a confidence score ≥ 900. Then, we combined interactions from the HPRD and STRING databases. The pathway data used in this study for functional analysis were obtained from the KEGG (Kyoto Encyclopedia of Genes and Genomes) database [29].

2.1.3. Drug and Drug Target Data

In this study, according to our research purpose, in order to improve the practicability of our study, the candidate drugs need to satisfy two requirements simultaneously. Firstly, existing gene targets and regulatory effects on miRNA have to be confirmed. Secondly, the drugs have to have been approved by US Food and Drug Administration (FDA, https://www.fda.gov/), which are prescribed for cancer treatment. We extracted drugs and drug targets from DrugBank [30] and SM2miR [20]. Finally, a total of 36 anticancer drugs were used in this study. The complete information of the 36 anticancer drugs can be found in Supplementary Table S1, including drug ID and drug targets.

2.2. Reconstructed KEGG Pathway Graphs

The reconstructed KEGG (Kyoto Encyclopedia of Genes and Genomes) pathway graphs contained both genes and miRNAs, replicating real biological pathways. We firstly collected 220 KEGG pathway data and converted them into undirected graphs with genes as nodes and their interactions as edges by using our previously developed R package "iSubpathway Miner" [31]. Then, we reconstructed these pathways by wiring miRNAs into these pathways through integrating miRNA-target relations and pathway data. More details, if target genes of a specific miRNA were over-represented within a pathway, the miRNA was wired into the pathway by connecting with target genes within the pathway. The hypergeometric test was used to evaluate the significance of enrichment. The formulas is as follows:

$$P = 1 - \sum_{t=0}^{q-1} \frac{\binom{l}{t}\binom{n-l}{m-t}}{\binom{n}{m}}$$

where n represents the number of background genes (all genome-wide genes), m is the number of genes involved in a given pathway, l is the number of target genes for a specific miRNA, and q is the number of miRNA target genes annotated in the given pathway.

2.3. Identification of Risk Genes and miRNAs Related to Breast Cancer Subtypes

For each breast cancer subtype, we identified significant differentially expressed genes/miRNAs by comparing the tumor with normal samples in each subtype. The unpaired Student's t-test and fold-change methods were simultaneously used to evaluate differentially expressed genes/miRNAs. Then, the significance p-values from the t-test were calibrated by Benjamini-Hochberg multiple tests to obtain the false discovery rate (FDR) values. Finally, we applied $p < 0.01$ and $|\log_2 FC| > 2$ as thresholds to identify differentially expressed genes/miRNAs. These significant differentially expressed genes/miRNAs were regarded as breast cancer subtype-associated genes, which were also defined by us as risk genes and miRNAs, respectively.

2.4. Mining Risk Pathways Associated with Breast Cancer Subtypes

In order to explore the roles of these risk genes and miRNAs in the occurrence and development of breast cancer, we performed them to conduct pathway enrichment analysis to dig out the pathways closely related to breast cancer. We identified pathways with significant enrichment results as risk pathways for each subtype based on risk genes and miRNAs. The cumulative hypergeometric test was used to calculate the significance of each pathway that enriched by risk genes and miRNAs. The formula of the cumulative hypergeometric test is as follows:

$$P = 1 - \sum_{k=0}^{m} \frac{\binom{n}{k}\binom{N-n}{M-k}}{\binom{N}{M}}$$

where N represents the number of background genes (all genome-wide genes), M is the number of a given pathway's genes and miRNAs that are annotated in the N genes, n is total number of the risk genes and miRNAs of a given subtype of breast cancer, and m is the number of risk genes and miRNAs in the given pathway.

2.5. Establishing the Risk Pathways' Crosstalk of Breast Cancer

In each breast cancer subtype, we calculated the crosstalk of each pair of risk pathways based on the correlation strength of genes and miRNAs between them according to previous studies [21]. The Pearson's product moment correlation coefficient and unpaired Student's t-test were performed to measure correlation strength for any two interrelated pathways. As for genes and miRNAs presenting both in pathway i and j, we reckoned their correlation strength only if they interact with other genes or miRNAs in the PPI network. Then, we used correlation strength to construct and assess risk pathways' crosstalk. The formula of calculating correlation strength is as follows:

$$CS(i,j) = F(P(i), P(j)|Exp_i, Exp_j) = -2 * (\log_e P(i) + \log_e P(j) + \log_e P(i,j))$$

where i is the gene that is annotated in pathway a is the gene that is annotated in pathway b; Exp_i and Exp_j are the expression values of genes i and j in samples, respectively; $P(i)$ and $P(j)$ are the differential significance p-values of genes i and j calculated using the unpaired Student's t-test, respectively; and $P(i, j)$ is the significant p-value of expression correlation coefficient between a and b genes/miRNAs based on the Pearson's product moment correlation coefficient.

The crosstalk of any pair of risk pathways was gained by adding up all the correlation strengths between them, and crosstalk of risk pathways i and j was developed based on formula as follows:

$$Crosstalk_{(a,b)} = \sum_{a}^{n} CS$$

where n presents the number of all gene–gene, gene–miRNA, and miRNA–miRNA interactions between any two pathways.

In order to strengthen the differences of risk pathways in different subtypes, we constructed specific dysfunctional crosstalk networks based on the specific crosstalk relationship in each subtype for subsequent calculation and research, which means that when a pair of crosstalk pathways only exist in a certain subtype, they will be selected to construct the subtype crosstalk network.

2.6. Evaluating the Impacts of Drugs on Crosstalk

We integrated the drug information from the DrugBank and SM2miR databases and screened them for Food and Drug Administration (FDA)-approved anticancer drugs that contain both target genes and target miRNAs, and a total of 36 anticancer drugs were screened. Research has shown that the crosstalk among the signaling pathways plays a key role in the occurrence and development of breast cancer. Thus, evaluating the impact of drugs on pathway crosstalk based on the expression of drug targets could help to optimize the treatment of various subtypes of breast cancer. From this standpoint, in order to assess the impacts of drug on dysfunction crosstalk network, for each drug, we first removed its target genes and miRNAs from the specific risk pathway crosstalk of a given subtype. Next, we recalculated the crosstalk to quantify the destructive effects of drugs on different subtypes. At the same time, a formula was designed and developed. The destructive score (DS) of drug to crosstalk was gained using the following formula:

$$DS(d) = \frac{\sum_{i}^{k} \left|1 - \frac{Crosstalk_d}{Crosstalk}\right|}{k}$$

where $Crosstalk_d$ is the crosstalk after drug action, and k presents the number of all specific crosstalks in the subtype.

We determined the destructive score (DS) of all anticancer drugs to specific crosstalk networks in each subtype to assess the impacts of drugs on pathway crosstalk of the drugs. A higher DS score indicates the greater effects of the drug on crosstalk between risk pathways. In each subtype, we only screened anticancer drugs that could impact the crosstalk between dysregulated pathways (DS score greater than zero) as candidate drugs, and we ranked candidate drugs of each subtype by DS score from high to low in various subtypes of breast cancer.

2.7. Survival Analysis

We performed survival analysis based on the targets of candidate drugs that were implicated in the specific pathway crosstalk of each subtypes of breast cancer to evaluate the effects for patient survival of candidate drugs. For a given drug, we extracted its target genes and miRNAs that target a specific crosstalk network as drug target signatures. Each candidate drug target signature was performed for survival analysis in patients of each subtype separately, and we used the K-mean clustering method to stratify patients into shorter survival time and longer survival time groups based on the level of these drug target molecules' expression. In this project, we used 100 as the maximum number of iterations of k means algorithm, and randomly started k means algorithm 20 times to return the best result. Then Kaplan–Meier estimate method was used to evaluate the survival difference of these two classified groups in each subtype, respectively. Finally, the significance p-value of survival difference was estimated using the log-rank test.

3. Results

3.1. Identifying Breast Cancer Subtype-Associated Risk Pathways

We identified the risk miRNAs and genes by comparing tumor samples in each subtype with normal controls, respectively. The differentially expressed genes and miRNAs were detected using t-test and fold-change methods, and then multiple testing correction by the Benjamini–Hochberg procedure was used. Genes/miRNAs with adjusted p-values < 0.01 and $|\log\_2 FC| > 2$ were identified as differential expression (risk genes/miRNAs). In total, we obtained 4096 risk genes (2284 from basal-like subtype, 2192 from her2-enriched subtype, 1831 from luminal A subtype, and 2487 from luminal B subtype) and 223 risk miRNAs (148 from basal-like subtype, 72 from her2-enriched subtype, 76 from luminal A subtype, and 116 from luminal B subtype). Unsupervised hierarchical clustering analysis was performed to observe discrepancy of the expression of risk genes and miRNAs between case samples and normal samples, as shown in Figure 2A. We also performed the degree of overlap of risk genes and miRNAs between subtypes, displayed in Figure 2B. These results indicate that genes and miRNAs exhibit widespread expression disorder in the various breast cancer subtypes.

Breast cancer is affected by multiple factors and pathways. In order to veritably and accurately reflect the changes of the pathways of breast cancer, we used the methods that we developed previously to reconstruct all biological pathways among KEGG, and miRNAs were added into the signaling pathway to form a more abundant signaling pathway. To discover the biological function of these risk genes and miRNAs, we used pathway enrichment analysis to identify risk pathways in each subtype. A pathway is identified as a risk pathway only if risk genes and miRNAs are enriched in it under the significance level $p < 0.05$. In total, there were 32 risk pathways in basal-like subtype, 29 risk pathways in her2-enriched subtype, 21 risk pathways in luminal A subtype, and 26 risk pathways in luminal B subtype. We show the top ten pathways of each breast cancer subtype in Figure 2C. We found that some risk pathways such as the Chemokine signaling pathway, ECM–receptor interaction, the PPAR signaling pathway, and Tyrosine metabolism were simultaneously identified in different breast cancer subtypes. Furthermore, we found some subtype-specific risk pathways in each subtype of breast cancer. Amoebiasis, drug metabolism–other enzymes, fatty acid metabolism, the p53 signaling pathway, and salivary secretion were found in basal-like, cell adhesion molecules (CAMs) in her2-enriched, histidine metabolism in Luminal A, and glycerolipid metabolism and TGF-beta signaling pathway in Luminal B subtypes. These subtype-specific risk pathways may be one of the reasons that resulted in distinct molecular mechanisms and clinical outcomes of breast cancer subtypes.

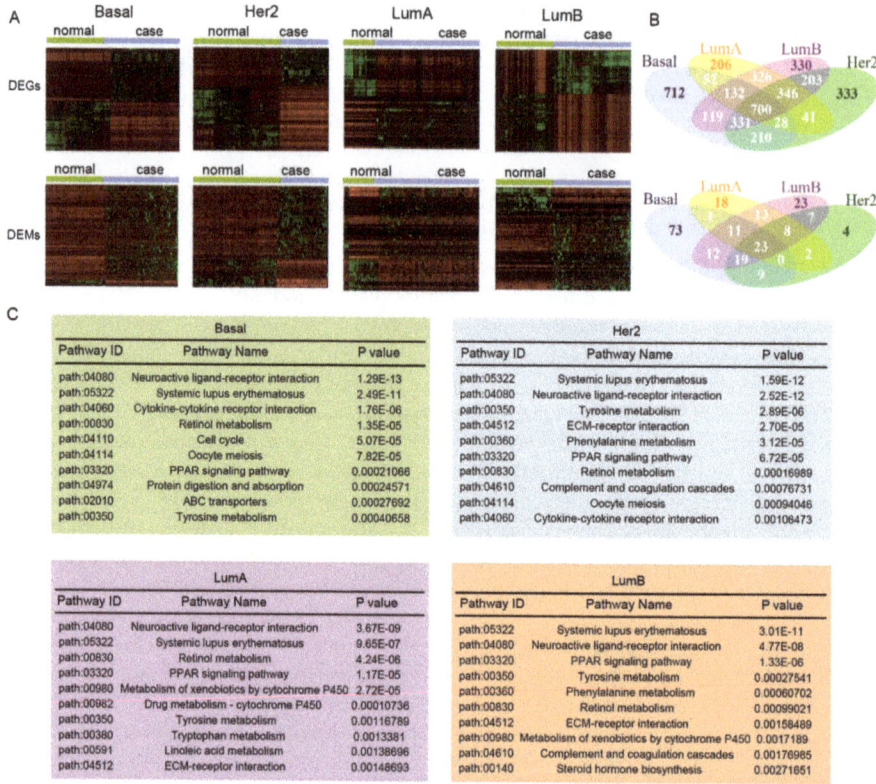

Figure 2. Global view of risk genes and miRNAs in each subtype of breast cancer. (**A**) Heat maps show risk genes and miRNAs in four breast cancer subtypes. Unsupervised hierarchical clustering analysis is used, which divided genes and miRNAs into two clusters, the lower and higher expression values are represented by green and the red colors, respectively. (**B**) Venn plots of risk genes and miRNAs associated with breast cancer subtypes separately. (**C**) Results of top 10 pathways with significant enrichment result of each subtype. Note: Basal, basal-like subtype; Her2, her2-enriched subtype; LumA, luminal A subtype; LumB, luminal B subtype.

3.2. Constructing Risk Pathway Crosstalk Networks for Various Subtypes of Breast Cancer

The occurrence of breast cancer is complex and there is crosstalk between different functional biological pathways in the process of cancer development. Thus, it is necessary to dissect the crosstalk of dysfunctional pathways related to breast cancer. To elucidate the molecular mechanism of various breast cancer subtypes, we analyzed the crosstalk between dysfunctional pathways that are related to breast cancer. In our study, the risk pathway crosstalk networks for each breast cancer subtype were constructed. The quantification of crosstalk was conducted by calculating both the correlation strength and the dysfunction degree of genes and miRNAs in any two risk pathways of each breast cancer subtype, and the expression correlation coefficient between genes and miRNAs and the unpaired Student's t-test of genes and miRNAs were used for assessment of crosstalk.

Our results showed that there were crosstalks with significant differences in the extent of crosstalk between risk pathways in each subtype (Figure 3). For example, 'calcium signaling pathway' and 'focal adhesion' have more crosstalk relationships with other pathways in basal-like subtype. 'Pathways in cancer' and 'focal adhesion' crosstalk more with other pathways in her2-enriched subtype. In luminal A subtype, 'Jak–STAT signaling pathway' has the greatest crosstalk with 'cytokine–cytokine receptor interaction'. In luminal B subtype, 'pathways in cancer' and 'cytokine–cytokine receptor interaction' possess larger crosstalk values with other pathways.

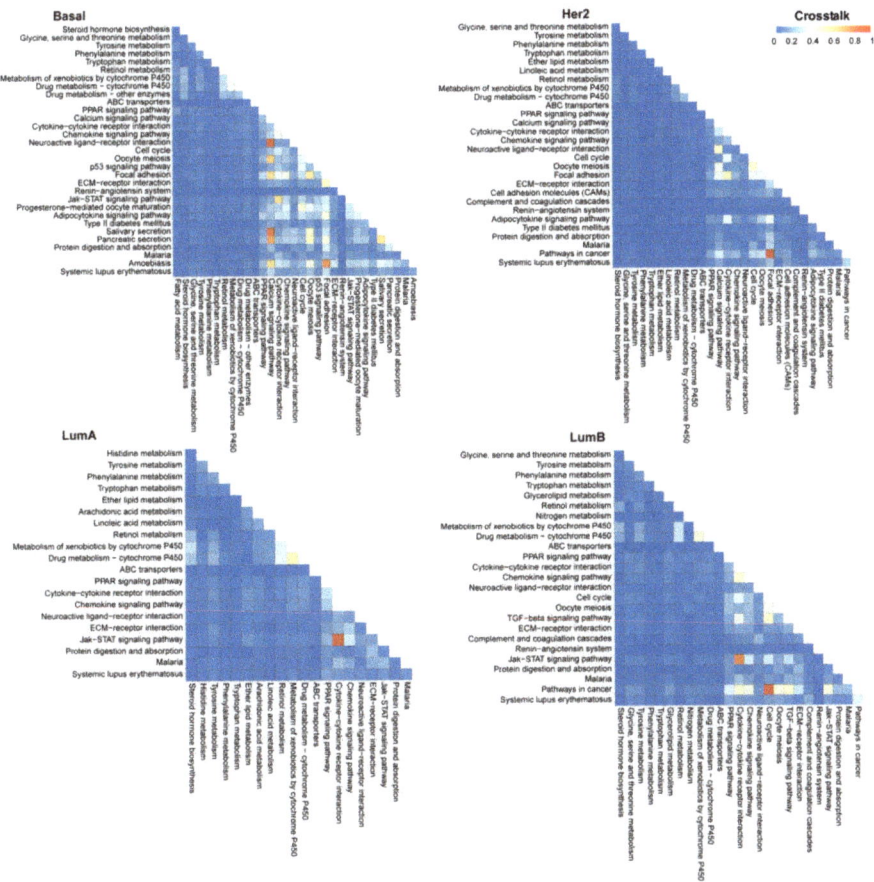

Figure 3. The crosstalk for each two interrelated risk pathways in breast cancer subtypes. Heat maps of crosstalk between risk pathways for comparing the heterogeneity of crosstalk across different subtypes of breast cancer. The color of the box represents the crosstalk between the two pathways, the lower and higher crosstalk are represented by blue and the red colors, respectively.

Moreover, we found some subtype-specific crosstalk of pathways in breast cancer. We extracted the specific crosstalk risk pathways of each subtype and used them to construct the specific crosstalk network of the risk pathway in four subtypes (Figure 4). There are 197 specific crosstalk relationships in basal like, 56 specific crosstalk relationships in her2-enriched, 41 specific crosstalk relationships in luminal A, and 74 specific crosstalk relationships in luminal B subtypes. The above results indicate that these subtype-specific crosstalks of risk pathways may be one of the molecular mechanisms that lead to distinct clinical outcomes of breast cancer patients, which will help us to understand the discrepancy between subtypes and points a new way to optimize the treatment of breast cancer patients.

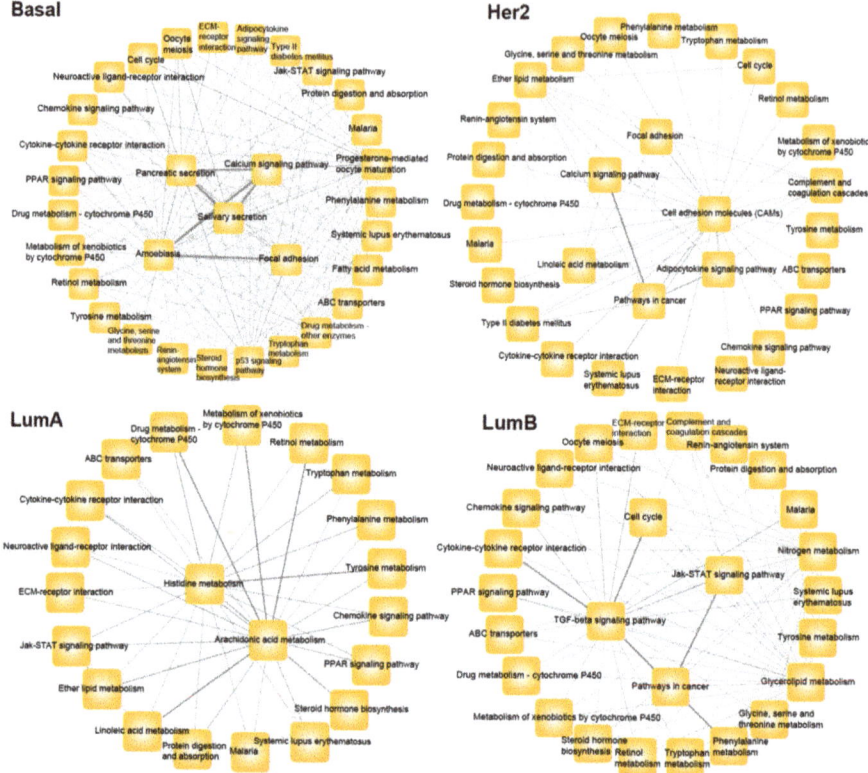

Figure 4. The specific crosstalk network of each breast cancer subtype. The yellow rectangle represents the pathways of the specific crosstalk network. The thickness of edges represents the intensity of crosstalk between pathways; the larger the crosstalk value, the thicker the edge.

3.3. Screening Candidate Therapeutic Drugs for Each Subtype of Breast Cancer Based on DS Score

Previous experimental studies have demonstrated that cancer cells could adapt signaling pathway circuits under drug treatment by establishing alternative signaling routes through crosstalk [32,33]. Based on this point of view, we developed an evaluation method to optimize the therapeutic drugs for each subtype of breast cancer by assessing the impact of drugs on crosstalk among risk pathways. The drug targets of each drug were removed from risk pathways and we reconstructed crosstalk networks targeted by drugs to evaluate the perturbance effects of those drugs. Next, we recalculated the crosstalk to measure the perturbance effects of drugs on different subtypes and optimize the drug use for each subtype of breast cancer. We obtained 36 anticancer drugs that target both genes and miRNAs, and the results of evaluation of anticancer drugs are shown in Table 1. We only screened anticancer drugs of each subtype with a *DS* score greater than zero as candidate drugs, and ranked candidate drugs of each subtype by *DS* score from high to low. A higher DS score indicates the greater effects of the drug on crosstalk between risk pathways. In total, there are 33 drugs in basal-like, 32 drugs in her2-enriched, 22 drugs in luminal A, and 30 drugs in luminal B subtypes.

Table 1. Screened candidate drugs for various subtypes of breast cancer based on DS score.

DS Score Ranking	Basal	Her2	LumA	LumB
1	5-Fluorouracil	Arsenic trioxide	Arsenic trioxide	Arsenic trioxide
2	Arsenic trioxide	Adriamycin	5-Fluorouracil	Adriamycin
3	Tamoxifen	5-Fluorouracil	Adriamycin	5-Fluorouracil
4	Trastuzumab	Trastuzumab	Trastuzumab	Trastuzumab
5	Etoposide	Paclitaxel	Etoposide	Etoposide
6	Cisplatin	Temozolomide	Tamoxifen	Cisplatin
7	Paclitaxel	Etoposide	Vorinostat	Topotecan
8	Vorinostat	Gemcitabine	Bicalutamide	Irinotecan
9	Gemcitabine	Everolimus	Cisplatin	Paclitaxel
10	Adriamycin	Sunitinib	Vemurafenib	Tamoxifen
11	Temozolomide	Tamoxifen	Medroxyprogesterone acetate	Vemurafenib
12	Cyclophosphamide	Vorinostat	Gemcitabine	Gemcitabine
13	Bicalutamide	Cisplatin	Temozolomide	Sunitinib
14	Sunitinib	Sorafenib	Everolimus	Vorinostat
15	Vemurafenib	Cyclophosphamide	Sunitinib	Temozolomide
16	Medroxyprogesterone acetate	Goserelin	Paclitaxel	Everolimus
17	Everolimus	Vemurafenib	Oxaliplatin	Lenalidomide
18	Vinblastine	Bicalutamide	Cyclophosphamide	Cyclophosphamide
19	Lenalidomide	Vinblastine	Sorafenib	Bicalutamide
20	Oxaliplatin	Lenalidomide	Irinotecan	Goserelin
21	Sorafenib	Imatinib mesylate	Topotecan	Rapamycin
22	Goserelin	Bortezomib	Lenalidomide	Oxaliplatin
23	Irinotecan	Oxaliplatin		Vinblastine
24	Mitoxantrone	Medroxyprogesterone acetate		Sorafenib
25	Topotecan	Melphalan		Vincristine
26	Imatinib mesylate	Gefitinib		Medroxyprogesterone acetate
27	Vincristine	Rapamycin		Bortezomib
28	Gefitinib	Vincristine		Imatinib mesylate
29	Docetaxel	Irinotecan		Mitoxantrone
30	Bortezomib	Topotecan		Melphalan
31	Melphalan	Mitoxantrone		
32	Rapamycin	Docetaxel		
33	Epirubicin			

3.4. Dissecting the Effects of Candidate Therapeutic Drugs for Patient Survival in Each Subtype of Breast Cancer

A drug could specifically interact with a target molecule to modulate a physiological process and further impact the progression of a disease [34]. In order to further screen drugs for breast cancer patients, we got the patients' clinical survival information in each breast cancer subtype. For each candidate therapeutic drug that was screened based on DS score in different subtypes, we evaluated the drug target signature's influence on patient survival. Patients from each subtype of breast cancer were divided into two groups (shorter survival time group and longer survival time group) based on the expression of drug target signatures. As shown in Figure 5, we found that there were, in total, six candidate therapeutic drugs screened based on DS score (DS score greater than zero) that significantly correlated with overall survival (OS) in the different subtypes of breast cancer patients. Paclitaxel, Vincristine, and Sorafenib in basal-like, Irinotecan in her2-enriched, Vemurafenib in luminal A, and Vorinostat in luminal B subtypes. These six dugs not only impacted the crosstalk of risk pathways, but they also had an effect on the patients' survival in their corresponding subtypes. This indicates that they may be more suitable treatment candidates for the corresponding subtypes of breast cancer. More details, according to drug target signatures of Paclitaxel and Sorafenib in the basal-like subtype, these 97 patients were divided into a shorter survival group ($n = 5$) and a longer survival group ($n = 92$), respectively. Vincristine drug target signatures divided 97 patients in the basal-like subtype into a shorter survival group ($n = 63$) and a longer survival group ($n = 55$). The 47 patients in the her2-enriched subtype were separated into a shorter survival group ($n = 10$) and a longer survival group ($n = 37$) by Irinotecan drug target signatures. Based on the drug target signatures of Vemurafenib in luminal A subtype, the 287 patients (survival information was missing in four patients) were stratified into a shorter survival group ($n = 78$) and a longer survival group ($n = 209$), and Vorinostat drug target signatures stratified 118 luminal B subtype patients into a shorter survival group ($n = 63$) and a longer survival group ($n = 55$). Here, drugs' signatures stratified the patients into two groups in a statistically significant manner and their expression direction were not considered.

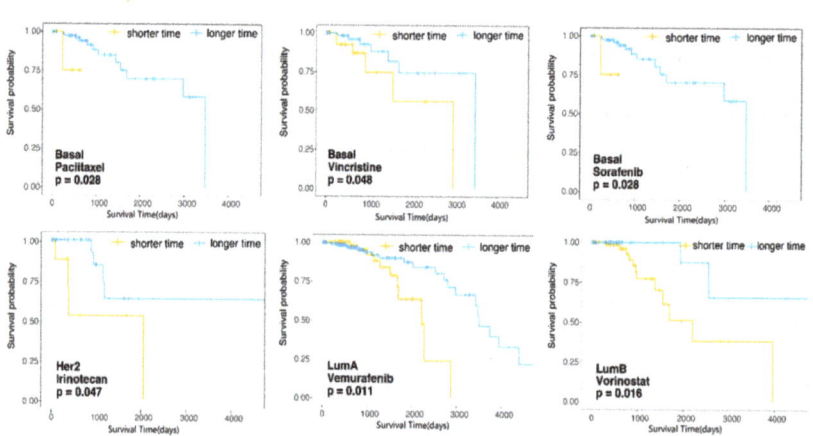

Figure 5. Kaplan-Meier survival curves of patients at shorter survival time group or longer survival time group stratified by drug target signatures of candidate drugs of each breast cancer subtype.

3.5. Dissecting the Mechanism of Candidate Drugs for Each Subtype

In our drugs' optimization results, Paclitaxel, Sorafenib, and Vincristine were found to have potential therapy effect in the basal-like subtype of breast cancer. Consistent with clinical findings, Paclitaxel and Vincristine were the optimal adjuvant therapy for triple-negative breast cancer [35,36]. Sorafenib is a multiple targeted agent which can inhibit tumor cell proliferation and angiogenesis by inhibiting the activation of multiple different kinases [37], and our results indicate that Sorafenib plays a therapeutic role in the basal-like subtype of breast cancer mainly through affecting specific risk pathway crosstalk mediated by hsa-miR-30a, hsa-miR-222, and hsa-miR-193a. Some studies have confirmed that hsa-miR-30a, hsa-miR-222, and hsa-miR-193a play key roles in breast cancer [38–40]. Irinotecan, an antitumor enzyme inhibitor mainly used for the treatment of colorectal cancer [41], is suitable for the her2-enriched subtype, which mediates the specific crosstalk among the risk pathways of the her2-enriched subtype through regulating hsa-miR-23a and hsa-miR-324. In accordance with the result of WT Kuo and Eissa [42,43], hsa-miR-324 and hsa-miR-23a have distinct biological functions in breast cancer. Vemurafenib has long been approved for the treatment of metastatic melanoma with BRAF mutation [44], and our results showed that this drug had a damaging effect on the specific crosstalk of risk pathway of the luminal A subtype through action on hsa-miR-145. Just as some researches have shown that miR-145 is a potential cancer biomarker and serves as a novel target for cancer therapy, including breast cancer [45]. Vorinostat as an anticancer agent that inhibits histone deacetylases, approved for cutaneous T-cell lymphoma [46], and plays a key role in the epigenetic regulation of gene expression. Vorinostat could act on the specific risk pathways crosstalk of the luminal B subtype via 14 miRNAs (Figure 6), which have been found to play important roles in the occurrence and development of breast cancer, such as hsa-miR-155, hsa-miR-34a, hsa-miR-17, hsa-miR-22, and hsa-miR-140 [47–51].

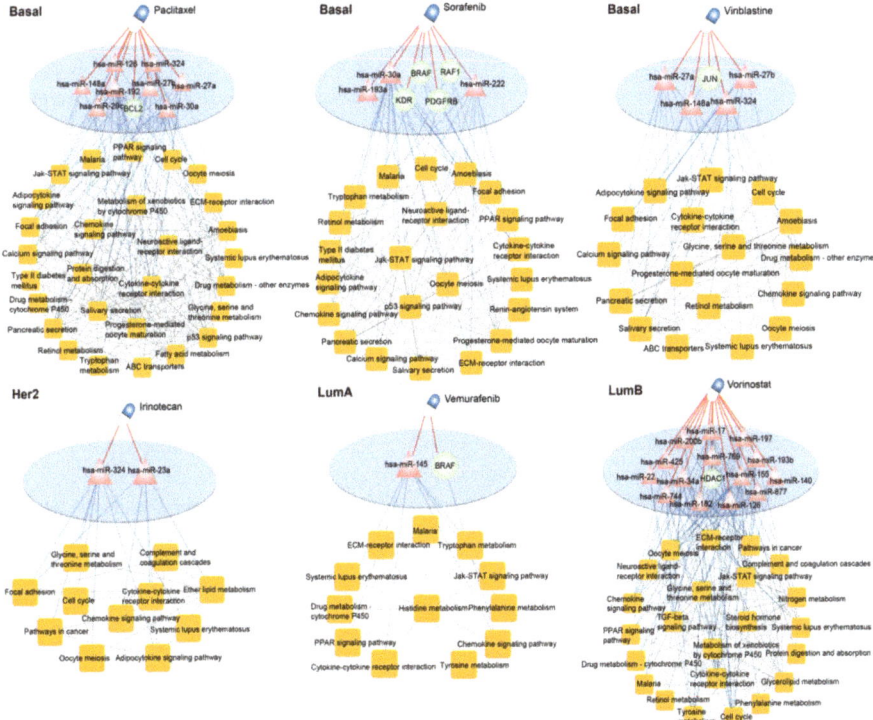

Figure 6. The mechanism of optimal therapeutic drugs in each subtype of breast cancer. Sorafenib, Paclitaxel, and Vincristine were applicable for the basal-like subtype treatment, Irinotecan was optimum for the her2-enriched subtype treatment, Vemurafenib was suitable for the luminal A subtype treatment, and Vorinostat was applied to the luminal B subtype treatment.

4. Discussion

Breast cancer is a complex disease with high heterogeneity in terms of the underlying molecular alterations, the cellular composition of tumors, and even the clinical outcomes. Different subtypes exhibit distinct biological behavior, prognosis, and usually different responses to drug treatment [52], yet identifing applicable drugs for each subtype still largely remains limited. Therefore, it is urgently needed to develop a systematic pipeline to identify medications for different subtypes of breast cancer.

The occurrence and development of tumors is a complex process involving many steps, links, and factors. It is mostly the action of a single molecule (gene or miRNA) that leads to poor therapeutic effect among many chemotherapeutic regimens [53]. In recent years, many researches have revealed that the occurrence of tumors is closely related to the abnormality of biological pathways, and crosstalk of abnormal pathways is one of the prime reasons for the poor outcomes of tumor treatment [54]. Studies have shown that regulatory molecules such as non-coding RNA participate in the anomaly of biological pathways through the regulation of genes, adding to the difficulty of cancer treatment [55]. In order to actually reflect the intricate crosstalk of pathways, we have developed a new method based on biological pathways—that is, reconstruction of biological pathways which include both genes and miRNAs. We have also identified the optimal drugs by quantifying the effect of candidate drugs on miRNA-mediated crosstalk of pathways. We have successfully identified the specific crosstalk of pathways in each subtype of breast cancer and revealed their pathogenesis respectively by applying this method. Moreover, we also screened applicable drugs for each subtype of breast cancer. We successfully screened the most suitable drugs for each subtype of breast cancer, including Paclitaxel and Vincristine, which are breast cancer treatment drugs in clinical application. On the basis of the original application, we accurately identified their applications in each subtype, such that Paclitaxel and Vincristine were best for basal-like, Irinotecan was suitable for her2-enriched, and Vorinostat was the optimal drug for luminal B subtypes. We also identified other anticancer drugs application in each subtypes of breast cancer. The results show that our approach could help doctors to further improve treatment strategies with the current menu of chemotherapy options.

Currently, several methods have been proposed to optimize drugs for human cancers. For example, Lamb et al. provided a computational method to connect diseases and their potential therapeutic small molecules based on gene expression profiles form disease and cultured human cells treated with bioactive small molecules respectively [56]. Gottlieb et al. predicted novel drug indications based on multiple drug–drug and disease–disease similarity measures [57]. Furthermore, Malas et al. prioritized drugs using the semantic information between drug and disease concepts [58]. Comparing with these methods, our study has some unique features. First, we considered the role of non-coding RNAs in our approach. Second, our study optimized anticancer drugs by measuring their effects for mediating the crosstalk between risk pathways, which was an important molecular mechanism in the initiation and progression of human cancers. Finally, we optimized candidate drugs for different breast cancer subtypes, which may further promote the precise use of drugs for human cancer.

There are also several limitations in our study. First of all, drugs targeting miRNAs for therapeutic purposes are limited, and there are many drugs without miRNA targets. Secondly, miRNAs affected by the drugs are required for further study. We believe that more and more drugs that regulate miRNAs and drug-regulated miRNAs will be discovered with the development of in-depth study on the interaction of drugs and miRNAs, and our method can identify the optimal therapeutic agent for complex diseases more accurately and comprehensively. In summary, the results in this study highlight that dissecting subtype-specific risk pathway crosstalk could provide novel insights into the underlying molecular mechanisms and thus promote the drug discovery for various breast cancer subtype. Moreover, we focused on breast cancer in this study, but the method proposed here could also be applied to many other complex diseases, as pathway crosstalk is widespread in biological systems and the dysregulation of which play a critical role in the occurrence of disease.

Supplementary Materials: The following are available online at http://www.mdpi.com/2073-4425/10/9/657/s1, Table S1: Detailed information of the 36 anticancer drugs and their targets.

Author Contributions: Conceptualization, Y.X. and Y.X.; data curation, J.W. and C.Z.; formal analysis, Y.X., H.Z., and C.H.; investigation, S.L., H.Z., and J.W.; methodology, Y.X.; supervision, Y.X. and L.W.; validation, H.Z. and Q.W.; visualization, S.L. and C.H.; writing—original draft, Y.X. and S.L; writing—review and editing, C.Z., Q.D., D.S., Y.X., and L.W.

Funding: This work was supported by the Fundamental Research Funds for the Provincial Universities (2017JCZX51,2017JCZX53, 2017JCZX54); the Heilongjiang Postdoctoral Science Foundation (LBHZ16123, LBH-Z17218, LBH-Z17110); the China Postdoctoral Science Foundation (2018M631943, 2016M600260); the China Postdoctoral Science Special Foundation (2019T120280); the National Natural Science Foundation of China (61903105, 31801115, 31801107, 61803129); and the Wu lien-teh Youth Science Fund Project of Harbin Medical University (WLD-QN1407)

Acknowledgments: Not applicable.

Conflicts of Interest: The authors declare no conflicts of interest.

References

1. Holm, J.; Eriksson, L.; Ploner, A.; Eriksson, M.; Rantalainen, M.; Li, J.; Hall, P.; Czene, K. Assessment of breast cancer risk factors reveals subtype heterogeneity. *Cancer Res.* **2017**, *77*, 3708–3717. [CrossRef] [PubMed]
2. Zardavas, D.; Irrthum, A.; Swanton, C.; Piccart, M. Clinical management of breast cancer heterogeneity. *Nat. Rev. Clin. Oncol.* **2015**, *12*, 381–394. [CrossRef] [PubMed]

3. Goldhirsch, A.; Wood, W.C.; Coates, A.S.; Gelber, R.D.; Thurlimann, B.; Senn, H.J.; Panel Members. Strategies for subtypes—Dealing with the diversity of breast cancer: Highlights of the st. Gallen international expert consensus on the primary therapy of early breast cancer 2011. *Ann. Oncol. Off. J. Eur. Soc. Med. Oncol.* **2011**, *22*, 1736–1747. [CrossRef] [PubMed]
4. Onitilo, A.A.; Engel, J.M.; Greenlee, R.T.; Mukesh, B.N. Breast cancer subtypes based on er/pr and her2 expression: Comparison of clinicopathologic features and survival. *Clin. Med. Res.* **2009**, *7*, 4–13. [CrossRef] [PubMed]
5. Cancer Genome Atlas Network. Comprehensive molecular portraits of human breast tumours. *Nature* **2012**, *490*, 61–70. [CrossRef]
6. Sorlie, T.; Perou, C.M.; Tibshirani, R.; Aas, T.; Geisler, S.; Johnsen, H.; Hastie, T.; Eisen, M.B.; van de Rijn, M.; Jeffrey, S.S.; et al. Gene expression patterns of breast carcinomas distinguish tumor subclasses with clinical implications. *Proc. Natl. Acad. Sci. USA* **2001**, *98*, 10869–10874. [CrossRef] [PubMed]
7. Cheung, P.S. Recent advances in breast cancer treatment. *Hong Kong Med. J. Xianggang Yi Xue Za Zhi* **2018**, *24*, 6–8. [CrossRef]
8. Wang, L.; Li, J.; Zhao, H.; Hu, J.; Ping, Y.; Li, F.; Lan, Y.; Xu, C.; Xiao, Y.; Li, X. Identifying the crosstalk of dysfunctional pathways mediated by lncRNAs in breast cancer subtypes. *Mol. BioSyst.* **2016**, *12*, 711–720. [CrossRef]
9. Restelli, M.; Magni, M.; Ruscica, V.; Pinciroli, P.; De Cecco, L.; Buscemi, G.; Delia, D.; Zannini, L. A novel crosstalk between ccar2 and akt pathway in the regulation of cancer cell proliferation. *Cell Death Dis.* **2016**, *7*, e2453. [CrossRef]
10. Brechbiel, J.M.-M.K.; Adjei, A.A. Crosstalk between hedgehog and other signaling pathways as a basis for combination therapies in cancer. *Cancer Treat. Rev.* **2014**, *40*, 750–759. [CrossRef]
11. Aksamitiene, E.; Kiyatkin, A.; Kholodenko, B.N. Cross-talk between mitogenic ras/mapk and survival pi3k/akt pathways: A fine balance. *Biochem. Soc. Focus. Meet.* **2012**, *40*, 139–146. [CrossRef] [PubMed]
12. Jaeger, S.; Igea, A.; Arroyo, R.; Alcalde, V.; Canovas, B.; Orozco, M.; Nebreda, A.R.; Aloy, P. Quantification of pathway cross-talk reveals novel synergistic drug combinations for breast cancer. *Cancer Res.* **2017**, *77*, 459–469. [CrossRef] [PubMed]
13. Godard, P.; van Eyll, J. Pathway analysis from lists of microRNAs: Common pitfalls and alternative strategy. *Nucleic Acids Res.* **2015**, *43*, 3490–3497. [CrossRef] [PubMed]
14. Mulrane, L.; McGee, S.F.; Gallagher, W.M.; O'Connor, D.P. miRNA dysregulation in breast cancer. *Cancer Res.* **2013**, *73*, 6554–6562. [CrossRef] [PubMed]
15. Anton, R.; Chatterjee, S.S.; Simundza, J.; Cowin, P.; Dasgupta, R. A systematic screen for micro-RNAs regulating the canonical wnt pathway. *PLoS ONE* **2011**, *6*, e26257. [CrossRef] [PubMed]
16. Kaboli, P.J.; Rahmat, A.; Ismail, P.; Ling, K.H. MicroRNA-based therapy and breast cancer: A comprehensive review of novel therapeutic strategies from diagnosis to treatment. *Pharmacol. Res.* **2015**, *97*, 104–121. [CrossRef] [PubMed]
17. Bai, F.; Yu, Z.; Gao, X.; Gong, J.; Fan, L.; Liu, F. Simvastatin induces breast cancer cell death through oxidative stress up-regulating mir-140-5p. *Aging (Albany NY)* **2019**, *11*, 3198–3219. [CrossRef]
18. Zhang, L.; Zhang, F.; Li, Y.; Qi, X.; Guo, Y. Triiodothyronine promotes cell proliferation of breast cancer via modulating mir-204/amphiregulin. *Pathol. Oncol. Res. POR* **2019**, *25*, 653–658. [CrossRef]
19. Shenoda, B.B.; Ramanathan, S.; Ajit, S.K. In vitro validation of miRNA-mediated gene expression linked to drug metabolism. *Curr. Protoc. Pharmacol.* **2017**, *79*, 9.26.1–9.26.15.
20. Liu, X.; Wang, S.; Meng, F.; Wang, J.; Zhang, Y.; Dai, E.; Yu, X.; Li, X.; Jiang, W. Sm2mir: A database of the experimentally validated small molecules' effects on microRNA expression. *Bioinformatics* **2013**, *29*, 409–411. [CrossRef]
21. Zhang, Y.; Xu, Y.; Li, F.; Li, X.; Feng, L.; Shi, X.; Wang, L.; Li, X. Dissecting dysfunctional crosstalk pathways regulated by miRNAs during glioma progression. *Oncotarget* **2016**, *7*, 25769–25782. [CrossRef] [PubMed]
22. Ciriello, G.; Gatza, M.L.; Beck, A.H.; Wilkerson, M.D.; Rhie, S.K.; Pastore, A.; Zhang, H.; McLellan, M.; Yau, C.; Kandoth, C.; et al. Comprehensive molecular portraits of invasive lobular breast cancer. *Cell* **2015**, *163*, 506–519. [CrossRef] [PubMed]
23. Hsu, S.D.; Lin, F.M.; Wu, W.Y.; Liang, C.; Huang, W.C.; Chan, W.L.; Tsai, W.T.; Chen, G.Z.; Lee, C.J.; Chiu, C.M.; et al. Mirtarbase: A database curates experimentally validated microRNA-target interactions. *Nucleic Acids Res.* **2011**, *39*, D163–D169. [CrossRef] [PubMed]

24. Jiang, Q.; Wang, Y.; Hao, Y.; Juan, L.; Teng, M.; Zhang, X.; Li, M.; Wang, G.; Liu, Y. Mir2disease: A manually curated database for microRNA deregulation in human disease. *Nucleic Acids Res.* **2009**, *37*, D98–D104. [CrossRef] [PubMed]
25. Xiao, F.; Zuo, Z.; Cai, G.; Kang, S.; Gao, X.; Li, T. Mirecords: An integrated resource for microRNA-target interactions. *Nucleic Acids Res.* **2009**, *37*, D105–D110. [CrossRef] [PubMed]
26. Vergoulis, T.; Vlachos, I.S.; Alexiou, P.; Georgakilas, G.; Maragkakis, M.; Reczko, M.; Gerangelos, S.; Koziris, N.; Dalamagas, T.; Hatzigeorgiou, A.G. Tarbase 6.0: Capturing the exponential growth of miRNA targets with experimental support. *Nucleic Acids Res.* **2012**, *40*, D222–D229. [CrossRef] [PubMed]
27. Keshava Prasad, T.S.; Goel, R.; Kandasamy, K.; Keerthikumar, S.; Kumar, S.; Mathivanan, S.; Telikicherla, D.; Raju, R.; Shafreen, B.; Venugopal, A.; et al. Human protein reference database—2009 update. *Nucleic Acids Res.* **2009**, *37*, D767–D772. [CrossRef] [PubMed]
28. Szklarczyk, D.; Franceschini, A.; Wyder, S.; Forslund, K.; Heller, D.; Huerta-Cepas, J.; Simonovic, M.; Roth, A.; Santos, A.; Tsafou, K.P.; et al. String v10: Protein-protein interaction networks, integrated over the tree of life. *Nucleic Acids Res.* **2015**, *43*, D447–D452. [CrossRef]
29. Kanehisa, M.; Goto, S.; Hattori, M.; Aoki-Kinoshita, K.F.; Itoh, M.; Kawashima, S.; Katayama, T.; Araki, M.; Hirakawa, M. From genomics to chemical genomics: New developments in kegg. *Nucleic Acids Res.* **2006**, *34*, D354–D357. [CrossRef]
30. Wishart, D.S.; Feunang, Y.D.; Guo, A.C.; Lo, E.J.; Marcu, A.; Grant, J.R.; Sajed, T.; Johnson, D.; Li, C.; Sayeeda, Z.; et al. Drugbank 5.0: A major update to the drugbank database for 2018. *Nucleic Acids Res.* **2018**, *46*, D1074–D1082. [CrossRef]
31. Li, C.; Li, X.; Miao, Y.; Wang, Q.; Jiang, W.; Xu, C.; Li, J.; Han, J.; Zhang, F.; Gong, B.; et al. Subpathwayminer: A software package for flexible identification of pathways. *Nucleic Acids Res.* **2009**, *37*, e131. [CrossRef] [PubMed]
32. Bernards, R. A missing link in genotype-directed cancer therapy. *Cell* **2012**, *151*, 465–468. [CrossRef] [PubMed]
33. Yamaguchi, H.; Chang, S.S.; Hsu, J.L.; Hung, M.C. Signaling cross-talk in the resistance to her family receptor targeted therapy. *Oncogene* **2014**, *33*, 1073–1081. [CrossRef] [PubMed]
34. Koscielny, G.; An, P.; Carvalho-Silva, D.; Cham, J.A.; Fumis, L.; Gasparyan, R.; Hasan, S.; Karamanis, N.; Maguire, M.; Papa, E.; et al. Open targets: A platform for therapeutic target identification and validation. *Nucleic Acids Res.* **2017**, *45*, D985–D994. [CrossRef] [PubMed]
35. Zeng, F.; Ju, R.J.; Liu, L.; Xie, H.J.; Mu, L.M.; Zhao, Y.; Yan, Y.; Hu, Y.J.; Wu, J.S.; Lu, W.L. Application of functional vincristine plus dasatinib liposomes to deletion of vasculogenic mimicry channels in triple-negative breast cancer. *Oncotarget* **2015**, *6*, 36625–36642. [CrossRef] [PubMed]
36. Wahba, H.A.; El-Hadaad, H.A. Current approaches in treatment of triple-negative breast cancer. *Cancer Biol. Med.* **2015**, *12*, 106–116. [PubMed]
37. Wilhelm, S.; Carter, C.; Lynch, M.; Lowinger, T.; Dumas, J.; Smith, R.A.; Schwartz, B.; Simantov, R.; Kelley, S. Discovery and development of sorafenib: A multikinase inhibitor for treating cancer. *Nat. Rev. Drug Discov.* **2006**, *5*, 835–844. [CrossRef]
38. Zhang, N.; Wang, X.; Huo, Q.; Sun, M.; Cai, C.; Liu, Z.; Hu, G.; Yang, Q. MicroRNA-30a suppresses breast tumor growth and metastasis by targeting metadherin. *Oncogene* **2014**, *33*, 3119–3128. [CrossRef]
39. Shah, M.Y.; Calin, G.A. MicroRNAs mir-221 and mir-222: A new level of regulation in aggressive breast cancer. *Genome Med.* **2011**, *3*, 56. [CrossRef]
40. Tsai, K.W.; Leung, C.M.; Lo, Y.H.; Chen, T.W.; Chan, W.C.; Yu, S.Y.; Tu, Y.T.; Lam, H.C.; Li, S.C.; Ger, L.P.; et al. Arm selection preference of microRNA-193a varies in breast cancer. *Sci. Rep.* **2016**, *6*, 28176. [CrossRef]
41. Vanhoefer, U.; Harstrick, A.; Achterrath, W.; Cao, S.; Seeber, S.; Rustum, Y.M. Irinotecan in the treatment of colorectal cancer: Clinical overview. *J. Clin. Oncol. Off. J. Am. Soc. Clin. Oncol.* **2001**, *19*, 1501–1518. [CrossRef] [PubMed]
42. Kuo, W.T.; Yu, S.Y.; Li, S.C.; Lam, H.C.; Chang, H.T.; Chen, W.S.; Yu, C.C. MicroRNA-324 in human cancer: Mir-324-5p and mir-324-3p have distinct biological functions in human cancer. *Anticancer Res.* **2016**, *36*, 5189–5196. [CrossRef] [PubMed]
43. Eissa, S.; Matboli, M.; Shehata, H.H. Breast tissue–based microRNA panel highlights microRNA-23a and selected target genes as putative biomarkers for breast cancer. *Transl. Res.* **2015**, *165*, 417–427. [CrossRef] [PubMed]

44. Bollag, G.; Tsai, J.; Zhang, J.; Zhang, C.; Ibrahim, P.; Nolop, K.; Hirth, P. Vemurafenib: The first drug approved for braf-mutant cancer. *Nat. Rev. Drug Discov.* **2012**, *11*, 873–886. [CrossRef] [PubMed]
45. Sachdeva, M.; Mo, Y.Y. Mir-145-mediated suppression of cell growth, invasion and metastasis. *Am. J. Transl. Res.* **2010**, *2*, 170–180. [PubMed]
46. Mann, B.S.; Johnson, J.R.; He, K.; Sridhara, R.; Abraham, S.; Booth, B.P.; Verbois, L.; Morse, D.E.; Jee, J.M.; Pope, S.; et al. Vorinostat for treatment of cutaneous manifestations of advanced primary cutaneous t-cell lymphoma. *Clin. Cancer Res. Off. J. Am. Assoc. Cancer Res.* **2007**, *13*, 2318–2322. [CrossRef]
47. Li, L.; Xie, X.; Luo, J.; Liu, M.; Xi, S.; Guo, J.; Tang, J. Targeted expression of mir-34a using the t-visa system suppresses breast cancer cell growth and invasion. *Mol. Ther.* **2012**, *20*, 2326–2334. [CrossRef]
48. Mattiske, S.; Suetani, R.J.; Neilsen, P.M.; Callen, D.F. The oncogenic role of mir-155 in breast cancer. *Cancer Epidemiol. Biomark. Prev. Publ. Am. Assoc. Cancer Res. Cosponsored Am. Soc. Prev. Oncol.* **2012**, *21*, 1236–1243. [CrossRef]
49. Hossain, A.; Kuo, M.T.; Saunders, G.F. Mir-17-5p regulates breast cancer cell proliferation by inhibiting translation of aib1 mRNA. *Mol. Cell. Biol.* **2006**, *26*, 8191–8201. [CrossRef]
50. Chen, B.; Tang, H.; Liu, X.; Liu, P.; Yang, L.; Xie, X.; Wei, W. Mir-22 as a prognostic factor targets glucose transporter protein type 1 in breast cancer. *Cancer Lett.* **2015**, *356*, 410–417. [CrossRef]
51. Li, Q.; Yao, Y.; Eades, G.; Liu, Z.; Zhang, Y.; Zhou, Q. Downregulation of mir-140 promotes cancer stem cell formation in basal-like early stage breast cancer. *Oncogene* **2014**, *33*, 2589–2600. [CrossRef] [PubMed]
52. DeSantis, C.E.; Ma, J.; Goding Sauer, A.; Newman, L.A.; Jemal, A. Breast cancer statistics, 2017, racial disparity in mortality by state. *CA Cancer J. Clin.* **2017**, *67*, 439–448. [CrossRef] [PubMed]
53. Ayers, D.; Vandesompele, J. Influence of microRNAs and long non-coding RNAs in cancer chemoresistance. *Genes* **2017**, *8*, 95. [CrossRef] [PubMed]
54. Burrell, R.A.; McGranahan, N.; Bartek, J.; Swanton, C. The causes and consequences of genetic heterogeneity in cancer evolution. *Nature* **2013**, *501*, 338–345. [CrossRef] [PubMed]
55. Zuzic, M.; Rojo Arias, J.E.; Wohl, S.G.; Busskamp, V. Retinal miRNA functions in health and disease. *Genes* **2019**, *10*, 377. [CrossRef] [PubMed]
56. Lamb, J.; Crawford, E.D.; Peck, D.; Modell, J.W.; Blat, I.C.; Wrobel, M.J.; Reich, M. The Connectivity Map: Using gene-expression signatures to connect small molecules, genes, and disease. *Science* **2006**, *313*, 1929–1935. [CrossRef] [PubMed]
57. Gottlieb, A.; Stein, G.Y.; Ruppin, E.; Sharan, R. PREDICT: A method for inferring novel drug indications with application to personalized medicine. *Mol. Syst. Biol.* **2011**, *7*, 496. [CrossRef] [PubMed]
58. Malas, T.B.; Vlietstra, W.J.; Kudrin, R.; Starikov, S.; Charrout, M.; Roos, M.; van Mulligen, E.M. Drug prioritization using the semantic properties of a knowledge graph. *Sci. Rep.* **2019**, *9*, 6281. [CrossRef] [PubMed]

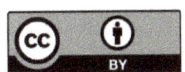

© 2019 by the authors. Licensee MDPI, Basel, Switzerland. This article is an open access article distributed under the terms and conditions of the Creative Commons Attribution (CC BY) license (http://creativecommons.org/licenses/by/4.0/).

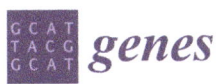

Article

Impact of *CYP2C9* and *VKORC1* Polymorphisms on Warfarin Sensitivity and Responsiveness in Jordanian Cardiovascular Patients during the Initiation Therapy

Laith N. AL-Eitan [1,2,*], Ayah Y. Almasri [1] and Rame H. Khasawneh [3]

1. Department of Applied Biological Sciences, Jordan University of Science and Technology, Irbid 22110, Jordan; ayalmasri13@sci.just.edu.jo
2. Department of Biotechnology and Genetic Engineering, Jordan University of Science and Technology, Irbid 22110, Jordan
3. Department of Hematopathology, King Hussein Medical Center (KHMC), Jordan Royal Medical Services (RMS), Amman 11118, Jordan; rami.khasawneh@jaf.mil.jo
* Correspondence: lneitan@just.edu.jo; Tel.: +962-2-7201000 (ext. 23464); Fax: +962-2-7201071

Received: 15 October 2018; Accepted: 21 November 2018; Published: 27 November 2018

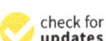

Abstract: Warfarin is an oral anticoagulant frequently used in the treatment of different cardiovascular diseases. Genetic polymorphisms in the *CYP2C9* and *VKORC1* genes have produced variants with altered catalytic properties. A total of 212 cardiovascular patients were genotyped for 17 Single Nucleotide Polymorphisms (SNPs) within the *CYP2C9* and *VKORC1* genes. This study confirmed a genetic association of the *CYP2C9*3* and *VKORC1* rs10871454, rs8050894, rs9934438, and rs17708472 SNPs with warfarin sensitivity. This study also found an association between *CYP2C9* and *VKORC1* genetic haplotype blocks and warfarin sensitivity. The initial warfarin dose was significantly related to the *CYP2C9*3* polymorphism and the four *VKORC1* SNPs ($p < 0.001$). There were significant associations between rs4086116 SNP and TAT haplotype within *CYP2C9* gene and rs17708472 SNP and CCGG haplotype within *VKORC1* gene and warfarin responsiveness. However, possessing a *VKORC1* variant allele was found to affect the international normalized ratio (INR) outcomes during initiation of warfarin therapy. In contrast, there was a loose association between the *CYP2C9* variant and INR measurements. These findings can enhance the current understanding of the great variability in response to warfarin treatment in Arabs.

Keywords: *CYP2C9*; *VKORC1*; warfarin; warfarin initiation phase of therapy; INR; pharmacogenetics study

1. Introduction

Warfarin is a commonly prescribed oral anticoagulant that is employed for the treatment of venous and arterial thromboembolic disorders and cardiac valve replacements [1]. However, interindividual genetic variation causes great variability in dosage requirements, making the latter a problematic issue for physicians. A higher or lower dose than needed could lead to bleeding and thrombotic risk, respectively [2,3]. Two-thirds of warfarin dose variation was due to environmental factors like age, body mass index, smoking status, gender, and diet, among others, while the remaining one-third is caused by genetic factors such as the *CYP2C9* and *VKORC1* genes [4–6].

Belonging to the cytochrome P450 superfamily, the *CYP2C9* gene is involved in the metabolism and clearance of S-warfarin, the latter of which is a racemic form of warfarin together with R-warfarin [7,8]. *CYP2C9* is located on the long arm of chromosome 10, and like other members of CYP2C, *CYP2C9* is highly polymorphic [9–11]. Although there are over 50 single nucleotide polymorphisms (SNPs) located in the regulatory and coding region of the *CYP2C9* sequence, the most studied *CYP2C9* polymorphisms are *CYP2C9*2* (R144C) and *CYP2C9*3* (I359L) [12,13]. It was found that individuals carrying the *CYP2C9* *2 *3 alleles reduced the elimination of S-warfarin and, therefore, plasma concentrations of the latter increased significantly compared to the wild-type allele and the individuals with these variant alleles need a lower warfarin maintenance dose [14].

Similarly, the *VKORC1* gene encodes the vitamin K epoxide reductase complex subunit 1 and it is a warfarin target [5]. The vitamin K epoxide reductase complex subunit 1 normally catalyzes the carboxylation reaction of the vitamin K-dependent protein glutamic acid residues in order to activate it, the latter of which are responsible for catalyzing the clotting factor pathway [15]. Several genetic studies conducted in different populations suggest that the G3673A (rs9923231), C6484T (rs9934438), and G9041A (rs7294) polymorphisms of the *VKORC1* gene are the most common and well-studied [7,16].

Analysis of *CYP2C9* and *VKORC1* gene polymorphisms revealed that they were responsible for 10% and 40% of warfarin dose requirement variance, respectively [17]. Combined with clinical data, both of the aforementioned genes can explain up to 60% of the warfarin variance [18,19]. More than 50 years ago, the dose of warfarin was determined by trial and error, with an initial dose (2–10 mg/day) dependent on the indication of warfarin and clinical factors, regardless of the effect of the genetic factor [20]. Patients are treated with warfarin in two stages, the first called the initiation phase of treatment, which is considered as the stage in which the initial international normalized ratio (INR) value of the patient is unstable and fluctuates up and down. With the second (maintenance) stage of the therapy, the patient is within the therapeutic INR for at least two consecutive visits [21]. However, pharmacogenetics for specific populations including Jordanian Arabs is necessary. Therefore, the objective of this study was to recognize genetic variations within the *CYP2C9* and *VKORC1* genes that are involved in warfarin sensitivity and responsiveness in Jordanian cardiovascular patients of Arab descent during initiation of treatment.

2. Materials and Methods

2.1. Patient Population and Study Design

The study population consisted of 212 unrelated warfarin intake patients selected from the Jordanian-Arab population, from the Anticoagulation Clinic at the Queen Alia Heart Institute (QAHI) in Amman, Jordan. Informed consent was obtained from all subjects. The study protocol was approved by the Human Ethics Committee at Jordan University of Science and Technology in Irbid, Jordan, and the Royal Medical Services in Amman, Jordan. Ethical approval code: 13/78/2014.

In this study, patients have cardiovascular diseases and are prescribed warfarin as an anticoagulant therapy. Inclusion criteria involved patients being 18 years or older and having received warfarin for at least three months. Patients who did not provide informed written consent, did not visit the anticoagulation clinic regularly, took *CYP2C9* inducers or inhibitors, or did not have a complete data set were excluded.

Initially, 350 patients were screened and, based on the aforementioned inclusion and exclusion criteria, 300 patients were approached to participate in this study (Figure 1). 80 patients were subsequently excluded because of inability to complete the treatment program or refusal. Of the remaining patients, 220 accepted to be part of this study, after which an additional eight patients were excluded from the final analysis because of a failure in genotyping. In total, whole sets of data were obtained from 212 patients with cardiovascular disease who were being treated with warfarin. Data was collected on demographic (age, gender, and body mass index) and lifestyle (smoking status and diet) characteristics as well as medical history (diseases and clinical features of warfarin therapy). Clinical features included the target INR, mean weekly warfarin doses required to reach the target INR, and the use of concomitant medication, all of which are required to be known in order to adjust warfarin doses. All data were blinded and obtained through semi-standardized interviews and medical records.

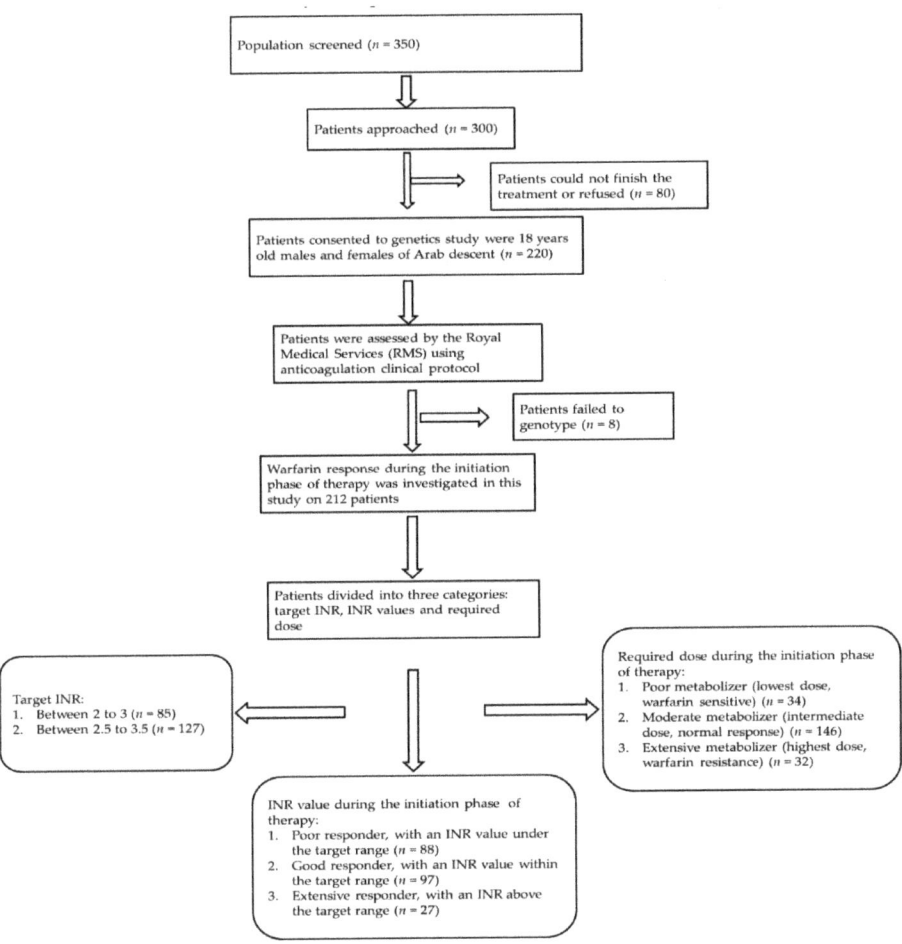

Figure 1. Flow chart depicting study design. INR: international normalized ratio.

All subjects in this study received warfarin anticoagulant therapy according to RMS anticoagulation protocol, which began with 2.5 to 10 mg nightly doses. INR monitoring is required at least once a week for the first three to four weeks after the initiation of therapy. After three consecutive visits, a patient with stable INR reaches the maintenance dose and is monitored for warfarin treatment administration by clinic protocol.

2.2. Outcome Measurement

Oral anticoagulant therapy was mandated by the prothrombin time (PT) that is, evaluated using an automated method over STAGO coagulometric unit in the QAHI laboratory. To calculate INR, there was a blood coagulation (clotting) test. INR monitoring for dose adjustments was determined by the physician and pharmacist. INR values between January 2014 and November 2015 were obtained from medical records, and these values were then used to divide the patients according to warfarin responsiveness into: (1) good responders, with an INR value within the target range; (2) poor responders, with an INR value under the target range; and (3) extensive responders, with an INR above the target range.

Further, based on their warfarin sensitivity, patients were divided into resistant, normal, or sensitive to warfarin as follows: (1) warfarin resistance (or Poor metabolizer), largest daily doses were required to keep a patient's INR within a therapeutic range (dose required > 49 mg/week); (2) warfarin normal patient (or Intermediate metabolizer), intermediate doses required (doses between 21–49 mg/week); and (3) warfarin sensitive patient (or Extensive metabolizer) lowest doses required (required dose <21 mg/week) [22].

2.3. SNP Selection, DNA Extraction, and Genotyping

In this study, 17 SNPs in the *CYP2C9* and *VKORC1* genes were selected from public databases and genotypes. Information about the aforementioned SNPs is shown in Table S1. Genomic DNA was extracted within one week of blood collection using the commercially available Wizard Genomic DNA Purification Kit (Promega Corporation, Madison, WI, USA) according to the manufacturer's instructions. After extraction, the DNA was diluted in 96-well plates using an automated robotic system to achieve concentrations of 20 ng/µL (50–500 µL). Concentrations were confirmed with the Nano-Drop ND-100 (Thermo Scientific, Wilmington, DE, USA). Genotyping was carried out by means of the MassARRAY®system (iPLEX GOLD) (Sequenom, San Diego, CA, USA), which was carried out at the Australian Genome Research Facility (AGRF) (Sequenom).

2.4. Statistical Analysis

Discrepancy and call rates were calculated using Microsoft Excel, and the deviation from Hardy Weinberg Equilibrium (HWE) was assessed using the Pearson X^2 test. Minor allele frequencies (MAF) and HWE *p*-values for genotypic distribution were calculated via the Court lab-HW calculator. To test which of the chosen SNPs is associated with warfarin response, various statistical genetic association analyses were conducted, such as the chi-square, nonparametric correlation tests (Kruskal-Wallis and Tukey Pairwise comparison) and haplotype genetic analysis test. The Statistical Package for the Social Sciences (SPSS) version 21.0 and the SNPStat Web Tool (https://www.snpstats.net/start.htm) were used to perform all analyses.

3. Results

3.1. Study Group

The study group comprised of 212 unrelated Jordanian-Arabs patients treated with warfarin, with a mean age (±SD) of 56.03 (±17.68) years, a median age of 60, and an age range of 18 to 85 years. There were 34 poor responders (16%), 146 moderate responders (68.9%), and 32 extensive responders (15.1%). Table 1 summarizes the demographic, lifestyle, and medical characteristics of each of the three groups.

In total, 17 SNPs (100%) passed the quality control measures for throughput genotyping and were analyzed by the MassARRAY®system (iPLEX GOLD) with high accuracy and a 97% average success rate. The genotypic discrepancy average (±SD) rate over the 17 loci was only 0.06% (±0.0004%) out of the entire cohort (212 subjects). Genotypic and allelic frequencies are shown in Table S2.

For the 17 SNPs examined in this study, all were in accordance with the HWE. Ten polymorphisms (rs104894539, rs104894540, rs104894541, rs104894542, and rs61742245 in *VKORC1*, and rs28371685, rs28371686, rs72558191, rs9332131, and rs9332239 in *CYP2C9*) were non-polymorphic. In contrast, the seven remaining SNPs (rs10871454, rs8050894, rs9934438, and rs17708472 located in *VKORC1*, and rs1799853, rs4086116, and rs1057910 located in *CYP2C9*) were polymorphic and thus included in the study. The minor alleles and their frequencies for the successful genotyped SNPs are shown in Table S3.

3.2. Effect of CYP2C9 and VKORC1 Polymorphisms on Warfarin Sensitivity during Initiation Phase of Therapy

Regarding the association of *VKORC1* and *CYP2C9* SNPs with warfarin sensitivity among the three inclusion groups, significant differences in proportions among genotypes were observed at all tested *VKORC1* SNPs ($p < 0.001$) (Table 2). Significant differences were also observed between two SNPs of the *CYP2C9* gene (rs4086116 ($p = 0.012$) and rs1057910 ($p < 0.001$)), as shown in Table 2. Moreover, there was a significant association observed between *VKORC1* and *CYP2C9* haplotypes and warfarin sensitivity ($p < 0.0001$) (Table 3).

Table 1. Descriptive analysis of demographics and clinical characteristics of 212 cardiovascular patients treated with warfarin at the Queen Alia Heart Institute.

Category	Subcategory	Extensive Metabolizer	Good Metabolizers	Poor Metabolizers
Demographics	Patients (N, %)	(32/212) 15.1%	(146/212) 68.9%	(34/212) 16%
	Age [a] (years)	56.0 (17.68)	55.0 (14.64)	48.29 (15.09)
	BMI [a]	27.87 (3.72)	27.7 (4.85)	27.42 (3.45)
	Smoking (N, %)	31.25%	18.6%	41.2%
	Male	59.4%	51.4%	67.6%
	Female	40.6%	48.6%	32.4%
Concomitant Disease	Co morbidity	56.3%	68.5%	55.9%
	Hypertension	34.4%	42.5%	23.5%
	Diabetes mellitus	18.8%	21.9%	26.5%
	CHD [b]	28.1%	25.3%	29.4%
	Thyroid	0%	3.4%	2.9%
	Lipid	3.1%	6.8%	2.9%
Medication	Aspirin	62.5%	65.8%	76.5%
Indication of Treatment	MVR [c]	18.8%	10.3%	20.6%
	AVR [d]	6.3%	24.0%	20.6%
	AF [e]	34.4%	19.2%	20.6%
	DVR [f]	9.4%	15.8%	11.8%
	Others	9.4%	7.5%	0.0%
Target INR	2–3	43.8%	39.7%	38.2%
	2.5–3.5	56.3%	60.3%	61.8%
Mean weakly dose [a]		16.699 (2.79)	35.896 (7.39)	67.44 (42.48)
Mean INR [a]		2.82 (0.72)	2.38 (0.75)	2.44 (0.83)

[a] Mean Standard deviation in square brackets. [b] CHD: Chronic heart disease. [c] MVR: Mitral valve replacement. [d] AVR: Aortic valve replacement. [e] AF: Atrial Fibrillation. [f] DVR: Double valve replacement.

Table 2. Association of *VKORC1* and *CYP2C9* single nucleotide polymorphism (SNPs) with warfarin sensitivity during the initiation phase of therapy of 212 cardiovascular patients.

Gene	SNP ID	Genotype	Sensitive	Moderate	Resistance	p-Value *
VKORC1	rs10871454	CC	4.3%	57.4%	38.3%	<0.001
		CT	10.0%	76.4%	13.6%	
		TT	34.5%	63.6%	1.8%	
	rs8050894	CC	2.3%	60.5%	37.2%	<0.001
		CG	10.9%	74.5%	14.5%	
		GG	32.2%	64.4%	3.4%	
	rs9934438	CC	4.2%	58.3%	37.5%	<0.001
		CT	9.9%	76.6%	13.5%	
		TT	35.8%	62.3%	1.9%	
	rs17708472	CC	18.1%	68.8%	13.1%	<0.001
		CT	6.1%	73.5%	20.4%	
		TT	0.0%	0.0%	100%	
CYP2C9	rs1799853	CC	14%	70.1%	15.9%	0.744
		CT	19.6%	63%	17.4%	
		TT	0.0%	100%	0.0%	
	rs4086116	CC	8.1%	73.2%	18.7%	0.012
		CT	24.1%	62.0%	13.9%	
		TT	30.0%	70.0%	0.0%	
	rs1057910	AA	8.8%	72.5%	18.7%	<0.001
		AC	41.5%	53.7%	4.9%	

* Chi-Square Test with p-value < 0.05 is considered significant.

Table 3. Frequencies of the haplotypes of *VKORC1* and *CYP2C9* genes among the 212 warfarin sensitive patients.

Gene	Haplotypes	Frequency * (%)	Odds Ratio (95% CI)	p-Value **
VKORC1	TGAG	0.512	0.00	—
	CCGG	0.324	0.32 (0.2–0.43)	<0.0001
	CCGA	0.129	0.38 (0.23–0.54)	<0.0001
	CGGG	0.028	0.34 (0.03–0.66)	0.034
	TCGG	0.007	0.21 (−0.38–0.8)	0.48
CYP2C9	CAC	0.767	0.00	—
	TAT	0.116	−0.05 (−0.21–0.11)	0.53
	TCC	0.094	−0.45 (−0.64−−0.27)	<0.0001
	TAC	0.021	0.01 (−0.34–0.37)	0.95
	TCT	0.002	−1.11 (−2.14−−0.08)	0.037

* Genetic haplotype frequency of 212 warfarin intake patients, ** p-value < 0.05 is considered significant.

3.3. Effect of CYP2C9 and VKORC1 Polymorphisms on Warfarin Required Dose during Initiation Phase of Therapy

Carriers of *CYP2C9* and *VKORC1* polymorphisms had a significantly increased required dose compared with wild-type subjects or carriers of only one polymorphism of *CYP2C9* or *VKORC1* (Table 4).

Table 4. Association of *VKORC1* and *CYP2C9* SNPs with variability on warfarin required doses and with INR treatment outcome.

SNP ID	Initiation Dose	p-Value *	Initiation INR	p-Value *
rs10871454		<0.001		0.006
rs8050894		<0.001		0.008
rs9934438		<0.001		0.009
rs17708472	38.1 (23.02)	<0.001	2.46 (0.77)	0.511
rs1799853		0.118		0.184
rs4086116		0.001		0.08
rs1057910		0.001		0.572

* Kurskal Wallis test with p-value < 0.05 is considered significant, Mean Standard deviation in square brackets.

3.4. Effect of CYP2C9 and VKORC1 Polymorphisms on Warfarin Responsiveness during Initiation of Therapy

There were no significant differences in patient responder groups regarding the *VKORC1* and *CYP2C9* SNPs except for the *VKORC1* rs17708472 ($p = 0.042$) and the *CYP2C9* rs4086116 ($p = 0.005$) SNPs (Table 5). However, significant associations were found between genetic haplotypes of CCGG *VKORC1* and TAT *CYP2C9* and warfarin sensitivity, with $p = 0.02$ and $p = 0.018$, respectively (Table 6).

3.5. Effect of CYP2C9 and VKORC1 Polymorphisms on INR Treatment Outcome

There were no significant differences observed between the *CYP2C9* SNP genotypes and INR values measured at start of treatment for 212 cardiovascular patients treated with warfarin. In contrast, significant differences were observed between INR values measured at the initiation phase of therapy and certain *VKORC1* SNPs, namely rs10871454 ($p = 0.006$), rs8050894 ($p = 0.007$), and rs9934438 ($p = 0.009$), as shown in Table 4.

Table 5. Association of *VKORC1* and *CYP2C9* SNPs with response to warfarin during the initiation phase of therapy of 212 cardiovascular patients.

Gene	SNP ID	Genotype	Poor Responder	Good Responder	Extensive Responder	p-Value *
VKORC1	rs10871454	CC	55.3%	36.2%	8.5%	0.171
		CT	40.9%	45.5%	13.6%	
		TT	30.9%	54.5%	14.5%	
	rs8050894	CC	53.5%	39.5%	7%	0.235
		CG	41.8%	43.6%	14.5%	
		GG	32.2%	54.2%	13.6%	
	rs9934438	CC	54.2%	37.5%	8.3%	0.226
		CT	40.5%	45%	14.4%	
		TT	32.1%	54.7%	13.2%	
	rs17708472	CC	38.1%	50.6%	11.3%	0.042
		CT	55.1%	28.6%	16.3%	
		TT	0.0%	66.7%	33.3%	
CYP2C9	rs1799853	CC	45.1%	44.5%	10.4%	0.076
		CT	28.3%	52.5%	19.6%	
		TT	50.0%	0.0%	50.0%	
	rs4086116	CC	45.5%	43.9%	10.6%	0.005
		CT	39.2%	49.4%	11.4%	
		TT	10.0%	40.0%	50.0%	
	rs1057910	AA	42.1%	45.0%	12.9%	0.910
		AC	39%	48.8%	12.2%	

* Chi-Square Test with p-value < 0.05 is considered significant.

Table 6. Frequencies of the haplotypes of *VKORC1* and *CYP2C9* genes among the 212 warfarin responsiveness patients.

Gene	Haplotypes	Frequency * (%)	Odds Ratio (95% CI)	p-Value **
VKORC1	TGAG	0.512	0.00	—
	CCGG	0.326	−0.18 (−0.33−−0.03)	0.02
	CCGA	0.129	−0.08 (−0.28−0.12)	0.46
	CGGG	0.026	−0.05 (−0.47−0.36)	0.8
	TCGG	0.007	0.55 (−0.22−1.32)	0.16
CYP2C9	CAC	0.767	0.00	—
	TAT	0.115	0.25 (0.04−0.45)	0.018
	TCC	0.094	0.06 (−0.17−0.3)	0.59
	TAC	0.021	0.44 (−0.01−0.89)	0.059
	TCT	0.003	0.4 (−0.9−1.71)	0.55

* Genetic haplotype frequency of 212 warfarin intake patients, ** p-value < 0.05 is considered significant.

3.6. Correlation Between Warfarin Dose and Clinical Data

Finally, there was no significant correlation between warfarin dose and body mass index, age, gender, co-morbidities, or the treatment indication ($p = 0.505$).

4. Discussion

Earlier studies on warfarin pharmacogenetics provide evidence that common *VKORC1* and *CYP2C9* polymorphisms with clinical and environmental factors are responsible for over half of the variability in warfarin required dose [23,24]. Genotyping patients who are carriers of *VKORC1* and

CYP2C9 variant alleles has been proven to reduce the risk of over-anticoagulation compared to the traditional initial dose approach [25,26].

In this study, our goal was to identify genetic factors associated with sensitivity and responsiveness to warfarin treatment during the initiation phase of treatment in Jordanian-Arab patients with cardiovascular disease. The results of the current pharmacogenetic study strongly suggest that there is a significant association of the VKORC1 rs8050894, rs10871454, rs9934438, and rs17708472 SNPs and the CYP2C9 rs4086116 and rs1057910 SNPs and their haplotypes with the required warfarin dosage and warfarin sensitivity. This study also reported that there is a genetic association between VKORC1 rs17708472 SNP and CCGG genetic haplotype block and CYP2C9 rs4086116 SNP and TAT genetic haplotype block with warfarin responsiveness during the initiation phase of therapy.

The allelic frequencies of CYP2C9 and VKORC1 SNPs in our population were similar to those found in other ethnic groups, as in the case of CYP2C9*2, with 10% in our population, 6% in American and European populations, and 1% in Africans [27]. However, allelic frequencies of VKORC1 SNPs were found to differ drastically from other populations. For example, rs10871454 was 52% in our population compared to 41% in Americans, 39% in Europeans, and 6% in African populations [27]. With regard to the association of CYP2C9 polymorphisms with warfarin sensitivity, our results are consistent with the study by Takahashi et al. (2001) which shows that CYP2C9 *2 and *3 polymorphisms reduce warfarin clearance [28] as CYP2C9 is the major metabolizing enzyme of warfarin, therefore, reduction of activity results in lower required doses needed to achieve the therapeutic INR. We found a strong association of CYP2C9*3 (rs1057910 A>C) and CYP2C9 (rs4086116 C>T) genotypes with warfarin sensitivity during the initiation stage of treatment with $p < 0.001$ and $p = 0.012$, respectively (Table 2). This study reported that individuals with one variant allele were associated with an increased risk of warfarin sensitivity. For example, 41.5% of the patients who carried the rs1057910 A>C variant allele were sensitive to warfarin, compared to 8.8% of the wild-type patients were sensitive. Moreover, carrying a CYP2C9 TCC genetic haplotype block was significantly associated with warfarin sensitivity with $p < 0.0001$ (Table 3).

In disagreement with other studies, the CYP2C9*2 variant did not show a significant association with warfarin sensitivity ($p = 0.744$). This can possibly be explained by the genotypic frequency having an impact on the association; in our population only two patients were homozygous for the variant allele (TT), 32 were heterozygous patients (CT), and 105 patients were homozygous for the wild-type allele (CC) (Table 2). Moreover, it has been proposed that patients who carry one CYP2C9* 2 allele results in a dose reduction compared with the wild-type dose [14,29,30]. Although the allelic frequency of CYP2C9*2 (rs1799853) in our samples was in agreement with the American and European populations [27], this study did not find significant differences between this SNP and variability in required doses in the initiation phase of therapy ($p = 0.366$) as shown in Table 4 and Figure 2.

Clinical pharmacogenetic studies suggested that patients who carry the CYP2C9*3 (rs1057910) C allele leads to a dose reduction of 28–41% [12,29,30] in the Caucasian American population and from 12–38% of the Asian population compared to the wild-type [31–34]. In alignment with the aforementioned studies, we revealed that there is a 34.3% reduction in warfarin dose. Patients carrying one variant allele (C) required 41.75 mg/week, in comparison with the wild-type allele which required 27.43 mg/week ($p < 0.001$), as shown in Table 4 and Figure 2. Therefore, in our study the CYP2C9*3 allele has a greater effect on variation in warfarin dose during the initiation phase of therapy compared with CYP2C9*2. In the case of individuals carrying rs4086116 C>T variant allele, this resulted in 23.9% and 37.9% reduction on warfarin dose compared to wild-type with $p = 0.016$, as shown in Table 4 and Figure 2.

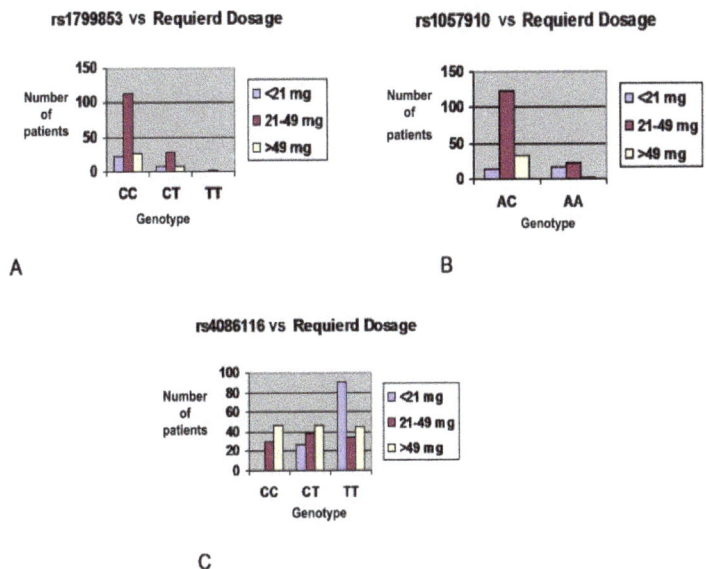

Figure 2. The distribution of warfarin dose by CYP2C9 genotypes during the initiation phase of therapy for 212 Jordanian cardiovascular patients: X axis represents different CYP2C9 genotypes, Y axis represents the proportion of patients across each genotype, Blue column represents a sensitive group who required the lowest warfarin dose (<21 mg/week), Purple column represents the intermediate group who required moderate warfarin dose ((21–49) mg/week), Yellow column represents a resistant group who required the highest warfarin dose (>49 mg/week). (**A**) Distribution of warfarin dose by rs1799853 variant. (**B**) Distribution of warfarin dose by rs1057910 variant. (**C**) Distribution of warfarin dose by rs4086116 variant.

For the four studied *VKORC1* SNPs, we observed a strong association of *VKORC1* SNPs with warfarin sensitivity ($p < 0.001$). For example, patients with the T allele for rs10871454 C>T showed a high risk of warfarin sensitivity with 25.5% (CT) and 48.3% (TT) reduction of the required dose, respectively. In this case, the drug target enzyme could be expressed in smaller amounts and, therefore, low doses of the drug can obtain a therapeutic INR in an initial phase of therapy (Table 2). Furthermore, *VKORC1* genetic haplotype analysis showed a significant association between three *VKORC1* genetic haplotype blocks and sensitivity to warfarin with $p < 0.0001$ (Table 3). Moreover, Schelleman et al. (2007) and Wadelius et al. (2005) reported that a correlation exists between *VKORC1* SNP 1173 C> T (rs9934438), and the variation in warfarin dose patients carrying the variant allele of this SNP is related to a reduction in the required dose compared to the wild-type [5,35]. In alignment with these results, we found that patients who carry one variant allele required an average dose of 39.47mg/week and two variant allele carriers needed an average of 26.82 mg/week, while patients carrying the wild type CC needed an average dose of 53.02 mg/week with $p < 0.001$ as shown in Figure 3. Limdi et al. (2007) and Shrif et al. (2011) showed that *VKORC1* rs8050894 (1542G>C) were associated with lower warfarin doses in European Americans and Sudanese patients, respectively [36,37]. Accordingly, our results found a significant association between lower required warfarin dose and this SNP at an initial phase of therapy with $p < 0.001$ as shown in Figure 3.

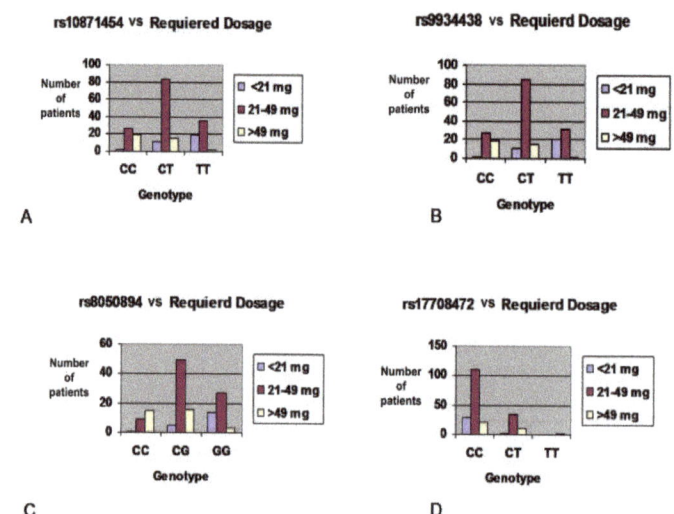

Figure 3. The distribution of warfarin dose by *VKORC1* genotypes during the initiation phase of therapy for 212 Jordanian cardiovascular patients: X axis represents different *VKORC1* genotypes, Y axis represents the proportion of patients across each genotype, Blue column represents a sensitive group who required the lowest warfarin dose (<21 mg/week), Purple column represents the intermediate group who required moderate warfarin dose ((21–49) mg/week), Yellow column represents a resistant group who required the highest warfarin dose (>49 mg/week). (**A**) Distribution of warfarin dose by rs10871454 variant. (**B**) Distribution of warfarin dose by rs9934438 variant. (**C**) Distribution of warfarin dose by rs8050894 variant. (**D**) Distribution of warfarin dose by rs17708472 variant.

For the last *VKORC1* SNP *VKORC1**4 C<T (rs17708472), our study is similar to the study by Haug et al. (2008), which reported that this SNP was associated with higher dose requirements [38]. Our results showed that this variant was associated with significant differences in initial warfarin required dose; patients who were homozygous for the variant allele (TT) genotype required an average dose of 57.8 mg/week, heterozygous (CT) patients required an average dose of 41.63 mg/week, while wild-type (CC) patients required an average dose of 33.65 with $p < 0.001$ (Table 4).

With regard to the correlation of *CYP2C9* and *VKORC1* SNPs and warfarin responsiveness, we compared SNP genotypes with the warfarin responder groups (poor, good, and extensive responders). Significant differences were found between *VKORC1* rs17708472 (C>T) genotypes and the three different responder groups (Table 5); 33.3% of the patients carrying the variant allele (TT) were within the extensive responder group (meaning this variant allele was associated with increased risk of over-anticoagulation), compared to 11.3% of the wild-type (CC) patients who were extensive responders ($p = 0.042$). Accordingly, Kringen et al. (2011) have also shown that patients who carry this SNP are associated with an increased risk of the existence of therapeutic INR (over-anticoagulation) [39]. Otherwise, *VKORC1* rs10871454, rs8050894, and rs9934438 alleles show no significant differences between SNP genotypes within the three responder groups in our population, with $p = 0.171, 0.235,$ and 0.226, respectively (Table 5). In contrast, *VKORC1* CCGG genetic haplotype block showed a significant association with warfarin responsiveness with $p = 0.02$ (Table 6).

Moreover, significant differences were observed between *VKORC1* rs10871454, rs8050894, and rs9934438 SNPs and INR value during the initiation phase of therapy ($p = 0.006, 0.007,$ and 0.009, respectively), while rs17708472 SNP showed no significant differences ($p = 0.493$). Therefore, in our population the *VKORC1* SNP genotypes are associated with the generation of a high or low INR during the initiation phase of therapy (Table 4).

Taube et al. (2000) reported that an individual carrying an allelic variant of *CYP2C9* was not associated with an increased incidence of severe over-coagulation during long-term treatment [40]. Correspondingly, our results show no significant differences between the *CYP2C9*2* and *3* genotypes within the three responder groups with $p = 0.076$ and 0.910, respectively (Table 5). Conversely, our study reported significant differences between the proportion of *CYP2C9* rs4086116 (C>T) genotype and the three different responder groups; 50% of TT carriers were within the extensive responder group compared with 10.6% of wild type CC carriers ($p = 0.005$), which means that TT carriers are associated with increased risk of over-anticoagulation (Table 5). Moreover, significant association was observed between *CYP2C9* TAT genetic haplotype block and warfarin responsiveness with $p = 0.018$ (Table 6).

In addition, we did not observe significant differences in the three studied SNPs (*CYP2C9*2, *3*, and *CYP2C9* (C> T) rs4086116) and the INR value during the initiation phase of therapy. Therefore, in our population *CYP2C9* is not associated with the generation of a high or low INR as shown in Table 4.

Confirmation of our results and ongoing research including additional factors will be accomplished in a larger patient cohort, including genetic factors such as *OATP* transporters (mediates the uptake of warfarin into hepatocytes), *CYP3A4*, *CYP1A1*, and *CYP1A2* enzymes (metabolizing of R-warfarin), or *GGCX* encoded *gamma-glutamyl carboxylase* (the reduced vitamin K–form to activate coagulation factors) [5,41]. Application for individualized warfarin treatment will be both beneficial and efficient for cardiovascular patients in the future. Finally, the majority of the population included in this study is elderly, with only 15% of the subjects under 40 years of age. Therefore, additional study is needed in children and young adults.

Supplementary Materials: The following are available online at http://www.mdpi.com/2073-4425/9/12/578/s1. Table S1: SNPs ID, their position and genotyping data based on whole cohort ($N = 220$). Table S2: List of SNPs, their minor allele frequencies, and HWE *p* values for genotypic distribution at each locus based on 220 patients. Table S3: The frequency of the allele and genotype for all polymorphisms in cardiovascular patients treated with warfarin.

Author Contributions: L.N.A.-E. designed the study. L.N.A.-E., A.Y.A. and R.H.K. were responsible for clinical data and blood samples collection. L.N.A.-E. and A.Y.A. analyzed and interpreted the data. L.N.A.-E. and A.Y.A. prepared the manuscript. All authors helped in reviewing the manuscript.

Funding: This work was supported by the Deanship of Research at Jordan University of Science and Technology under grant number 203/2014.

Acknowledgments: We are grateful to Pharmacist Nadia Al-Omary, and engineer of Nutrition Miss Hanna from anticoagulation clinic for cooperation and providing excellent samples for this study and for coordinating the Anticoagulant Service, and Miss Diana, laboratory technician, for the blood collection and INR measurements.

Conflicts of Interest: The authors declare no conflict of interest, financial or otherwise.

References

1. Kim, Y.; Smith, A.; Wu, A. C3435T polymorphism of *MDR1* gene with warfarin resistance. *Clin. Chim. Acta* **2013**, *425*, 34–36. [CrossRef] [PubMed]
2. Motulsky, A.G.; Qi, M. Pharmacogenetics, pharmacogenomics and ecogenetics. *J. Zhejiang Univ. Sci. B.* **2006**, *7*, 169–170. [CrossRef] [PubMed]
3. Eriksson, N.; Wadelius, M. Prediction of warfarin dose: Why, when and how? *Pharmacogenomics* **2012**, *13*, 429–440. [CrossRef] [PubMed]
4. Sconce, E.A.; Khan, T.I.; Wynne, H.A.; Avery, P.; Monkhouse, L.; King, B.P.; Wood, P.; Kesteven, P.; Daly, A.K.; Kamali, F. The impact of *CYP2C9* and *VKORC1* genetic polymorphism and patient characteristics upon warfarin dose requirements: Proposal for a new dosing regimen. *Blood* **2005**, *106*, 2329–2333. [CrossRef] [PubMed]
5. Wadelius, M.; Chen, L.Y.; Downes, K.; Ghori, J.; Hunt, S.; Eriksson, N.; Wallerman, O.; Melhus, H.; Wadelius, C.; Bentley, D. Common *VKORC1* and *GGCX* polymorphisms associated with warfarin dose. *Pharmacogen. J.* **2005**, *5*, 262–270. [CrossRef] [PubMed]

6. Eichelbaum, M.; Ingelman-Sundberg, M.; Evans, W. Pharmacogenomics and individualized drug therapy. *Annu. Rev. Med.* **2006**, *57*, 119–137. [CrossRef] [PubMed]
7. D'Andrea, G.; D'Ambrosio, R.L.; Di Perna, P.; Chetta, M.; Santacroce, R.; Brancaccio, V.; Grandone, E.; Margaglione, M. A polymorphism in the *VKORC1* gene is associated with an interindividual variability in the dose-anticoagulant effect of warfarin. *Blood* **2005**, *105*, 645–649. [CrossRef] [PubMed]
8. Muszkat, M.; Blotnik, S.; Elami, A.; Krasilnikov, I.; Caraco, Y. Warfarin metabolism and anticoagulant effect: A prospective, observational study of the impact of *CYP2C9* genetic polymorphism in the presence of drug-disease and drug-drug interactions. *Clin. Ther.* **2007**, *29*, 427–437. [CrossRef]
9. Rendic, S. Summary of information on human CYP enzymes: Human P450 metabolism data. *Drug Metab. Rev.* **2002**, *34*, 83–448. [CrossRef] [PubMed]
10. Dean, L. *Warfarin Therapy and VKORC1 and CYP Genotype*; National Center for Biotechnology Information: Bethesda, MD, USA, 2012.
11. Zhou, S.; Zhou, Z.; Yang, L.; Cai, J. Substrates, inducers, inhibitors and structure-activity relationships of human cytochrome P450 2C9 and implications in drug development. *Curr. Med. Chem.* **2009**, *16*, 3480–3675. [CrossRef] [PubMed]
12. Kirchheiner, J.; Brockmoller, J. Clinical consequences of cytochrome P450 2C9 polymorphisms. *Clin. Pharmacol. Ther.* **2005**, *77*, 1–16. [CrossRef] [PubMed]
13. Zhou, Y.; Ingelman-Sundberg, M.; Lauschke, V.M. Worldwide distribution of cytochrome P450 alleles: A meta-analysis of population-scale sequencing projects. *Clin. Pharmacol. Ther.* **2017**, *102*, 688–700. [CrossRef] [PubMed]
14. Linder, M.W.; Homme, M.B.; Reynolds, K.K.; Gage, B.F.; Eby, C.; Silvestrov, N.; Valdes, R. Interactive modeling for ongoing utility of pharmacogenetic diagnostic testing: Application for warfarin therapy. *Clin. Chem.* **2009**, *55*, 1861–1868. [CrossRef] [PubMed]
15. Tie, J.K.; Stafford, D.W. Structural and functional insights into enzymes of the vitamin K cycle. *J. Thromb. Haemost.* **2016**, *14*, 236–247. [CrossRef] [PubMed]
16. Loebstein, R.; Dvoskin, I.; Halkin, H.; Vecsler, M.; Lubetsky, A.; Rechavi, G.; Amariglio, N.; Cohen, Y.; Ken-Dror, G.; Almog, S.; et al. A coding VKORC1 Asp36Tyr polymorphism predisposes to warfarin resistance. *Blood* **2007**, *109*, 2477–2480. [CrossRef] [PubMed]
17. Schalekamp, T.; De Boer, A. Pharmacogenetics of oral anticoagulant therapy. *Curr. Pharm. Des.* **2010**, *16*, 187–203. [CrossRef] [PubMed]
18. Wadelius, M.; Chen, L.Y.; Lindh, J.D.; Eriksson, N.; Ghori, M.J.; Bumpstead, S.; Holm, L.; McGinnis, R.; Rane, A.; Deloukas, P. The largest prospective warfarin-treated cohort supports genetic forecasting. *Blood* **2009**, *113*, 784–792. [CrossRef] [PubMed]
19. Lenzini, P.; Wadelius, M.; Kimmel, S.; Anderson, J.L.; Jorgensen, A.L.; Pirmohamed, M.; Caldwell, M.D.; Limdi, N.; Burmester, J.K.; Dowd, M.B.; et al. Integration of genetic, clinical, and INR data to refine warfarin dosing. *Clin. Pharmacol. Ther.* **2010**, *87*, 572–578. [CrossRef] [PubMed]
20. Gage, B.; Lesko, L. Pharmacogenetics of warfarin: Regulatory, scientific, and clinical issues. *J. Thromb. Thrombolysis* **2007**, *25*, 45–51. [CrossRef] [PubMed]
21. Kuruvilla, M.; Gurk-Turner, C. A review of warfarin dosing and monitoring. *Proc. Bayl. Univ. Med. Cent.* **2001**, *14*, 305–306. [CrossRef] [PubMed]
22. Hylek, E.; D'Antonio, J.; Evans-Molina, C.; Shea, C.; Henault, L.; Regan, S. Translating the results of randomized trials into clinical practice: The challenge of warfarin candidacy among hospitalized elderly patients with atrial fibrillation. *Stroke* **2006**, *37*, 1075–1080. [CrossRef] [PubMed]
23. Wiedermann, C.J.; Stockner, I. Warfarin-induced bleeding complications—Clinical presentation and therapeutic options. *Thromb. Res.* **2008**, *122*, S13–S18. [CrossRef]
24. Borgiani, P.; Ciccacci, C.; Forte, V.; Romano, S.; Federici, G.; Novelli, G. Allelic variants in the *CYP2C9* and *VKORC1* loci and interindividual variability in the anticoagulant dose effect of warfarin in Italians. *Pharmacogenomics* **2007**, *8*, 1545–1550. [CrossRef] [PubMed]
25. Hamberg, A.; Dahl, M.L.; Barban, M.; Scordo, M.G.; Wadelius, M.; Pengo, V.; Padrini, R.; Jonsson, E.N. A PK-PD model for predicting the impact of age, *CYP2C9*, and *VKORC1* genotype on individualization of warfarin therapy. *Clin. Pharmacol. Ther.* **2007**, *81*, 529–538. [CrossRef] [PubMed]

26. Teichert, M.; Van Schaik, R.H.N.; Hofman, A.; Uitterlinden, A.G.; de Smet, P.A.G.M.; Stricker, B.; Visser, L.E. Genotypes associated with reduced activity of *VKORC1* and *CYP2C9* and their modification of acenocoumarol anticoagulation during the initial treatment period. *Clin. Pharmacol. Ther.* **2009**, *85*, 379–386. [CrossRef] [PubMed]
27. 1000 Genomes Project Consortium. An integrated map of genetic variation from 1092 human genomes. *Nature* **2012**, *491*, 56–65. [CrossRef] [PubMed]
28. Takahashi, H.; Echizen, H. Pharmacogenetics of warfarin elimination and its clinical implications. *Clin. Pharmacokinet.* **2001**, *40*, 587–603. [CrossRef] [PubMed]
29. Kealey, C.; Chen, Z.; Christie, J.; Thorn, C.F.; Whitehead, A.S.; Price, M.; Samaha, F.F.; Kimmel, S.E. Warfarin and cytochrome P450 2C9 genotype: Possible ethnic variation in warfarin sensitivity. *Pharmacogenomics* **2008**, *8*, 217–225. [CrossRef] [PubMed]
30. Limdi, N.; McGwin, G.; Goldstein, J.; Beasley, T.; Arnett, D.; Adler, B.; Baird, M.; Acton, R. Influence of *CYP2C9* and *VKORC1 1173C/T* genotype on the risk of hemorrhagic complications in African-American and European-American patients on warfarin. *Clin. Pharmacol. Ther.* **2007**, *83*, 312–321. [CrossRef] [PubMed]
31. Ohno, M.; Yamamoto, A.; Ono, A.; Miura, G.; Funamoto, M.; Takemoto, Y.; Otsu, K.; Kouno, Y.; Tanabe, T.; Masunaga, Y.; et al. Influence of clinical and genetic factors on warfarin dose requirements among Japanese patients. *Eur. J. Clin. Pharmacol.* **2009**, *65*, 1097–1103. [CrossRef] [PubMed]
32. Huang, S.W.; Chen, H.S.; Wang, X.Q.; Huang, L.; Xu, D.L.; Hu, X.J.; Huang, Z.H.; He, Y.; Chen, K.M.; Xiang, D.K.; et al. Validation of *VKORC1* and *CYP2C9* genotypes on interindividual warfarin maintenance dose: A prospective study in Chinese patients. *Pharmacogenet. Genomics* **2009**, *19*, 226–234. [CrossRef] [PubMed]
33. Gan, G.; Phipps, M.; Ku, C.; Teh, A.; Sangkar, V. Genetic polymorphism of the CYP2C9 subfamily of 3 different races in warfarin maintenance dose. *Int. J. Hematol.* **2004**, *80*, 295–296. [CrossRef] [PubMed]
34. Tanira, M.; Al-Mukhaini, M.; Al-Hinai, A.; Al Balushi, K.; Ahmed, I. Frequency of CYP2C9 genotypes among Omani patients receiving warfarin and its correlation with warfarin dose. *Community Genet.* **2007**, *10*, 32–37. [CrossRef] [PubMed]
35. Schelleman, H.; Chen, Z.; Kealey, C.; Whitehead, A.S.; Christie, J.; Price, M.; Brensinger, C.M.; Newcomb, C.W.; Thorn, C.F.; Samaha, F.F.; et al. Warfarin response and vitamin K epoxide reductase complex 1 in African Americans and Caucasians. *Clin. Pharmacol. Ther.* **2007**, *81*, 742–747. [CrossRef] [PubMed]
36. Limdi, N.A.; Arnett, D.K.; Goldstein, J.A.; Beasley, T.M.; McGwin, G.; Adler, B.K.; Acton, R.T. Influence of *CYP2C9* and *VKORC1* on warfarin dose, anticoagulation attainment and maintenance among European Americans and African Americans. *Pharmacogenomics* **2008**, *9*, 511–526. [CrossRef] [PubMed]
37. Shrif, N.; Won, H.H.; Lee, S.T.; Park, J.H.; Kim, K.K.; Kim, M.J.; Kim, S.; Lee, S.Y.; Ki, C.S.; Osman, I.M.; et al. Evaluation of the effects of *VKORC1* polymorphisms and haplotypes, *CYP2C9* genotypes, and clinical factors on warfarin response in Sudanese patients. *Eur. J. Clin. Pharmacol.* **2011**, *67*, 1119–1130. [CrossRef] [PubMed]
38. Haug, K.B.; Sharikabad, M.N.; Kringen, M.K.; Narum, S.; Sjaatil, S.T.; Johansen, P.W.; Kierulf, P.; Seljeflot, I.; Arnesen, H.; Brørs, O. Warfarin dose and INR related to genotypes of CYP2C9 and VKORC1 in patients with myocardial infarction. *Thromb. J.* **2008**, *6*, 7. [CrossRef] [PubMed]
39. Kringen, M.K.; Haug, K.B.F.; Grimholt, R.M.; Stormo, C.; Narum, S.; Opdal, M.S.; Fosen, J.T.; Piehler, A.P.; Johansen, P.W.; Seljeflot, I.; et al. Genetic variation of VKORC1 and CYP4F2 genes related to warfarin maintenance dose in patients with myocardial infarction. *J. Biomed. Biotechnol.* **2011**, *2011*, 739–751. [CrossRef] [PubMed]
40. Taube, J.; Halsall, D.; Baglin, T. Influence of cytochrome P-450 CYP2C9 polymorphisms on warfarin sensitivity and risk of over-anticoagulation in patients on long-term treatment. *Blood* **2000**, *96*, 1816–1819. [PubMed]
41. Frymoyer, A. Effect of single-dose rifampin on the pharmacokinetics of warfarin in healthy volunteers. *Clin. Pharmacol. Ther.* **2010**, *88*, 540–547. [CrossRef] [PubMed]

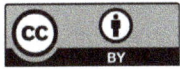

© 2018 by the authors. Licensee MDPI, Basel, Switzerland. This article is an open access article distributed under the terms and conditions of the Creative Commons Attribution (CC BY) license (http://creativecommons.org/licenses/by/4.0/).

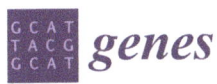

Article

Azathioprine Biotransformation in Young Patients with Inflammatory Bowel Disease: Contribution of Glutathione-S Transferase M1 and A1 Variants

Marianna Lucafò [1,2], Gabriele Stocco [3,*], Stefano Martelossi [2], Diego Favretto [2], Raffaella Franca [4], Noelia Malusà [5], Angela Lora [2,4], Matteo Bramuzzo [2], Samuele Naviglio [2], Erika Cecchin [1], Giuseppe Toffoli [1], Alessandro Ventura [2,4] and Giuliana Decorti [2,4]

1. Centro di Riferimento Oncologico, IRCCS, 33081 Aviano, Italy; mlucafo@units.it (M.L.); ececchin@cro.it (E.C.); gtoffoli@cro.it (G.T.)
2. Institute for Maternal and Child Health IRCCS Burlo Garofolo, 34137 Trieste, Italy; stefano.martelossi@aulss2.veneto.it (S.M.); dieg.o@libero.it (D.F.); angelalora86@gmail.com (A.L.); matteo.bramuzzo@burlo.trieste.it (M.B.); samuele.naviglio@burlo.trieste.it (S.N.); alessandro.ventura@burlo.trieste.it (A.V.); decorti@units.it (G.D.)
3. Department of Life Sciences, University of Trieste, 34127 Trieste, Italy
4. Department of Medical, Surgical and Health Sciences, University of Trieste, 34149 Trieste, Italy; rfranca@units.it
5. Sanitary Services Agency 1, 34129 Trieste, Italy; tossicologia.forense@asuits.sanita.fvg.it
* Correspondence: stoccog@units.it; Tel.: +39-04-0558-8634

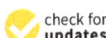

Received: 19 February 2019; Accepted: 1 April 2019; Published: 4 April 2019

Abstract: The contribution of candidate genetic variants involved in azathioprine biotransformation on azathioprine efficacy and pharmacokinetics in 111 young patients with inflammatory bowel disease was evaluated. Azathioprine doses, metabolites thioguanine-nucleotides (TGN) and methylmercaptopurine-nucleotides (MMPN) and clinical effects were assessed after at least 3 months of therapy. Clinical efficacy was defined as disease activity score below 10. Candidate genetic variants (*TPMT* rs1142345, rs1800460, rs1800462, *GSTA1* rs3957357, *GSTM1*, and *GSTT1* deletion) were determined by polymerase chain reaction (PCR) assays and pyrosequencing. Statistical analysis was performed using linear mixed effects models for the association between the candidate variants and the pharmacological variables (azathioprine doses and metabolites). Azathioprine metabolites were measured in 257 samples (median 2 per patient, inter-quartile range IQR 1-3). Clinical efficacy at the first evaluation available resulted better in ulcerative colitis than in Crohn's disease patients (88.0% versus 52.5% responders, $p = 0.0003$, linear mixed effect model, LME). TGN concentration and the ratio TGN/dose at the first evaluation were significantly higher in responder. *TPMT* rs1142345 variant (4.8% of patients) was associated with increased TGN (LME $p = 0.0042$), TGN/dose ratio (LME $p < 0.0001$), decreased azathioprine dose (LME $p = 0.0087$), and MMPN (LME $p = 0.0011$). *GSTM1* deletion (58.1% of patients) was associated with a 18.5% decrease in TGN/dose ratio (LME $p = 0.041$) and 30% decrease in clinical efficacy (LME $p = 0.0031$). *GSTA1* variant (12.8% of patients) showed a trend ($p = 0.046$, LME) for an association with decreased clinical efficacy; however, no significant effect on azathioprine pharmacokinetics could be detected. In conclusion, GSTs variants are associated with azathioprine efficacy and pharmacokinetics.

Keywords: azathioprine; inflammatory bowel disease; glutathione-S transferase; pharmacogenetics; pharmacokinetics

1. Introduction

Inflammatory bowel disease (IBD) is a chronic, relapsing and remitting disease of the gastrointestinal tract that comprises two main entities, Crohn's disease (CD) and ulcerative colitis (UC). The disease has a peak onset in subjects 15 to 30 years old, and its incidence is rising in the pediatric population [1]. Despite the recent introduction in therapy of biologicals, thiopurines continue to be widely used in this disease; indeed, these are cheap drugs, and maintain at least 20% of patients in a state of stable long term steroid free clinical remission [2]. Among thiopurines, azathioprine is mainly used as an immunosuppressant in IBD, and, although it has a well described risk benefit profile, adverse drug reactions are relatively common, occurring in 15–18% of patients, and can be severe enough to require the withdrawal of therapy [3,4] In addition, a significant proportion of patients does not respond to therapy with this agent [5–7]. The reasons of this high heterogeneity in clinical response is not clear yet [8]; however, variability in azathioprine metabolism can be important; indeed, azathioprine is a prodrug that requires metabolic conversion to its active form. The first step in this metabolic conversion is mediated by conjugation with glutathione, resulting in the formation of mercaptopurine. This reaction is in part nonenzymatic but it is even controlled, as demonstrated by recent publications, by the enzyme glutathione S-transferase (GST in particular by the isoforms A and M [9]. The latter is also inactive and is converted by the enzymes of the purine salvage pathway to the active thioguanine nucleotides, which are responsible of the cytotoxic and apoptotic effect of these drugs [10]. Mercaptopurine is metabolized by the enzyme xanthine oxidase in the liver, and by thiopurine methyltransferase (TPMT) and inosine triphosphatase (ITPA), mainly in extra hepatic tissues [10]. Polymorphisms in genes involved in azathioprine metabolism can hence influence the efficacy and toxicity of this drug [6].

In this study, we aimed to evaluate the contribution of candidate genetic variants involved in azathioprine biotransformation on azathioprine efficacy and pharmacokinetics in young patients with IBD.

2. Materials and Methods

2.1. Patient Characteristics

111 patients with IBD were enrolled by the Gastroenterology Unit of the Pediatric Hospital "Burlo Garofolo" in Trieste, Italy between March 2004 and February 2015. The study was conducted in accordance with the Declaration of Helsinki, and the protocol was approved by the Institutional Ethics Committee (Projects RC 23/2005 and 12/2013). All subjects and parents gave their informed consent for inclusion before they participated in the study. The inclusion criteria were age less than 30 years, previous diagnosis of IBD and treatment with azathioprine for at least 3 months. The patients enrolled are all the patients taking azathioprine at "Burlo Garofolo" in Trieste in the time-frame of the study. Blood samples for azathioprine metabolites measurement and for genotyping were taken at the appropriate clinic visit. Timing of metabolite level measurement was determined by the clinical setting of azathioprine administration at the hospital: generally, azathioprine metabolites levels were measured after 3, 6, and 12 months of treatment and then every year. Patients were treated with a dose-escalating strategy to reduce the risk of adverse events starting, however, from a relatively high dose (median of 2 mg/kg). At subsequent follow-up visits (every 3 months), the dose was increased or reduced so as to obtain the optimal clinical response; the criteria used to increase or reduce the dose of azathioprine were the level of disease activity and laboratory parameters used to monitor azathioprine toxicity (in particular leukocyte, erythrocyte and platelet counts, hemoglobin concentration, mean corpuscular volume, liver enzymes alanine aminotransferase, aspartate aminotransferase and γ-glutamyltransferase, and amylase levels). According to current guidelines, genotyping information was shared with the clinicians only for patients presenting *TPMT* variant alleles, in order to allow increased monitoring of adverse events.

Clinical response was assessed using Pediatric Crohn's Disease Activity Index and Pediatric Ulcerative Colitis Activity Index, respectively [11], for CD and UC patients at the time of blood sample collection for the first metabolites' measurement, which occurred at least 3 months since the beginning of therapy. The disease was considered inactive if the disease activity index was <10 at the time of sample collection.

2.2. Measurement of Azathioprine Metabolites

Metabolites (TGN and MMPN) were measured in patients' erythrocytes using the high performance liquid chromatography assay by Dervieux and Boulieu [12]. The ratio between TGN and the dose of azathioprine was calculated considering, for each individual measurement of the metabolites, the dose the patients took the day the blood sample was recorded.

2.3. Genotypes

Genomic DNA was extracted from peripheral blood samples using a commercial kit (Sigma, Milan, Italy), to characterize genetic polymorphisms in the candidate genes *TPMT* (rs1142345, rs1800460 and rs1800462), *GSTA1* (rs3957357), *GSTM1* (deletion), and *GSTT1* (deletion). The considered genotypes and method of analysis are described in Table 1. Genotypes for *TPMT* rs1800462 was determined by polymerase chain reaction (PCR) with allele specific oligonucleotides (ASO). Primers used were, for the wild-type allele, as forward P2W 5'-GTATGATTTTATGCAGGTTTG-3' and as reverse P2C 5'-TAAATAGGAACCATCGGACAC-3'; primers. For the variant allele, a second tube was used with P2M 5'-GTATGATTTTATGCAGGTTTC-3' as forward primer and the above-mentioned P2C 5'-TAAATAGGAACCATCGGACAC-3' as reverse. PCR protocol for these primers were: initial denaturation 5 min at 94 °C, followed by 37 cycles with 30 s at 94 °C, 30 s at 57 °C, and 2 min at 72 °C, with a final extension for 10 min at 72 °C. PCR product was visualized on a 2% agarose gel. In case of a patient carrying the wild type allele, the product (254 bp) was present with the P2W and P2C primers; in case of patients carrying the variant allele, with the P2M and P2C primers for *TPMT* rs1800460 and rs1142345, PCR- restriction fragment length polymorphism (RFLP) was used. For rs1800460, primers used were: forward 5'-AGGCAGCTAGGGAAAAAGAAAGGTG-3' and reverse 5'-CAAGCCTTATAGCCTTACACCCAGG-3'. PCR protocol for these primers was: initial denaturation 5 min at 94 °C, followed by 37 cycles with 30 s at 94 °C, 30 s at 55 °C, and 2 min at 72 °C, with a final extension for 10 min at 72 °C. The DNA amplification produces an amplicon of 694 bp, which is subsequently digested enzymatically with the enzyme MwoI (concentration of 1 U/10 μl) incubated for 90 min at 60 °C. The enzyme recognizes the wild-type site and cuts the DNA strand into two fragments of 443 bp and 251 bp, while it does not cut the variant fragment. A 2% agarose gel was prepared for visualization. For rs1142345, primers used were forward 5'-AATCCCTGCTGTCATTCTTCATAGTATTT-3' and reverse 5'-CACATCATAATCTCCTCTCC-3'. PCR protocol was the same as *TPMT* rs1800460. PCR produces a 401 bp amplicon, which is subsequently digested enzymatically with the AccI enzyme (concentration 1 U/10 μl) and incubated for 90 min at 37 °C. The enzyme recognizes the variant site and cuts the DNA strand into two 252 pb and 149 pb fragments while the wild-type strand is not cut. A 2% agarose gel was prepared for visualization. *GSTM1* and *GSTT1* genotypes were determined by MULTIPLEX-PCR-ASO as previously described [13], in which three pairs of primers were used simultaneously: a specific pair for the T isoform, one for the M isoform and one for the β-globin gene, which acts as an internal positive control in order to verify the amplification. The three pairs of primers lead to three fragments of different sizes: 480 bp (*GSTT*), 286 bp (β-globin), and 219 bp (*GSTM*). The primers used have the following sequence: GSTM Forward: 5'-GAACTCCCTGAAAAGCTAAAGC-3'; GSTM Reverse: 5'-GTTGGGCTCAAATATACGGTGC-3'; β-GlobinForward: 5'-GAAGAGCCAAGGACAGGT-3'; β-Globin Reverse: 5'-CAACTTCATCCACGTTCACC-3'; GSTT Forward: 5'-TTCCTTACTGGTCCTCACATCTC-3'; GSTT Reverse: 5'-TCACCGGATCATGGCCAGCA-3'. PCR protocol for these primers were: initial denaturation 5 min at 94 °C, followed by 37 cycles with 30 s at 94 °C, 30 s at 57 °C, and 2 min at 72 °C, with a final extension for 7 min at 72 °C. All PCR reactions described were carried out using RedTaq polymerase (Sigma, Milan, Italy), with the addition of dNTPs 0,25 nM and with a primer concentration of 1 mM.

Table 1. Assay used for genotyping of the considered variants.

Gene	Polymorphism		
	rs Number	Primary Locus Alleles [14]	Genotyping Method
TPMT	rs1800462	C > G missense	PCR-ASO [13]
	rs1800460	C > T missense	PCR-RFLP [13]
	rs1142345	T > C missense	PCR-RFLP [13]
GSTM1	No rs number	Deletion	MULTIPLEX-PCR-ASO [13]
GSTT1	No rs number	Deletion	MULTIPLEX-PCR-ASO [13]
GSTA1	rs3957357	A > G (5′-UTR)	Pyrosequencing [15]

ASO: allele specific oligonucleotides; GST: glutathione-S-transferase, TPMT: thiopurine-S-methyl transferase; RFLP: restriction fragment length polymorphism. PCR: polymerase chain reaction.

For GSTA1, pyrosequencing was employed (Table 1), since this genotyping method was already validated in the laboratory. The primers used for the pyrosequencing were: forward 5′-ATCCAGTAGGTGGCCCCTTG-3′, reverse 5′-ACCGTCCTGGCTCGACAA-3′ (biotinylated). Sequencing primer was: 5′-GCTTTTCCCTAACTTGAC-3′. PCR protocol for these primers were: initial denaturation 10 min at 95 °C, followed by 40 cycles with 30 s at 95 °C, 30 s at 66 °C, and 30 s at 72 °C and with a final extension for 10 min at 72 °C. PCR produces a 148 bp amplicon. For pyrosequencing, we used PSQ96MA (Qiagen, Hilden, Germany). PCR amplifications were performed in an Eppendorf Mastercycler gradient, with TaqGold DNA Polymerase (AB Applied Biosystems, Foster City, CA, USA).

2.4. Statistical Analysis

Statistical analysis was performed using the software R (version 2.15). The association between pharmacological phenotypes of interest (i.e., clinical efficacy of treatment, dose of azathioprine, TGN metabolites concentrations, MMPN metabolites concentrations, ratio TGN/dose) and the considered demographic variables, IBD type, cotreatment or genotypes in a univariate analysis, was evaluated using linear mixed effects model built using the phenotype as the dependent variable, each covariate as the fixed effect and the patients as the random effect in the model. For clinical efficacy, the first available measurement was used, while for other pharmacological variables, all available measurements were used.

Multivariate analysis was carried out to test the independence of the effects of the genotypes significant in the univariate analysis on the phenotypes considered (i.e., TGN or MMPN concentrations, dose of azathioprine, ratio TGN/dose); for this multivariate analysis generalized linear models of the Gaussian family were used considering individually each phenotype from the univariate analysis as the dependent variable and the covariates significant in the univariate analysis as the independent variables. Normality of the phenotype was tested by the Shapiro test and log10 transformation was applied if needed, in order to adjust the normality of the distribution.

3. Results

3.1. Patients Enrolled and Samples Collected

111 patients were enrolled from March 2004 to February 2015; median age was 15.05 years (IQR 12.28–16-82), 52 (46.8%) were females. Clinical and demographic characteristics of the enrolled patients are reported in Table 2.

Table 2. Demographic and clinical characteristics of the patients enrolled in the study.

		All Patients (n = 111)
Age (Years) at Time of Sample Collection		15.1, 12.3–16.8
Gender	Female (%)	52 (46.8%)
	Male (%)	59 (53.2%)
Type of IBD	Crohn's disease (%)	61 (55.0%)
	Ulcerative colitis (%)	50 (45.0%)
Length (days) of treatment with azathioprine		533, 245–917

For continuous variables, median, 1st–3rd quartiles values are reported. To report age and length of treatment median and interquartile range are provided; for patients with more than one measurement of azathioprine metabolites, median age and length of treatment were used.

Azathioprine metabolites were measured in 257 samples (median 2 per patient, IQR 1-3). Among these, 89 were obtained during treatment with azathioprine alone and 161 during treatment with azathioprine and other medications and in particular: 93 with an aminosalicylate, 18 with an aminosalicylate and a glucocorticoid, 15 with infliximab, 10 with an antibiotic, 4 with an aminosalicylate and an antibiotic, 4 with an antibiotic and a glucocorticoid, 3 with an aminosalicylate, an antibiotic and a glucocorticoid, 2 with an infliximab and a glucocorticoid, and 1 with an aminosalicylate and infliximab; for 7 patients, information about concomitant treatment could not be retrieved.

3.2. Measurement of Azathioprine Metabolites: Association with Demographic and Clinical Covariates

Results of measurements together with azathioprine dose are shown in Table 3.

Table 3. Summary of azathioprine's dose and metabolites' concentrations.

	TGN (pmol/8 × 10^8 Erythrocytes)	MMPN (pmol/8 × 10^8 Erythrocytes)	Dose (mg/kg)	TGN/Dose ((pmol/8 × 10^8 Erythrocytes)/(mg/kg))
Mean	361.6	1698.1	2.0	192.8
Median	345.0	1044.0	2.1	179.4
Interquartile range	240.1–465.1	431.2–2079.7	1.7–2.3	120.1–227.9

MMPN indicated methylated nucleotides, TGN indicates thioguanine nucleotides.

Concentration of TGN metabolites were associated with IBD type, with UC patients showing slightly increased concentrations (Supplementary Figure S1, LME $p = 0.047$), but not with gender or treatment length. Azathioprine dose was strongly associated with age, with younger patients taking higher doses (Supplementary Figure S2, LME $p = 0.0001$), but not with gender, IBD type or treatment length. Concentration of MMPN metabolites or the ratio between TGN concentration and azathioprine dose were not associated with IBD type, gender, or treatment length. Interestingly, the ratio between TGN concentration and azathioprine dose was strongly associated with azathioprine dose when the analysis was limited to pediatric patients (i.e., with age less than 18, Supplementary Figure S3, LME $p = 0.0043$). Clinical efficacy, defined as disease activity score below 10 at the time of first sample collection for measurement of azathioprine metabolites, was assessed in all patients. Azathioprine was more effective in UC than in CD patients (88.0% versus 52.5% responders, LME $p = 0.0003$), while gender, age, and duration of azathioprine treatment were not associated with azathioprine efficacy. A higher concentration of TGN metabolites at the first evaluation was observed in patients in remission (Figure 1, LME $p = 0.0099$), similarly a positive correlation was observed with TGN/dose ratio (Figure 1, LME $p = 0.0023$).

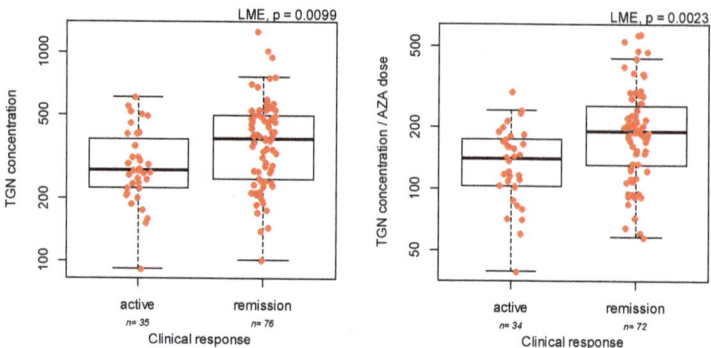

Figure 1. Response to azathioprine (AZA) and thioguanine nucleotides (TGN) concentration, as pmol/8 × 10^8 erythrocytes (left panel) or ratio between TGN concentration/daily azathioprine dose as pmol/8 × 10^8 erythrocytes/mg/kg/day (right panel). *p*-values are from linear mixed effect model (LME).

On the contrary, azathioprine dose and the concentration of MMPN metabolites were not associated with a clinical response (data not shown).

3.3. Genotyping

Results of genotyping are reported in Table 4.

Table 4. Genotype distribution in the 111 patients enrolled in the study.

Gene	Polymorphism		Genotyping Result			
	rs Number	Wild-Type	Hetero-zygous	Homozygous Variant	Not Available	*p*-value Hardy Weinberg
TPMT	rs1800462	105 (100%)	0	0	6	NA
TPMT	rs1800460	101 (97.1%)	3 (2.9%)	0	7	0.88
TPMT	rs1142345	100 (95.2%)	5 (4.8%)	0	6	0.81
GSTA1	rs3957357	38 (44.2%)	37 (43.0%)	11 (12.8%)	25	0.77
Gene	Polymorphism		Genotyping Result			
			Not Deleted	Deleted	Not Available	
GSTM1	Deletion		42 (41.9%)	61 (58.1%)	8	
GSTT1	Deletion		78 (75.7%)	25 (24.3%)	8	

GST indicates glutathione-S-transferase, TPMT indicates thiopurine-S-methyl transferase.

All polymorphisms evaluated respected Hardy-Weinberg equilibrium and their distribution was in accordance with literature data for subjects of Caucasian ethnicity. For the association between genetic variants and azathioprine pharmacokinetics, *TPMT* rs1142345 variant (4.8% of patients) was associated with increased TGN (LME $p = 0.0042$), TGN/dose ratio (LME $p < 0.0001$), decreased azathioprine dose (LME $p = 0.0087$) and MMPN (LME $p = 0.0011$; Figure 2), as well established [2]. Interestingly, all patients with variant *TPMT* were in remission at the first evaluation of thiopurine metabolites, in comparison to 65% of patients with wild-type *TPMT* (LME $p = 0.041$, Figure 2).

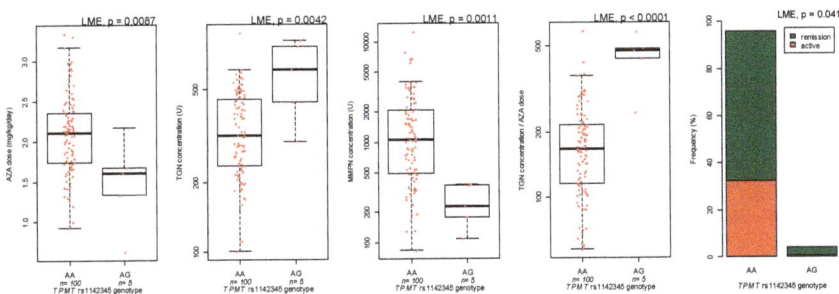

Figure 2. *TPMT* rs1142345 and azathioprine (AZA) dose, thioguanine (TGN) and methylmercaptopurine (MMPN) metabolites and efficacy. Concentration of azathioprine metabolites is expressed as pmol/8 × 10^8 erythrocytes (U). *p*-values are from linear mixed effect model (LME).

GSTM1 deletion (58.1% of patients) was associated with a 18.5% decrease in TGN/dose ratio (LME *p* = 0.041, Figure 3) and 30% decrease in clinical efficacy (LME *p* = 0.0031; Figure 3). Additionally, MMPN was reduced in patients with deletion of *GSTM1* (LME *p* = 0.039; Figure 3).

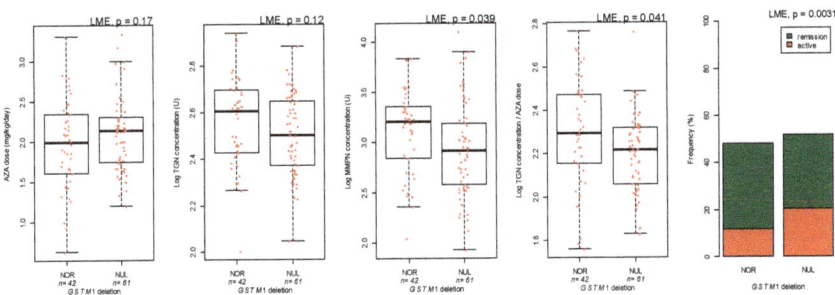

Figure 3. *GSTM1* deletion and azathioprine (AZA) dose, thioguanine (TGN), and methylmercaptopurine (MMPN) metabolites and efficacy. Concentration of azathioprine metabolites is expressed as pmol/8 × 10^8 erythrocytes (U). *p*-values are from linear mixed effect model (LME).

GSTA1 variant (12.8% of patients) showed a trend for an association with decreased clinical efficacy (LME *p* = 0.046, Figure 4); however, no significant effect on azathioprine pharmacokinetics could be detected (Figure 4).

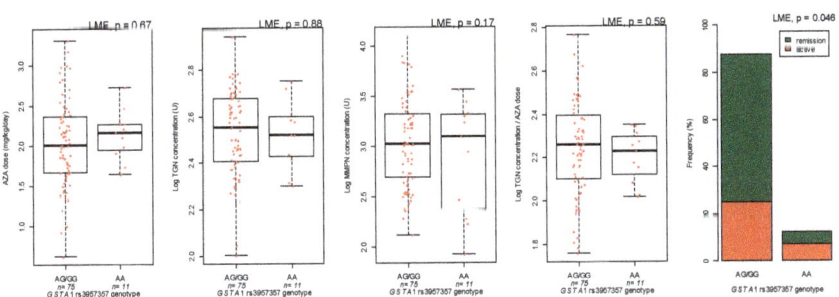

Figure 4. *GSTA1* rs3957357 variant and azathioprine (AZA) dose, thioguanine (TGN) and methylmercaptopurine (MMPN) metabolites and efficacy. Concentration of azathioprine metabolites is expressed as pmol/8 × 10^8 erythrocytes (U). *p*-values are from linear mixed effect model (LME).

GSTT1 deletion was not associated with azathioprine pharmacokinetics and efficacy (data not shown). Multivariate analysis supported the results of the univariate analysis (Table 5).

Table 5. Multivariate analysis considering for each pharmacological dependent variable covariate significant in the univariate analysis.

Azathioprine Related Pharmacological Phenotype (Dependent Variable)	Independent Variable in Multivariate Generalized Linear Model	Comparison	Effect	*p*-Value
Efficacy of azathioprine at the first metabolite measurement	IBD type	UC versus CD	1.96	0.0019
	GSTM1 genotype	Deletion versus Normal	−1.49	0.019
	GSTA1 genotype	AA versus GG/GA	−1.30	0.095
	TPMT genotype	AG versus GG	24.7	0.43
TGN metabolites concentrations	IBD type	UC versus CD	0.061	0.074
	TPMT genotype	AG versus GG	0.23	0.0049
MMPN metabolites concentration	*GSTM1* genotype	Deletion versus Normal	−0.21	0.014
	TPMT genotype	Heterozygous versus wild-type	−0.72	0.0004
Azathioprine dose	Age	Each year	−0.035	<0.0001
	TPMT genotype	Heterozygous versus wild-type	−0.58	0.0056
Ratio TGN/dose	*TPMT* genotype	Heterozygous versus wild-type	0.41	0.0001
	GSTM1 genotype	Deletion versus Normal	−0.072	0.055

GST: glutathione-S-transferase, IBD: inflammatory bowel disease, UC: ulcerative colitis, CD: Crohn's disease, MMPN: methylated nucleotides, TGN: thioguanine nucleotides, *TPMT*: thiopurine-S-methyl transferase. The effect size represents the increase (positive value) or decrease (negative value) in the value of the dependent variable for each independent variable listed. *p*-values are from linear mixed-effect models.

4. Discussion

Despite the introduction of new and effective biologics in the therapy of IBD, the thiopurine drugs azathioprine and mercaptopurine continue to be frequently used for maintaining remission in these diseases. The problem with these drugs is that they are ineffective in a significant percentage of patients, and also induce side effects that can be severe [2]. The reasons for this variability are not clear; however, a number of studies have suggested that variations in enzymes involved in their metabolism can be involved.

For azathioprine, this agent is the prodrug of mercaptopurine, and has to be converted to produce its pharmacological activity. This conversion can occur spontaneously, but is also catalyzed by the enzymes GST, in particular the A and M isoforms [16]. In rat liver homogenates, Kaplowitz et al. have demonstrated that, while at high pH (pH = 8.0) the nonenzymatic and enzymatic reactions occur at similar levels, at pH closer to physiological values, the enzymatic reaction prevails [17]. In addition, in homogenates of human livers obtained from transplant donors, treatment with furosemide, an inhibitor of soluble GSTs [18], inhibited the conversion of azathioprine to mercaptopurine [19]. Additional evidence of a role of GSTs in azathioprine metabolism has been obtained in animal models; indeed, pretreatment of rats with the GST inhibitor probenecid increased the proportion of azathioprine in rat liver and reduced GSH consumption. Similarly, less hepatic GSH depletion was observed after azathioprine treatment in Gunn rats, a model of hyperbilirubinemic rat [17]. Of interest, bilirubin is also a GST inhibitor, with some studies indicating a stronger inhibitory effect of bile acids on GSTM1 in comparison to other isoforms [20].

We previously showed that the frequency of *GSTM1* deletion was significantly lower in patients that developed an adverse event in comparison to patients that tolerated azathioprine treatment, in agreement with a model in which patients with *GSTM1* deletion are less sensitive to the effects of azathioprine, putatively because of the contribution of this enzyme on the conversion of azathioprine to mercaptopurine [13]. Moreover, in a recent previous study [21], we evaluated the effects of GST polymorphisms on azathioprine biotransformation in a cohort of young patients with IBD, tolerant to azathioprine therapy and taking the drug for more than 3 months. Patients with the deletion of *GSTM1* tolerated a dose of azathioprine significantly higher in comparison to patients with normal

GSTM1. Moreover, the amount of active TGNs generated in patients with the deletion of *GSTM1* was significantly decreased in comparison to patients with a normal genotype. Multivariate analysis confirmed that this effect was independent from that of other genes with a significant effect, such as *TPMT*, the main gene known to influence mercaptopurine metabolism [22].

The present study is the first report of an association between azathioprine efficacy and *GSTM1* and *GSTA1* variants in young patients with IBD. Moreover, we confirmed the reduced TGN/azathioprine dose ratio in patients with *GSTM1* deletion we previously reported, which may be associated with the described lower efficacy of azathioprine in patients with this genotype. This could support the need for genotype adjusted tailored therapy, possibly testing the efficacy of strategies leading to higher TGN concentration in patients with *GSTM1* deletion, such as increased azathioprine dose or co-treatment with an aminosalyciclate [23], even if prospective studies are needed to further support these strategies.

Therefore, all these studies support a role of *GSTM1* on azathioprine efficacy, mediated by an increased conversion of azathioprine to mercaptopurine. The reaction catalyzed by GSTM1 likely occurs after oral administration mainly in the intestine and the liver, modulating the amount of mercaptopurine and TGNs that are released in the main circulation [24].

Azathioprine dose is strongly associated with patients' age in the present study, an observation consistent with our previous results in children with IBD, showing that these patients require higher doses of azathioprine to achieve similar therapeutic efficacy and TGN concentration [25]. *TPMT* activity indeed is significantly higher in children than in adults [26]; interestingly, in pediatric patients (age less than 18 years), we could observe a lower ratio of TGN/azathioprine dose, as in our previous report. However, when the analysis was extended to young adults (age less than 30 years), the correlation between age and the TGN/dose ratio was lost. This may be related to environmental factors, including epigenetic determinants, even if more studies are needed to elucidate the mechanisms underlying these observations [27].

Considering studies by other groups, our results are in agreement with a recently published paper describing a lower efficacy of azathioprine in patients with *GSTM1* deletion, even if the results were not fully significant [28]. Moreover, in our study, we observed reduced concentration of MMPN nucleotides during azathioprine treatment in patients with *GSTM1* deletion: this result is consistent with a recent study by Broekman et al. [29]; this study also supports a lack of effect of *GSTA1* variants on azathioprine TGN and MMPN concentrations. The clinical implications of these observations need to be further explored. Additionally, age may affect the association of GSTs variants with thiopurine effects; indeed, studies in adult patients could not identify a consistent effect of *GSTM1* variants on thiopurines induced adverse effects [30], and therefore, other studies in the pediatric population are needed.

A recent study investigated the association among *GST* polymorphism, enzyme activity and azathioprine-related adverse drug reactions in Chinese Han patients with IBD, finding that the patients who became neutropenic had a significantly higher GSTs activity when compared with patients who did not develop toxicity [31]. The authors found, in the univariate analysis, that *GSTM1* wildtype genotype had a relationship with leukopenia and flue like symptoms, while *GSTP1* variant was strongly associated with leukopenia. Following adjustment for other potential risk factors, it was shown that *GSTP1* variants only were associated with increased risks of leukopenia. In our current study, we did not consider the effect of *GSTP1* polymorphisms on azathioprine effects and metabolism, since in our previous studies no significant association with adverse effect [13] or biotransformation [21] could be detected. The lack of association may be due to the tissue distribution of *GSTP1* and *GSTT1*, which are not highly expressed in the liver, but even to the lack of specific activity of these enzymes toward the catalysis of the reaction of azathioprine with glutathione [9,16]. Since the GSTP isoform does not catalyze the biotransformation of azathioprine to mercaptopurine [16], other mechanisms could be involved in the association observed by Liu and collaborators, such as induction of oxidative stress or modulation of apoptosis [24]. The study by Liu et al. reporting an effect of *GSTP1* variants on azathioprine induced adverse events, with a milder effect of *GSTM1*, seems to underline that the effects of GSTs on azathioprine pharmacogenetics may be influenced by ethnicity. Indeed, it is already known that variants frequent in Asian patients but uncommon in other ethnic groups, are associated with increased sensitivity to thiopurines, such as *MRP4* and *NUDT15* [32,33].

One limitation of our study is its retrospective design and the consequent difficulty of properly assessing phenomena such as drug interaction, which should rely on data collection from patients' charts. Drug interactions between azathioprine and other agents employed in IBD have been described; in particular, a significant decrease in TGN levels after discontinuation of aminosalicylates has been previously reported [23]. Moreover, for *GSTA1*, a marginal effect on thiopurine efficacy was observed but this was not supported by an effect on thiopurine pharmacokinetics: this may be related to the limited number of patients homozygous for the *GSTA1* variant enrolled. Another limitation is the fact that the current assay for thiopurine metabolites quantifies two main species (thioguanine nucleotides and methyl-mercaptopurine nucleotides), without distinguishing between monophosphate, diphosphate, and triphosphate nucleotides. Innovative mass spectrometry based assays are now available to quantify thiopurine metabolites [34], allowing quantification of phosphorylation of thionucleotides [35] and they could be applied to evaluate differences in thiopurine biotransformation in patients with various GST genotypes. Evaluation of the combined effects of genotypes in this study is limited. Indeed, multivariate analysis indicates independency in the effects of the candidate genotypes considered on the pharmacological variables in the present cohort. A larger cohort is needed to detect significant effects by combined genotypes. For demographic covariates, in particular gender, no significant effect was identified in the univariate analysis; to further evaluate interactive effect of gender and the considered genotypes, a larger cohort is needed.

In conclusion, GSTs variants were associated with azathioprine efficacy and pharmacokinetics; more studies, both clinical and molecular are still needed to apply this evidence to improve outcomes of therapy with azathioprine in young patients with IBD.

Supplementary Materials: The following are available online at http://www.mdpi.com/2073-4425/10/4/277/s1, Figure S1: inflammatory bowel disease (IBD type) and azathioprine thioguanine nucleotide (TGN) metabolites, Figure S2: Patient's age and azathioprine daily dose, Figure S3: Patient's age and ratio between concentration of azathioprine thioguanine-nucleotide metabolites and azathioprine daily dose.

Author Contributions: Conceptualization, M.L., G.S., E.C., G.T., A.V., and G.D.; Data curation, M.L., G.S., A.L., M.B., S.N., E.C., and G.D.; Formal analysis, M.L., G.S., D.F., N.M., E.C., and G.D.; Funding acquisition, S.M., M.B.; Methodology, M.L., S.M., D.F., R.F., N.M., A.L., M.B., S.N., and E.C.; Supervision, S.M., N.M., E.C., G.T., A.V., and G.D.; Writing—original draft, M.L., G.S. and G.D.; Writing—review & editing, M.L., G.S., S.M., E.C., A.V., and G.D.

Funding: This study was supported by the Italian Ministry of Health (Progetti Ricerca Corrente 23/2005, 12/2013 and 21/17).

Conflicts of Interest: The authors declare no conflict of interest.

References

1. Ponder, A.; Long, M.D. A clinical review of recent findings in the epidemiology of inflammatory bowel disease. *Clin. Epidemiol.* **2013**, *5*, 237–247. [CrossRef]
2. Louis, E.; Irving, P.; Beaugerie, L. Use of azathioprine in IBD: Modern aspects of an old drug. *Gut* **2014**, *63*, 1695–1699. [CrossRef] [PubMed]
3. Barabino, A.; Torrente, F.; Ventura, A.; Cucchiara, S.; Castro, M.; Barbera, C. Azathioprine in paediatric inflammatory bowel disease: An Italian multicentre survey. *Aliment. Pharmacol. Ther.* **2002**, *16*, 1125–1130. [CrossRef] [PubMed]
4. Prefontaine, E.; Macdonald, J.K.; Sutherland, L.R. Azathioprine or 6-mercaptopurine for induction of remission in Crohn's disease. *Cochrane Database Syst Rev.* **2010**, *6*, CD000545. [CrossRef]
5. Colombel, J.F.; Sandborn, W.J.; Reinisch, W.; Mantzaris, G.J.; Kornbluth, A.; Rachmilewitz, D.; Lichtiger, S.; D'Haens, G.; Diamond, R.H.; Broussard, D.L.; et al. Infliximab, azathioprine, or combination therapy for Crohn's disease. *N. Engl. J. Med.* **2010**, *362*, 1383–1395. [CrossRef]

6. Chouchana, L.; Narjoz, C.; Beaune, P.; Loriot, M.A.; Roblin, X. Review article: The benefits of pharmacogenetics for improving thiopurine therapy in inflammatory bowel disease. *Aliment. Pharmacol. Ther.* **2012**, *35*, 15–36. [CrossRef] [PubMed]
7. Lucafò, M.; Franca, R.; Selvestrel, D.; Curci, D.; Pugnetti, L.; Decorti, G.; Stocco, G. Pharmacogenetics of treatments for inflammatory bowel disease. *Expert Opin. Drug Metab. Toxicol.* **2018**, *14*, 1209–1223. [CrossRef]
8. Stocco, G.; De Iudicibus, S.; Franca, R.; Addobbati, R.; Decorti, G. Personalized therapies in pediatric inflammatory and autoimmune diseases. *Curr. Pharm. Des.* **2012**, *18*, 5766–5775. [CrossRef] [PubMed]
9. Modén, O.; Mannervik, B. Glutathione transferases in the bioactivation of azathioprine. *Adv. Cancer Res.* **2014**, *122*, 199–244. [CrossRef]
10. Zaza, G.; Cheok, M.; Krynetskaia, N.; Thorn, C.; Stocco, G.; Hebert, J.M.; McLeod, H.; Weinshilboum, R.M.; Relling, M.V.; Evans, W.E.; et al. Thiopurine pathway. *Pharm. Genom.* **2010**, *20*, 573–574. [CrossRef] [PubMed]
11. Turner, D.; Otley, A.R.; Mack, D.; Hyams, J.; de Bruijne, J.; Uusoue, K.; Walters, T.D.; Zachos, M.; Mamula, P.; Beaton, D.E.; et al. Development, validation, and evaluation of a pediatric ulcerative colitis activity index: A prospective multicenter study. *Gastroenterology* **2007**, *133*, 423–432. [CrossRef] [PubMed]
12. Dervieux, T.; Boulieu, R. Simultaneous determination of 6-thioguanine and methyl 6-mercaptopurine nucleotides of azathioprine in red blood cells by HPLC. *Clin Chem.* **1998**, *44*, 551–555. [PubMed]
13. Stocco, G.; Martelossi, S.; Barabino, A.; Decorti, G.; Bartoli, F.; Montico, M.; Gotti, A.; Ventura, A. Glutathione-S-transferase genotypes and the adverse effects of azathioprine in young patients with inflammatory bowel disease. *Inflamm. Bowel Dis.* **2007**, *13*, 57–64. [CrossRef] [PubMed]
14. Whirl-Carrillo, M.; McDonagh, E.M.; Hebert, J.M.; Gong, L.; Sangkuhl, K.; Thorn, C.F.; Altman, R.B.; Klein, T.E. Pharmacogenomics knowledge for personalized medicine. *Clin. Pharmacol. Ther.* **2012**, *92*, 414–417. [CrossRef] [PubMed]
15. De Mattia, E.; Cecchin, E.; Polesel, J.; Bignucolo, A.; Roncato, R.; Lupo, F.; Crovatto, M.; Buonadonna, A.; Tiribelli, C.; Toffoli, G. Genetic biomarkers for hepatocellular cancer risk in a caucasian population. *World J. Gastroenterol.* **2017**, *23*, 6674–6684. [CrossRef] [PubMed]
16. Eklund, B.I.; Moberg, M.; Bergquist, J.; Mannervik, B. Divergent activities of human glutathione transferases in the bioactivation of azathioprine. *Mol. Pharmacol.* **2006**, *70*, 747–754. [CrossRef]
17. Kaplowitz, N.; Kuhlenkamp, J. Inhibition of hepatic metabolism of azathioprine in vivo. *Gastroenterology* **1978**, *74*, 90–92.
18. Ahokas, J.T.; Davies, C.; Ravenscroft, P.J.; Emmerson, B.T. Inhibition of soluble glutathione S-transferase by diuretic drugs. *Biochem. Pharmacol.* **1984**, *33*, 1929–1932. [CrossRef]
19. Von Bahr, C.; Glaumann, H.; Gudas, J.; Kaplowitz, N. Inhibition of hepatic metabolism of azathioprine by furosemide in human liver in vitro. *Biochem. Pharmacol.* **1980**, *29*, 1439–1441. [CrossRef]
20. Singh, S.V.; Leal, T.; Awasthi, Y.C. Inhibition of human glutathione S-transferases by bile acids. *Toxicol. Appl. Pharmacol.* **1988**, *95*, 248–254. [CrossRef]
21. Stocco, G.; Cuzzoni, E.; De Iudicibus, S.; Franca, R.; Favretto, D.; Malusà, N.; Londero, M.; Cont, G.; Bartoli, F.; Martelossi, S.; et al. Deletion of glutathione-s-transferase m1 reduces azathioprine metabolite concentrations in young patients with inflammatory bowel disease. *J. Clin. Gastroenterol.* **2014**, *48*, 43–51. [CrossRef] [PubMed]
22. Relling, M.V.; Gardner, E.E.; Sandborn, W.J.; Schmiegelow, K.; Pui, C.H.; Yee, S.W.; Stein, C.M.; Carrillo, M.; Evans, W.E.; Hicks, J.K.; et al. Clinical pharmacogenetics implementation consortium guidelines for thiopurine methyltransferase genotype and thiopurine dosing: 2013 update. *Clin. Pharmacol. Ther.* **2013**, *93*, 324–325. [CrossRef] [PubMed]
23. Stocco, G.; Cuzzoni, E.; De Iudicibus, S.; Favretto, D.; Malusà, N.; Martelossi, S.; Pozzi, E.; Lionetti, P.; Ventura, A.; Decorti, G. Thiopurine metabolites variations during co-treatment with aminosalicylates for inflammatory bowel disease: Effect of N-acetyl transferase polymorphisms. *World J. Gastroenterol.* **2015**, *21*, 3571–3578. [CrossRef] [PubMed]
24. Stocco, G.; Pelin, M.; Franca, R.; De Iudicibus, S.; Cuzzoni, E.; Favretto, D.; Martelossi, S.; Ventura, A.; Decorti, G. Pharmacogenetics of azathioprine in inflammatory bowel disease: A role for glutathione-S-transferase? *World J. Gastroenterol.* **2014**, *20*, 3534–3541. [CrossRef] [PubMed]
25. Stocco, G.; Martelossi, S.; Arrigo, S.; Barabino, A.; Aloi, M.; Martinelli, M.; Miele, E.; Knafelz, D.; Romano, C.; Naviglio, S.; et al. Multicentric Case-Control Study on Azathioprine Dose and Pharmacokinetics in Early-onset Pediatric Inflammatory Bowel Disease. *Inflamm. Bowel Dis.* **2017**, *23*, 628–634. [CrossRef] [PubMed]

26. Serpe, L.; Calvo, P.L.; Muntoni, E.; D'Antico, S.; Giaccone, M.; Avagnina, A.; Baldi, M.; Barbera, C.; Curti, F.; Pera, A.; et al. Thiopurine S-methyltransferase pharmacogenetics in a large-scale healthy Italian-Caucasian population: Differences in enzyme activity. *Pharmacogenomics* **2009**, *10*, 1753–1765. [CrossRef] [PubMed]
27. De Iudicibus, S.; Lucafò, M.; Vitulo, N.; Martelossi, S.; Zimbello, R.; De Pascale, F.; Forcato, C.; Naviglio, S.; Di Silvestre, A.; Gerdol, M.; et al. High-Throughput Sequencing of microRNAs in Glucocorticoid Sensitive Paediatric Inflammatory Bowel Disease Patients. *Int. J. Mol. Sci.* **2018**, *19*, 1399. [CrossRef]
28. Al-Judaibi, B.; Schwarz, U.I.; Huda, N.; Dresser, G.K.; Gregor, J.C.; Ponich, T.; Chande, N.; Mosli, M.; Kim, R.B. Genetic Predictors of Azathioprine Toxicity and Clinical Response in Patients with Inflammatory Bowel Disease. *J. Popul. Ther. Clin. Pharmacol.* **2016**, *23*, e26–e36.
29. Broekman, M.M.T.J.; Wong, D.R.; Wanten, G.J.A.; Roelofs, H.M.; van Marrewijk, C.J.; Klungel, O.H.; Verbeek, A.L.M.; Hooymans, P.M.; Guchelaar, H.J.; Scheffer, H.; et al. The glutathione transferase Mu null genotype leads to lower 6-MMPR levels in patients treated with azathioprine but not with mercaptopurine. *Pharm. J.* **2018**, *18*, 160–166. [CrossRef]
30. Mazor, Y.; Koifman, E.; Elkin, H.; Chowers, Y.; Krivoy, N.; Karban, A.; Efrati, E. Risk factors for serious adverse effects of thiopurines in patients with Crohn's disease. *Curr. Drug Saf.* **2013**, *8*, 181–185. [CrossRef]
31. Liu, H.; Ding, L.; Zhang, F.; Zhang, Y.; Gao, X.; Hu, P.; Bi, H.; Huang, M. The impact of glutathione S-transferase genotype and phenotype on the adverse drug reactions to azathioprine in patients with inflammatory bowel diseases. *J. Pharmacol. Sci.* **2015**, *129*, 95–100. [CrossRef] [PubMed]
32. Moriyama, T.; Nishii, R.; Perez-Andreu, V.; Yang, W.; Klussmann, F.A.; Zhao, X.; Lin, T.N.; Hoshitsuki, K.; Nersting, J.; Kihira, K.; et al. NUDT15 polymorphisms alter thiopurine metabolism and hematopoietic toxicity. *Nat. Genet.* **2016**, *48*, 367–373. [CrossRef] [PubMed]
33. Ban, H.; Andoh, A.; Imaeda, H.; Kobori, A.; Bamba, S.; Tsujikawa, T.; Sasaki, M.; Saito, Y.; Fujiyama, Y. The multidrug-resistance protein 4 polymorphism is a new factor accounting for thiopurine sensitivity in Japanese patients with inflammatory bowel disease. *J. Gastroenterol.* **2010**, *45*, 1014–1021. [CrossRef] [PubMed]
34. Hofmann, U.; Heinkele, G.; Angelberger, S.; Schaeffeler, E.; Lichtenberger, C.; Jaeger, S.; Reinisch, W.; Schwab, M. Simultaneous quantification of eleven thiopurine nucleotides by liquid chromatography-tandem mass spectrometry. *Anal. Chem.* **2012**, *84*, 1294–1301. [CrossRef] [PubMed]
35. Pelin, M.; Genova, E.; Fusco, L.; Marisat, M.; Hofmann, U.; Favretto, D.; Lucafò, M.; Taddio, A.; Martelossi, S.; Ventura, A.; et al. Pharmacokinetics and pharmacodynamics of thiopurines in an in vitro model of human hepatocytes: Insights from an innovative mass spectrometry assay. *Chem. Biol. Interact.* **2017**, *275*, 189–195. [CrossRef] [PubMed]

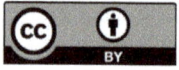

© 2019 by the authors. Licensee MDPI, Basel, Switzerland. This article is an open access article distributed under the terms and conditions of the Creative Commons Attribution (CC BY) license (http://creativecommons.org/licenses/by/4.0/).

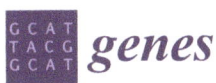

Article

MicroRNAs Mediated Regulation of Expression of Nucleoside Analog Pathway Genes in Acute Myeloid Leukemia

Neha S. Bhise [1,2], Abdelrahman H. Elsayed [1], Xueyuan Cao [3], Stanley Pounds [4] and Jatinder K. Lamba [1,*]

1. Department of Pharmacotherapy and Translational Research, Center for Pharmacogenomics, University of Florida, Gainesville, FL 32610, USA; Neha.bhise@gmail.com (N.S.B.); aelsayed@ufl.edu (A.H.E.)
2. Department of Experimental and Clinical Pharmacology, University of Minnesota, Minneapolis, MN 55455, USA
3. Department of Acute and Tertiary Care, University of Tennessee Health Science Center, Memphis, TN 38163, USA; xcao12@uthsc.edu
4. Department of Biostatistics, St. Jude Children's Research Hospital, Memphis, TN 38105, USA; stanley.pounds@stjude.org
* Correspondence: jlamba@cop.ufl.edu

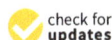

Received: 26 March 2019; Accepted: 20 April 2019; Published: 24 April 2019

Abstract: Nucleoside analog, cytarabine (ara-C) is the mainstay of acute myeloid leukemia (AML) chemotherapy. Cytarabine and other nucleoside analogs require activation to the triphosphate form (ara-CTP). Intracellular ara-CTP levels demonstrate significant inter-patient variation and have been related to therapeutic response in AML patients. Inter-patient variation in expression levels of drug transporters or enzymes involved in the activation or inactivation of cytarabine and other analogs is a prime mechanism contributing to development of drug resistance. Since microRNAs (miRNAs) are known to regulate gene-expression, the aim of this study was to identify miRNAs involved in regulation of messenger RNA expression levels of cytarabine pathway genes. We evaluated miRNA and gene-expression levels of cytarabine metabolic pathway genes in 8 AML cell lines and The Cancer Genome Atlas (TCGA) data base. Using correlation analysis and functional validation experiments, our data demonstrates that miR-34a-5p and miR-24-3p regulate DCK, an enzyme involved in activation of cytarabine and DCTD, an enzyme involved in metabolic inactivation of cytarabine expression, respectively. Further our results from gel shift assays confirmed binding of these mRNA-miRNA pairs. Our results show miRNA mediated regulation of gene expression levels of nucleoside metabolic pathway genes can impact interindividual variation in expression levels which in turn may influence treatment outcomes.

Keywords: nucleoside analogs; microRNAs; gene expression; drug resistance; AML

1. Introduction

Nucleoside analogs (NA) are a class of chemotherapeutic agents that structurally resemble the endogenous purine or pyrimidine nucleosides. These therapeutic agents mimic the endogenous nucleosides with respect to their uptake and metabolism and are incorporated into the newly synthesized DNA leading to inhibition of DNA synthesis and chain termination. Some of the nucleoside analogs also inhibit or block the enzymes that are required for the synthesis of purine or pyrimidine nucleotides and RNA synthesis, leading to the activation of the caspase cascade and cell death. The nucleoside analogs are extensively used for the treatment of both hematological malignancies and solid tumors.

The pyrimidine nucleoside analog, cytarabine, is one of the most widely used chemotherapeutic drugs for the treatment of acute myeloid leukemia (AML).

One of the major obstacles in the treatment of AML is development of resistance to nucleoside analogs. There is a growing need to understand the mechanisms that lead to development of resistance to these nucleoside analogs in order to help identify strategies that would effectively treat patients with relapsing or refractory diseases. One of the primary mechanisms of resistance to nucleoside analogs is insufficient intracellular concentration of the active triphosphate metabolite. This insufficient triphosphate levels could be due to inefficient cellular uptake of the drug, reduced levels of the activating enzyme, increased levels of inactivating enzymes and/or due to increased levels of endogenous deoxynucleotide (dNTP) pools [1–4]. Resistance could also develop due to inability to achieve sufficient alterations in the DNA strands or the dNTP pools, either due to altered interaction with DNA polymerases or by a lack of inhibition of ribonucleotide reductases, or due to inadequate p53 exonuclease activity. Since the expression and activity of drug transporters and metabolizing enzymes in the activation pathway of nucleoside analogs plays an important role in development of resistance to the NAs, it is essential to understand the factors influencing the expression and activity of these proteins.

MicroRNAs (miRNAs) are a group of novel gene regulators, which have been recently recognized to play an important role in cancers due to their tumor suppressive and oncogenic functions [5]. MiRNAs are known to regulate the expression of the target genes by binding to the specific sequence mainly on the 3′ untranslated region on the genes. Role of miRNAs in regulating the expression of various drug-metabolizing enzymes like cytochrome P450 3A4 (CYP3A4) etc., drug transporters like BCRP and various drug targets [6–8] have been established. However, there have not been any studies that have comprehensively evaluated the effect of miRNAs on the important genes involved in the transport, activation and inactivation of nucleoside analogs. Hence, the aim of this study was to assess the effect of miRNAs on the expression of nucleoside analog pharmacokinetic (PK) and pharmacodynamic (PD) pathway genes and in turn assessing their potential impact on resistance to nucleoside analogs.

2. Materials and Methods

2.1. Cell culture and Reagents

The AML cell lines HL-60, MV-4-11, Kasumi-1, THP-1, AML-193 and KG-1 cell lines were obtained from American Type Culture Collection (ATCC) (Manassas, VA, USA), while MOLM-16 and ME-1 cell lines were obtained from DSMZ (Braunschweig, Germany). Kasumi-1, ME-1 and MOLM-16 cell lines were cultured in Roswell Park Memorial Institute (RMPI)-1640 medium supplemented with 20% fetal bovine serum (FBS), THP-1 cell line was cultured in RPMI-1640 medium supplemented with 10% FBS, HL-60 and KG-1 cell lines were cultured in IMDM medium supplemented with 20% FBS, while AML-193 cell lines was cultured in IMDM medium supplemented with 5% FBS, 0.005 mg/mL insulin, 0.005 mg/mL transferrin and 5 ng/mL granulocyte/macrophage colony stimulating factor (GM-CSF). All the cell lines were maintained in a 37 °C humidified incubator with 5% CO_2. The cells were passaged every two to three days in order to maintain them in logarithmic growth phase.

2.2. RNA Isolation

Total RNA was isolated from the AML cell pellets using RNeasy Plus Mini Kit (Qiagen, Valencia, CA, USA) according to the manufacturer's protocol and stored in −80 °C until further analysis. The RNA quality and concentration were measured using NanoDrop 2000 UV-Vis spectrophotometer (Thermo Scientific, Wilmington, DE, USA). The ratio of absorbance at 260 nm and 280 nm was used to assess RNA sample purity and A260/A280 ratio of 1.8–2.1 was considered to be indicative of highly purified RNA. RNA was normalized to 0.2 µg/µL with nuclease-free water before being used for performing reverse transcription reactions, as recommended by the manufacturer. The total RNA was reverse transcribed to complementary DNA (cDNA) using High Capacity cDNA Reverse Transcription Kit (Applied Biosystems, Foster City, CA, USA) according to manufacturer's protocol.

2.3. Gene Expression Analysis

The expression of nucleoside analog genes was determined using the TaqMan® Low Density Array (TLDA) cards (Applied Biosystems). Each TLDA card was custom designed with pre-loaded gene expression assays for measuring the messenger RNA (mRNA) expression of selected nucleoside analog metabolic pathway genes- (n = 14) deoxycytidine kinase (*DCK*), cytidine deaminase (*CDA*), solute carrier family 29, member 1 (*SLC29A1*), solute carrier family 28, member 1 (SLC28A1), solute carrier family 28, member 3 (SLC28A3), deoxycytidylate deaminase (*DCTD*), 5'-nucleotidase, cytosolic II (*NT5C2*), 5'-nucleotidase cytosolic III (*NT5C3*), cytidine 5'-triphosphate synthase (*CTPS*), cytidine monophosphate kinase (*CMPK*), nucleoside diphosphate kinase 1 (*NME1*), ribonucleotide reductase M1 (*RRM1*), ribonucleotide reductase M2 (*RRM2*), ribonucleotide reductase M2B (*RRM2B*). Each TLDA card consists of eight separate loading ports that fill into 48 separate wells, for a total of 384 wells per card. Thus, each card could analyze the expression of 24 different genes for eight different samples in duplicates. Each cDNA sample was added to equal volume of 2X TaqMan Universal PCR Master Mix (Thermo Scientific) and 100 µL of the sample-specific PCR mix was added to the fill reservoir on the TLDA card. The card was centrifuged twice for one minute at 1200 rpm to distribute the sample-specific PCR reaction mix to the reaction wells. The card was sealed using the TaqMan Array Micro Fluidic Card Sealer (Thermo Scientific) and placed on microfluidic card thermal cycling block of Applied Biosystems 7900HT Fast Real-time PCR System (Applied Biosystems). Thermal cycling conditions were as follows: 2 min at 50 °C, 10 min at 94.5 °C, 30 s at 97 °C, 1 min at 59.7 °C for 40 cycles. The target mRNA expression levels were normalized to GAPDH and the expression values of nucleoside analogs pathway genes were calculated using $\Delta\Delta C_T$ method [9].

2.4. MicroRNA Expression Analysis

For determination of miRNA expression, total RNA was isolated using mirVana™ miRNA Isolation kit (Life Technologies, Carlsbad, CA, USA) as per the manufacturer's protocol. The RNA quality and concentration were measured using NanoDrop 2000 UV-Vis spectrophotometer (Thermo Scientific). A total of 100 ng of purified total RNA was used for nCounter miRNA sample preparation reactions according to manufacturer's instructions and was assayed for determination of 800 human miRNA expression using the nCounter Human v2 miRNA Expression Assay kit (Nanostring Technologies, Seattle, WA, USA). Preparation of small RNA samples involved multiplexed ligation of specific tags (miRtags) to the target miRNAs that provide unique identification for each miRNA species. After ligation, the detection was done by hybridization to microRNA: tag specific nCounter capture and barcoded reporter probes. Data collection was carried out using the nCounter Digital Analyzer (Nanostring Technologies) at The University of Minnesota Genomics Center, following manufacturer's instructions to count individual fluorescent barcodes and quantify the target miRNA molecules present in each sample. MiRNA expression data normalization was performed using the nSolver™ Analysis Software (Nanostring Technologies) according to the manufacturer's instructions. In particular, initially the data was normalized using the expression of the top 100 code sets. Further, to account for the background correction, mean of negative controls plus two-standard deviation (SD) method was used. In order to avoid using the miRNAs with a very low expression, we further filtered out the miRNAs with expression counts < 30 (2 times the mean ± 2 SD of negative control value), in order to account for the background noise. Total 412 miRNAs with expression counts > 30 were included for further analysis.

2.5. Acute Myeloid Leukemia Patient Sample Data from The Cancer Genome Atlas

The miRNA expression and mRNA expression of the nucleoside analog pathway genes in AML patients was extracted from The Cancer Genome Atlas (TCGA) Data Portal (cancergenome.nih.gov) [10].

Out of the 200 AML patients in TCGA database, 197 patients had gene expression profiling data available and 187 patients had miRNA expression data available. 186 patients had both gene expression and miRNA expression data available.

2.6. Electrophoretic Mobility Shift Assays

The functional validation for binding efficiencies between miRNAs and mRNAs was performed using the electrophoretic mobility shift assays (EMSAs). The binding free energy between the respective mRNA and miRNA pair was predicted using the RNAhybrid software. The miRNA oligonucleotides were labeled with cy5™ dye on their 5′ ends. The 2′ O-methyl-modified mRNA oligonucleotides were labeled with IRDye®800 (LI-COR Biosciences, Lincoln, NE, USA) dye on their 5′ ends. The labeled oligonucleotides were synthesized by Integrated DNA Technologies (Coralville, IA, USA). RNA EMSA experiment was performed using the LightShift Chemiluminescent RNA EMSA Kit (Thermo Scientific) according to the manufacturer's protocol. The mRNA oligonucleotide was heated for 10 min at 80 °C and then placed on ice in order to relax the secondary structures. In each 20 µL binding reaction, 200 nM miRNA oligonucleotide and/or mRNA oligonucleotide were mixed with RNA EMSA binding buffer and incubated at 25 °C for 25 min. The reaction mixtures were separated on a 12% polyacrylamide gel by electrophoresis at 4 °C. The binding reactions were transferred onto nylon membrane and the resulting mobility shifts were imaged using and Odyssey CLx Infrared System (LI-COR Biosciences).

2.7. Bioinformatic Analysis

Prediction of miRNA binding sites was performed using multiple prediction programs, which use different criteria for prediction of binding sites: TargetScan (www.targetscan.org), miRanda (www.microRNA.org), PICTAR (pictar.mdc-berlin.de), miRWalk (www.umm.uni-heidelberg.de/apps/zmf/mirwalk). Binding free energy calculations were performed using RNAhybrid software [11]. The 3′UTR (3′ untranslated region) sequence of mRNA was obtained from the UCSC Genome browser (https://genome.ucsc.edu/) and miRNA sequence was obtained from miRBase software (http://www.mirbase.org/).

2.8. Statistical Analysis

The nonparametric Spearman correlation was used to measure the correlation of mRNA expression with miRNA expression. Statistical significance was determined when p-value was < 0.01.

3. Results

3.1. Effect of Micro RNA on the Expression of Nucleoside Analog Pathway Genes in Acute Myeloid Leukemia Cell Lines

We determined expression of 800 miRNAs and 13 genes involved in PK/PD pathway of nucleoside analogs (Figure 1) in cytogenetically different AML cell lines ($n = 8$). In order to identify the miRNAs associated with the expression of nucleoside analog pathway genes, we correlated the miRNA expression and mRNA expression using the spearman correlation analysis. Table 1 lists the negative correlations of nucleoside analog pathway genes and respective miRNAs at p <0.01. We further used CyTargetLinker software [12] to establish the network of miRNAs correlated with the respective PK/PD pathway genes of the nucleoside analogs. Figure 2 shows the miRNA-mRNA pairs identified by CyTargetLinker.

The expression of *DCK* (the rate-limiting enzyme in the nucleoside analog pathway) correlated with the expression of miR-34a-5p expression (spearman $r = -0.88$; p-value < 0.01) and miR-96-5p expression (spearman $r = -0.91$; p-value < 0.01). The expression of deactivating enzyme *DCTD* was found to be correlated with miR-24-3p expression (spearman $r = -0.93$; p-value < 0.01). Interestingly, in our previous study, we identified that expression of miRNA miR-24-3p was correlated with cytarabine-induced cell cytotoxicity (spearman $r = -0.81$, p-value < 0.05) [13] which is in agreement with the current observation. The expression of *CMPK*, a kinase responsible for phosphorylation of the monophosphate form of nucleoside analog was negatively correlated with the expression of miR-1301, miR-1323, miR-320e, miR-381, miR-507, miR-584-5p, miR-605, miR-762, miR-769-3p, miR-891a (all p-values < 0.01). RRM2 expression was found to be negatively associated with the expression of miR-151a-3p (p-value < 0.01). Figure 3 shows correlation plots between *DCTD*-miR-24, *DCK*-miR34 and *NT5C3*-miR149 pairs.

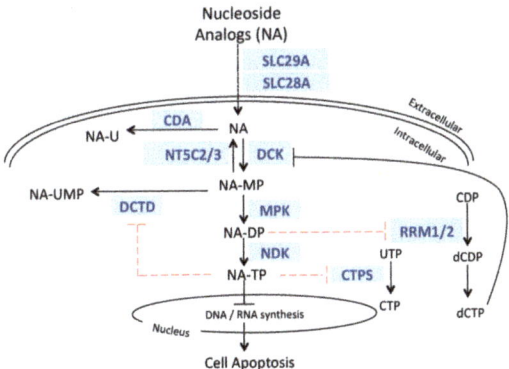

Figure 1. Disposition pathway of nucleoside analogs, cytarabine and clofarabine. DCTD: Deoxycytidylate deaminase, DCK: Deoxycytidine kinase, CDA: Cytidine deaminase, NT5C2/3: 5′-Nucleotidase, cytoplasmic, CTPS: CTP synthase, RRM1/2: Ribonucleotide reductase, SLC29A: Solute carrier family 29, SLC28A: Solute carrier family 28, MPK: Monophosphate kinase, NDK: Nucleoside diphosphate kinase

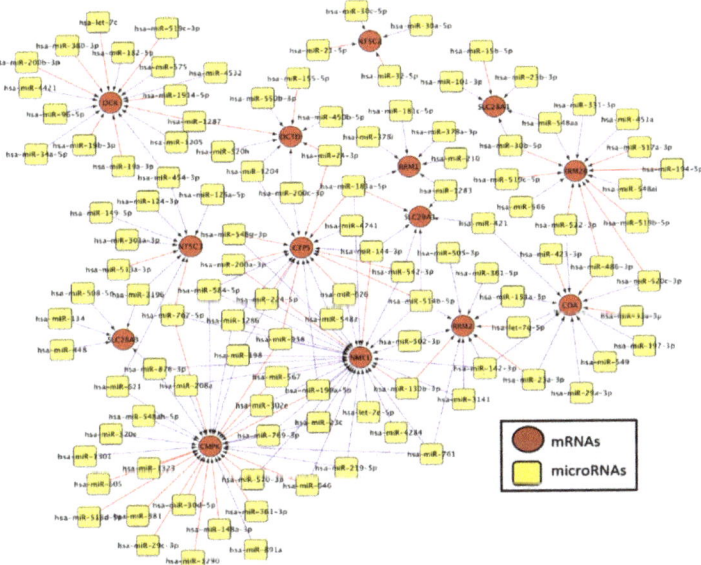

Figure 2. MicroRNA-mRNA network constructed using CyTargetLinker [12]. MiRNAs associated with the nucleoside analog metabolic pathway genes are shown in yellow and the mRNAs are depicted in red. Blue lines indicated positive and red indicated negative associations.

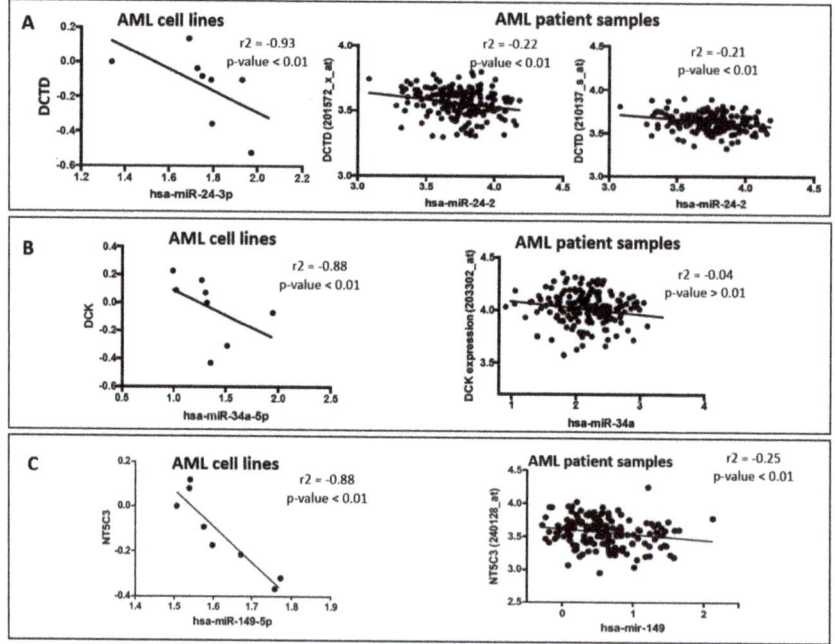

Figure 3. Correlation of miRNAs with nucleoside analog pathway gene expression in acute myeloid leukemia (AML) cell lines and patient samples from The Cancer Genome Atlas (TCGA) database. (**A**) Correlation between DCTD and hsa-miR-24a-3p. (**B**) Correlation between DCK and hsa-miR-34a-5p. (**C**) Correlation between NT5C3 and hsa-miR-149.

3.2. Bioinformatic Prediction of Binding of Micro RNAs and Messenger RNAs

MiRNAs are known to guide the RNA-induced silencing complex (RISC) to the specific sequence (usually in located in the 3'UTR) on the target mRNA. Using various bioinformatic prediction programs (TargetScan, miRanda, PICTAR, miRWalk) we determined if the miRNAs that were correlated with gene expression had binding sites on 3'-UTR of target genes. MiRNAs miR-1323, miR-30d-5p, miR-381, and miR-605 were predicted to have binding sites on *CMPK* gene, while miRNA miR-24-3p was found to have binding site on *DCTD* by multiple prediction programs. Supplementary Figure S1 shows comparisons of different miRNA prediction programs for genes involved in nucleoside analog pathways.

3.3. Effect of Micro RNAs on the Expression of Nucleoside Analog Pathway Genes in Acute Myeloid Leukemia Patients

In order to validate the significant correlations between miRNAs and mRNAs identified in AML cell lines, we evaluated the correlation between miRNA expression and nucleoside analog pathway gene expression in AML patient samples from TCGA database ($n = 186$). We extracted the miRNA expression data and nucleoside analog pathway gene expression data for AML patients from TCGA database and performed spearman correlation to identify the significant mRNA-miRNA pairs. Consistent with results from AML cell lines miR-24-3p was inversely correlated with the expression of both the probes for *DCTD* in AML patient samples ($r = -0.22$; p-value < 0.01 and $r = -0.21$; p-value < 0.01, Figure 3A). *DCK*-mir-34a pair unfortunately did not show significant association within the TCGA data-set. miR-149 was significantly correlated with expression of *NT5C3* in AML patients ($r = -0.25$; p-value < 0.01, Figure 3C).

Validation of Binding Efficiencies between Messenger RNAs and Micro RNAs

MiRNAs are known to bind to the specific seed sequence on the 3'UTR of the mRNAs, thereby regulating the expression of their target genes. In order to validate the binding between the mRNA-miRNAs identified from the in vitro studies and in AML patient samples, we performed RNA EMSA assays. We validated the interaction between *DCTD* and miR-24, since we identified this mRNA-miRNA pair to be significantly inversely correlated in both AML cell line and AML patient samples. In addition, various prediction databases predicted miRNA miR-24 to have binding site on the 3'UTR of *DCTD* mRNA. In silico analysis predicted miR-24-3p and miR-34a-5p might form complexes with target sequences in the 3'UTR of *DCTD* and *DCK* respectively with minimum free energies of binding of −27.2 kcal/mol for *DCTD* and miR-24-3p (Figure 4A and Table 1) and -25.6 kcal/mol for *DCK* and miR-34a-5p (Figure 5A and Table 1). The RNA EMSA results for IRD-800®-labeled *DCTD* and Cy-5-labeled miR-24-3p show miR-24a-3p was able to bind to its target sequence on *DCTD* 3'UTR (Figure 4B, lane 3) as seen by the band shift. The thermodynamic stability of this complex correlated with binding observed in the RNA EMSA assays. In addition, we found that mRNA-miRNA complex formed by *DCTD* and miR-24a-3p could be eliminated by adding excess unlabeled hsa-miR-24a-3p probe (Figure 4B, lane 4), but not by adding excess unlabeled non-specific probe (Figure 4B, lane 6). Adding excess unlabeled mRNA probe resulted in binding of all the labeled miRNA giving a greater intensity signal (Figure 4B, lane 5).

Similar to the interaction observed between *DCTD* and miR-24a-3p, we observed that miR-34a-5p binds to *DCK* 3'UTR as seen by shift in the band (Figure 5B, lane 3) and this interaction was eliminated by addition of unlabeled probe (Figure 5B, lane 4). Since the minimum free energy of binding for *NT5C3*- miR-149 pair was not strong (Table 1), we did not pursue EMSA assays for this pair.

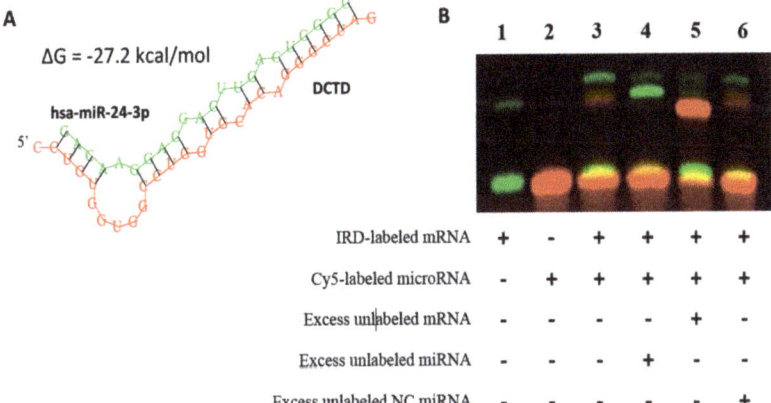

Figure 4. Validation of binding interaction between DCTD mRNA and has-miR-24-3p by RNA electrophoretic mobility shift assays (EMSAs). RNA EMSA with cy5-labeled has-miR-24-3p oligonucleotide and 2'-O-methyl modified and IRD-800 labeled DCTC mRNA oligonucleotide. Lanes 1 and 2 show the mobility of the labeled mRNA or miRNA oligonucleotide. Lane 3 shows the mobility of the labeled has-miR-24-3p oligonucleotide with *DCTD* mRNA oligonucleotide. Lanes 4 and 6 show the mobility of labeled *DCTD* mRNA oligonucleotide in presence of unlabeled excess specific competitor (has-miR-24-3p) ad excess unlabeled non-specific competitor (NC).

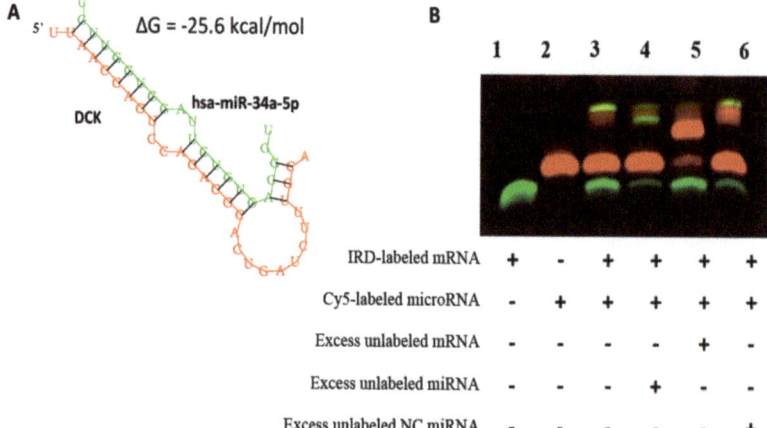

Figure 5. Validation of binding interactions between *DCK* and mRNA and has-miR-34a-5p by RNA EMSAs. RNA EMSA with cys5-labeled has-miR-34a-5p oligonucleotide and 2′-O-methyl modified and IRD-800 labeled DCK mRNA oligonucleotide. Lanes 1 and 2 show the mobility of the labeled mRNA or miRNA oligonucleotide. Lane 3 shows the mobility of the labeled has-miR-34a-5p oligonucleotide with DCK mRNA oligonucleotide. Lanes 4 and 6 show the mobility of labeled DCK mRNA oligonucleotide in presence of unlabeled excess specific competitor (has-miR-34a-5p) and excess unlabeled non-specific competitor (NC).

Table 1. MiRNAs with significant negative association (as reflected by *r* value) with nucleoside analog pathway genes in AML Cell lines.

Pathway Genes	MiRNAs	Spearman *r*	*p* Value	Minimum Free Energy (mfe) mRNA-miRNA Pair (kcal/mol)
DCTD	hsa-miR-24-3p	−0.9341	0.0011	−27.2
DCK	hsa-miR-96-5p	−0.9048	0.0046	−25.6
DCK	hsa-miR-34a-5p	−0.881	0.0072	−24.3
NT5C3	hsa-miR-149-5p	−0.881	0.0072	−21.4
RRM2	hsa-miR-151a-3p	−0.9524	0.0011	−26.4
RRM2B	hsa-miR-194-5p	−0.881	0.0072	−21.6
CMPK	hsa-miR-1301	−0.9762	0.0004	−23.6
CMPK	hsa-miR-320e	−0.9524	0.0011	−20.1
CMPK	hsa-miR-1323	−0.9286	0.0022	−22.3
CMPK	hsa-miR-584-5p	−0.9286	0.0022	−23.7
CMPK	hsa-miR-381	−0.881	0.0072	−25.8
CMPK	hsa-miR-507	−0.881	0.0072	−19.1
CMPK	hsa-miR-605	−0.881	0.0072	−23.1
CMPK	hsa-miR-762	−0.881	0.0072	−29.2
CMPK	hsa-miR-769-3p	−0.881	0.0072	−27.6
CMPK	hsa-miR-891a	−0.881	0.0072	−22.9
NME1	hsa-miR-514b-5p	−0.9286	0.0022	−22
NME1	hsa-miR-542-3p	−0.9286	0.0022	−19.3
NME1	hsa-miR-570-3p	−0.9048	0.0046	−22.2
NME1	hsa-miR-646	−0.9048	0.0046	−25.9
NME1	hsa-miR-224-5p	−0.881	0.0072	−17.9
NME1	hsa-miR-761	−0.881	0.0072	−24.3
NME1	hsa-miR-767-5p	−0.881	0.0072	−28.8
SLC28A1	hsa-miR-548aa	−0.9643	0.0028	−16.3
SLC28A3	hsa-miR-448	−0.9643	0.0028	−23.8

We further evaluated the association of the in vitro chemosensitivity of ara-C (defined previously Bhise et al, 2015 [13] with the three top miRNAs in the AML cell lines. As shown in Supplementary Figure S2. consistent with our results of miR-24-DCTD pair, we observed cell lines that were sensitive to ara-C has significantly higher levels of miR-24 as compared to cell lines that are resistant to ara-C ($p = 0.03$). These results suggest that high miR-24 in ara-C sensitive cell lines might be resulting in lowering DCTD levels and given that DCTD is involved in inactivation of ara-C, its low levels will result in better response.

4. Discussion

Nucleoside analogs are synthetic analogs of endogenous nucleosides that largely used for the treatment of hematological malignancies and solid tumors. Cytarabine, a pyrimidine nucleoside analog is the backbone of AML chemotherapy, while clofarabine is a second-generation purine nucleoside analog that is currently being investigated for treatment of AML in various clinical trials. Both cytarabine and clofarabine require active transport into the cell by nucleoside transporters, followed by activation by various kinases to form active di- and tri-phosphate metabolites that are incorporated in growing DNA strand and/or inhibit various enzymes involved in synthesis of endogenous nucleotides (Figure 1). However, despite being the backbone of treatment regimen used in AML patients, there is variability in response to cytarabine and other nucleoside analogs. In our previous study, we have demonstrated that miRNA expression is predictive of response to cytarabine therapy in AML patients and is also significantly associated with in vitro chemosensitivity of cytarabine in AML cell lines [13]. Recent studies are expanding on therapeutic relevance of miRNAs in AML. Recent review article by Wallace et al, 2017, have summarized the miRNAs that are deregulated in AML and thus hold potential as AML biomarkers. Further, mimics for miR-22, miR29b and miR-181 and antagomiRs for miR-21/miR-196b and miR-126 are currently under investigation for their therapeutic potential in AML [14]. However, given that cytarabine a nucleoside analog is the mainstay of AML chemotherapy for decades, in the current study, we wanted to determine if miRNA mediated regulation of expression of the transporters, activating and inactivating genes involved in the metabolic pathway of nucleoside analogs, could contribute to development of resistance to nucleoside analogs in AML patients. We hypothesized that miRNAs could bind to the 3'UTR of the mRNAs of nucleoside analog metabolic pathway genes, thereby altering their expression, which in turn would result in lower intracellular levels of active nucleoside analog triphosphate, resulting in chemo-resistance.

In our current study, DCK expression was negatively correlated with the expression of hsa-miR-34a-5p and hsa-miR-96-5p in AML cell lines (p-value < 0.01). DCK is a rate-limiting enzyme that is involved in activation of cytarabine and clofarabine. Studies have reported that decreased or complete loss of DCK activity results in cellular resistance to cytarabine [15–17]. Also, DCK mRNA expression has been shown to be positively associated with AML patient outcome, AML patients with higher DCK mRNA expression demonstrated longer event free survival than those with lower DCK mRNA expression [18]. Using EMSA, we were able to show that hsa-miR-34a-5p by binding to the 3'-UTR regulates expression of DCK. MiRNA hsa-miR-34a has been extensively studied in various cancers [19–23] and it has been shown to play an important role as a tumor suppressor by targeting various genes. However, the effect of miR-34a on DCK expression has not yet been studied. Identification of this additional regulatory mechanism for an important enzyme in the activation of nucleoside analogs could help in better prediction of chemosensitivity of these drugs. Unfortunately, we did not observe any significant correlation between DCK mRNA and miR-34a levels in TCGA dataset.

We also identified hsa-miR-24-3p to be negatively correlated with the expression of DCTD in both AML cell lines and in AML patient samples (p-value < 0.01). In addition, multiple bioinformatic prediction programs identified a binding site for hsa-miR-24-3p on the 3'UTR of DCTD. Our RNA EMSA results confirmed the binding interaction between DCTD and miR-24-3p. DCTD is an enzyme involved in deamination of the monophosphate form of the nucleoside analog, thus inactivating the drug. The levels of DCTD could thus affect the levels of the intracellular active triphosphate metabolites of nucleoside analogs. However, the role of DCTD in chemosensitivity of nucleoside analogs is poorly defined. Various studies have demonstrated a significant role of DCTD in metabolism of the monophosphate metabolite of the nucleoside analogs in human leukemia cells [24–26]. Sequencing of this gene identified a nonsynonymous SNP affecting the activity of DCTD in vitro [27]. Hence, the limited data on the regulation of DCTD gene warrants the need to evaluate additional mechanism regulating gene-expression. MiRNA miR-24 is has also been extensively studied in various cancers [28–34] and has been shown to enhance metastasis and invasion. Increased expression of miR-24 has been associated with increased risk of relapse and poor survival in acute lymphoblastic leukemia (ALL) [32]. In addition to miR-24 and hsa-miR-34a-5p, we also identified multiple other miRNAs that correlated with multiple genes in the PK/PD pathway (Table 1). We acknowledge the limitation of use of different platforms of miRNA and mRNA quantification between cell lines and the TCGA data-set which warrant the need for future prospective study to validate our results. Additionally, given that gel-shift assays do not consider interactions with argonaute which can impact thermodynamics of target recognition future in-depth mechanistic validation considering these factors are needed to establish miRNA-mRNA regulatory pairs of significant therapeutic implications in AML.

In summary, we identified several miRNAs, which were significantly associated with the expression of nucleoside analog pathway genes. Identification of these additional mechanisms of regulation would help provide a better understanding of the variability in the expression of these enzymes and transporters and in turn, help in better prediction of therapeutic response in AML patients. While additional functional studies are required to gain mechanistic understanding of these miRNA-mRNA interactions and its effect on the protein levels and activity, this study helps identify candidate miRNAs for further studies.

Supplementary Materials: The following are available online at http://www.mdpi.com/2073-4425/10/4/319/s1, Figure S1: Comparison of microRNA prediction programs for predicting binding sites on nucleoside analog pathway genes. Figure S2: A) Eight AML cell lines were treated with varying concentration of ara-C for 48 hrs followed by measuring cell viability using MTT assays using as described previously (Bhise et al, 2015). Area under the survival was calculated using Graphpad Prism and cell lines were classified as sensitive or resistant to ara-C. B) miR24-3p levels were observed to be higher in cell lines sensitive to ara-C as compared to ara-C resistant cell lines.

Author Contributions: J.K.L. and N.S.B. were involved in designing the study; N.S.B., J.K.L., A.H.E., X.C. and S.P. performed statistical analysis. All authors contributed to manuscript writing. All authors read and approved the final manuscript.

Funding: This research was funded by National Institutes of Health-National Cancer Institute R01-CA132946 (Lamba and Pounds).

Conflicts of Interest: The authors declare no conflict of interest. The funders had no role in the design of the study; in the collection, analyses, or interpretation of data; in the writing of the manuscript, or in the decision to publish the results.

References

1. Galmarini, C.M.; Clarke, M.L.; Jordheim, L.; Santos, C.L.; Cros, E.; Mackey, J.R.; Dumontet, C. Resistance to gemcitabine in a human follicular lymphoma cell line is due to partial deletion of the deoxycytidine kinase gene. *BMC Pharmacol.* **2004**, *4*, 8. [CrossRef] [PubMed]
2. Galmarini, C.M.; Thomas, X.; Calvo, F.; Rousselot, P.; Rabilloud, M.; El Jaffari, A.; Cros, E.; Dumontet, C. In vivo mechanisms of resistance to cytarabine in acute myeloid leukaemia. *Br. J. Haematol.* **2002**, *117*, 860–868. [CrossRef] [PubMed]
3. Lotfi, K.; Juliusson, G.; Albertioni, F. Pharmacological basis for cladribine resistance. *Leuk. Lymphoma* **2003**, *44*, 1705–1712. [CrossRef]
4. Mansson, E.; Flordal, E.; Liliemark, J.; Spasokoukotskaja, T.; Elford, H.; Lagercrantz, S.; Eriksson, S.; Albertioni, F. Down-regulation of deoxycytidine kinase in human leukemic cell lines resistant to cladribine and clofarabine and increased ribonucleotide reductase activity contributes to fludarabine resistance. *Biochem. Pharmacol.* **2003**, *65*, 237–247. [CrossRef]

5. Kent, O.A.; Mendell, J.T. A small piece in the cancer puzzle: MicroRNAs as tumor suppressors and oncogenes. *Oncogene* **2006**, *25*, 6188–6196. [CrossRef]
6. Rieger, J.K.; Reutter, S.; Hofmann, U.; Schwab, M.; Zanger, U.M. Inflammation-associated microRNA-130b down-regulates cytochrome P450 activities and directly targets CYP2C9. *Drug Metab. Dispos.* **2015**, *43*, 884–888. [CrossRef]
7. Pan, Y.Z.; Morris, M.E.; Yu, A.M. MicroRNA-328 negatively regulates the expression of breast cancer resistance protein (BCRP/ABCG2) in human cancer cells. *Mol. Pharmacol.* **2009**, *75*, 1374–1379. [CrossRef]
8. Mishra, P.J.; Humeniuk, R.; Mishra, P.J.; Longo-Sorbello, G.S.; Banerjee, D.; Bertino, J.R. A miR-24 microRNA binding-site polymorphism in dihydrofolate reductase gene leads to methotrexate resistance. *Proc. Natl. Acad. Sci. USA* **2007**, *104*, 13513–13518. [CrossRef] [PubMed]
9. Livak, K.J.; Schmittgen, T.D. Analysis of relative gene expression data using real-time quantitative PCR and the $2^{-\Delta\Delta C_T}$ Method. *Methods* **2001**, *25*, 402–408. [CrossRef] [PubMed]
10. Cancer Genome Atlas Research Network. Genomic and epigenomic landscapes of adult de novo acute myeloid leukemia. *N. Engl. J. Med.* **2013**, *368*, 2059–2074. [CrossRef] [PubMed]
11. Kruger, J.; Rehmsmeier, M. RNAhybrid: microRNA target prediction easy, fast and flexible. *Nucleic Acids Res.* **2006**, *34*, W451–W454. [CrossRef] [PubMed]
12. Kutmon, M.; Kelder, T.; Mandaviya, P.; Evelo, C.T.; Coort, S.L. CyTargetLinker: A cytoscape app to integrate regulatory interactions in network analysis. *PLoS ONE* **2013**, *8*, e82160. [CrossRef]
13. Bhise, N.S.; Chauhan, L.; Shin, M.; Cao, X.; Pounds, S.; Lamba, V.; Lamba, J.K. MicroRNA-mRNA Pairs Associated with outcome in AML: From in vitro cell-based studies to AML patients. *Front. Pharmacol.* **2015**, *6*, 324. [CrossRef] [PubMed]
14. Wallace, J.A.; O'Connell, R.M. MicroRNAs and acute myeloid leukemia: Therapeutic implications and emerging concepts. *Blood* **2017**, *130*, 1290–1301. [CrossRef]
15. Dumontet, C.; Fabianowska-Majewska, K.; Mantincic, D.; Callet Bauchu, E.; Tigaud, I.; Gandhi, V.; Lepoivre, M.; Peters, G.J.; Rolland, M.O.; Wyczechowska, D.; et al. Common resistance mechanisms to deoxynucleoside analogues in variants of the human erythroleukaemic line K562. *Br. J. Haematol.* **1999**, *106*, 78–85. [CrossRef]
16. Bhalla, K.; Nayak, R.; Grant, S. Isolation and characterization of a deoxycytidine kinase-deficient human promyelocytic leukemic cell line highly resistant to 1-β-D-arabinofuranosylcytosine. *Cancer Res.* **1984**, *44*, 5029–5037.
17. Verhoef, V.; Sarup, J.; Fridland, A. Identification of the mechanism of activation of 9-β-D-arabinofuranosyladenine in human lymphoid cells using mutants deficient in nucleoside kinases. *Cancer Res.* **1981**, *41*, 4478–4483.
18. Galmarini, C.M.; Thomas, X.; Calvo, F.; Rousselot, P.; El Jafaari, A.; Cros, E.; Dumontet, C. Potential mechanisms of resistance to cytarabine in AML patients. *Leuk. Res.* **2002**, *26*, 621–629. [CrossRef]
19. Garofalo, M.; Jeon, Y.J.; Nuovo, G.J.; Middleton, J.; Secchiero, P.; Joshi, P.; Alder, H.; Nazaryan, N.; di Leva, G. Correction: MiR-34a/c-dependent PDGFR-α/β downregulation inhibits tumorigenesis and enhances TRAIL-induced apoptosis in lung cancer. *PLoS ONE* **2015**, *10*, e0131729. [CrossRef]
20. Hong, J.H.; Roh, K.S.; Suh, S.S.; Lee, S.; Sung, S.W.; Park, J.K.; Byun, J.H.; Kang, J.I.I. The expression of microRNA-34a is inversely correlated with c-MET and CDK6 and has a prognostic significance in lung adenocarcinoma patients. *Tumour Biol.* **2015**, *36*, 9327–9337. [CrossRef]
21. Lu, G.; Sun, Y.; An, S.; Xin, S.; Ren, X.; Zhang, D.; Wu, P.; Liao, W.; Ding, Y.; Liang, L. MicroRNA-34a targets FMNL2 and E2F5 and suppresses the progression of colorectal cancer. *Exp. Mol. Pathol.* **2015**, *99*, 173–179. [CrossRef] [PubMed]
22. Qiao, P.; Li, G.; Bi, W.; Yang, L.; Yao, L.; Wu, D. microRNA-34a inhibits epithelial mesenchymal transition in human cholangiocarcinoma by targeting Smad4 through transforming growth factor-beta/Smad pathway. *BMC Cancer* **2015**, *15*, 469. [CrossRef]
23. Wang, X.; Li, J.; Dong, K.; Lin, F.; Long, M.; Ouyang, Y.; Wei, J.; Chen, X.; Weng, Y.; He, T.; et al. Tumor suppressor miR-34a targets PD-L1 and functions as a potential immunotherapeutic target in acute myeloid leukemia. *Cell. Signal.* **2015**, *27*, 443–452. [CrossRef]
24. Capizzi, R.L.; White, J.C.; Powell, B.L.; Perrino, F. Effect of dose on the pharmacokinetic and pharmacodynamic effects of cytarabine. *Semin. Hematol.* **1991**, *28* (Suppl. 4), 54–69. [PubMed]

25. Fridland, A.; Verhoef, V. Mechanism for ara-CTP catabolism in human leukemic cells and effect of deaminase inhibitors on this process. *Semin. Oncol.* **1987**, *14* (Suppl. 1), 262–268. [PubMed]
26. Liliemark, J.O.; Plunkett, W. Regulation of 1-β-D-arabinofuranosylcytosine 5′-triphosphate accumulation in human leukemia cells by deoxycytidine 5′-triphosphate. *Cancer Res.* **1986**, *46*, 1079–1083.
27. Gilbert, J.A.; Salavaggione, O.E.; Ji, Y.; Pelleymounter, L.L.; Eckloff, B.W.; Wieben, E.D.; Ames, M.M.; Weinshilboum, R.M. Gemcitabine pharmacogenomics: Cytidine deaminase and deoxycytidylate deaminase gene resequencing and functional genomics. *Clin. Cancer Res.* **2006**, *12*, 1794–1803. [CrossRef] [PubMed]
28. Xu, L.; Chen, Z.; Xue, F.; Chen, W.; Ma, R.; Cheng, S.; Cui, P. MicroRNA-24 inhibits growth, induces apoptosis, and reverses radioresistance in laryngeal squamous cell carcinoma by targeting X-linked inhibitor of apoptosis protein. *Cancer Cell Int.* **2015**, *15*, 61. [CrossRef] [PubMed]
29. Lu, K.; Wang, J.; Song, Y.; Zhao, S.; Liu, H.; Tang, D.; Pan, B.; Zhao, H.; Zhang, Q. miRNA-24-3p promotes cell proliferation and inhibits apoptosis in human breast cancer by targeting p27Kip1. *Oncol. Rep.* **2015**, *34*, 995–1002. [CrossRef] [PubMed]
30. Manvati, S.; Mangalhara, K.C.; Kalaiarasan, P.; Srivastava, N.; Bamezai, R.N. miR-24-2 regulates genes in survival pathway and demonstrates potential in reducing cellular viability in combination with docetaxel. *Gene* **2015**, *567*, 217–224. [CrossRef]
31. Zhao, G.; Liu, L.; Zhao, T.; Jin, S.; Jiang, S.; Cao, S.; Han, J.; Xin, Y.; Dong, Q.; Liu, X.; et al. Upregulation of miR-24 promotes cell proliferation by targeting NAIF1 in non-small cell lung cancer. *Tumour Biol.* **2015**, *36*, 3693–3701. [CrossRef] [PubMed]
32. Organista-Nava, J.; Gomez-Gomez, Y.; Illades-Aguiar, B.; del Carmen Alarcon-Romero, L.; Saavedra-Herrera, M.V.; Rivera-Ramirez, A.B.; Garzón-Barrientos, V.H.; Leyva-Vázquez, M.A. High miR-24 expression is associated with risk of relapse and poor survival in acute leukemia. *Oncol. Rep.* **2015**, *33*, 1639–1649. [CrossRef]
33. Gao, Y.; Liu, Y.; Du, L.; Li, J.; Qu, A.; Zhang, X.; Wang, L.; Wang, C. Down-regulation of miR-24-3p in colorectal cancer is associated with malignant behavior. *Med. Oncol.* **2015**, *32*, 362. [CrossRef]
34. Pan, B.; Chen, Y.; Song, H.; Xu, Y.; Wang, R.; Chen, L. Mir-24-3p downregulation contributes to VP16-DDP resistance in small-cell lung cancer by targeting ATG4A. *Oncotarget* **2015**, *6*, 317–331. [CrossRef] [PubMed]

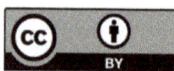

© 2019 by the authors. Licensee MDPI, Basel, Switzerland. This article is an open access article distributed under the terms and conditions of the Creative Commons Attribution (CC BY) license (http://creativecommons.org/licenses/by/4.0/).

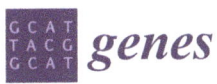

Article

Diagnostic and Therapeutic Strategies for Fluoropyrimidine Treatment of Patients Carrying Multiple *DPYD* Variants

Carin A. T. C. Lunenburg [1], Linda M. Henricks [2,3], André B. P. van Kuilenburg [4], Ron H. J. Mathijssen [5], Jan H. M. Schellens [2,3], Hans Gelderblom [1], Henk-Jan Guchelaar [6] and Jesse J. Swen [6,*]

1. Department of Medical Oncology, Leiden University Medical Center, 2333 ZA Leiden, The Netherlands; c.a.t.c.lunenburg@lumc.nl (C.A.T.C.L.); a.j.gelderblom@lumc.nl (H.G.)
2. Department of Clinical Pharmacology, Division of Medical Oncology, The Netherlands Cancer Institute, 1066 CX Amsterdam, The Netherlands; l.henricks@nki.nl (L.M.H.); j.schellens@gmail.com (J.H.M.S.)
3. Division of Pharmacology, The Netherlands Cancer Institute, 1066 CX Amsterdam, The Netherlands
4. Department of Clinical Chemistry, Amsterdam University Medical Centre, 1105 AZ Amsterdam, The Netherlands; a.b.vankuilenburg@amc.uva.nl
5. Department of Medical Oncology, Erasmus MC Cancer Institute, 3015 GD Rotterdam, The Netherlands; a.mathijssen@erasmusmc.nl
6. Department of Clinical Pharmacy & Toxicology, Leiden University Medical Center, 2333 ZA Leiden, The Netherlands; h.j.guchelaar@lumc.nl
* Correspondence: j.j.swen@lumc.nl; Tel.: +31-71-5262790

Received: 9 November 2018; Accepted: 26 November 2018; Published: 28 November 2018

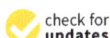

Abstract: *DPYD* genotyping prior to fluoropyrimidine treatment is increasingly implemented in clinical care. Without phasing information (i.e., allelic location of variants), current genotype-based dosing guidelines cannot be applied to patients carrying multiple *DPYD* variants. The primary aim of this study is to examine diagnostic and therapeutic strategies for fluoropyrimidine treatment of patients carrying multiple *DPYD* variants. A case series of patients carrying multiple *DPYD* variants is presented. Different genotyping techniques were used to determine phasing information. Phenotyping was performed by dihydropyrimidine dehydrogenase (DPD) enzyme activity measurements. Publicly available databases were queried to explore the frequency and phasing of variants of patients carrying multiple *DPYD* variants. Four out of seven patients carrying multiple *DPYD* variants received a full dose of fluoropyrimidines and experienced severe toxicity. Phasing information could be retrieved for four patients. In three patients, variants were located on two different alleles, i.e., in *trans*. Recommended dose reductions based on the phased genotype differed from the phenotype-derived dose reductions in three out of four cases. Data from publicly available databases show that the frequency of patients carrying multiple *DPYD* variants is low (< 0.2%), but higher than the frequency of the commonly tested *DPYD**13 variant (0.1%). Patients carrying multiple *DPYD* variants are at high risk of developing severe toxicity. Additional analyses are required to determine the correct dose of fluoropyrimidine treatment. In patients carrying multiple *DPYD* variants, we recommend that a DPD phenotyping assay be carried out to determine a safe starting dose.

Keywords: pharmacogenomics; pharmacogenetics; genotype; phenotype; alleles; precision medicine

1. Introduction

Fluoropyrimidines (including 5-fluorouracil (5-FU) and capecitabine) are the cornerstone of treatment for various types of cancer and are used by millions of patients worldwide each year [1–3].

However, up to one-third of treated patients experience severe toxicity (Common Terminology Criteria for Adverse Events (CTC-AE) grade ≥ 3), such as diarrhea, hand–foot syndrome, or mucositis upon treatment with fluoropyrimidines [4,5]. These adverse events can lead to mortality in approximately 1% of patients who experience severe toxicity [4,6]. Dihydropyrimidine dehydrogenase (DPD) is the key enzyme in the metabolism of 5-FU and its decreased activity is strongly associated with toxicity [7,8]. Variants in *DPYD*, the gene encoding DPD, can lead to decreased DPD enzyme activity [9–12]. Prospective *DPYD* genotyping of four main *DPYD* variants followed by dose reductions in patients carrying any of these four *DPYD* variants is safe, cost-effective, and feasible in clinical practice [13–15]. These *DPYD* variants are *DPYD**2A (rs3918290, c.1905+1G>A, IVS14+1G>A); *DPYD**13 (rs55886062, c.1679T>G, I560S); c.1236G>A/HapB3 (rs56038477, E412E); and c.2846A>T (rs67376798, D949V). For these four variants, convincing evidence has been provided warranting implementation in clinical practice [4,5,12,15–17].

An increasing number of hospitals apply prospective *DPYD* genotyping when treating patients with fluoropyrimidines [18]. Individual dosing guidelines for the abovementioned four *DPYD* variants are provided by the Dutch Pharmacogenetics Working Group (DPWG) and the Clinical Pharmacogenetics Implementation Consortium (CPIC) [19,20]. Dosing guidelines are based on the expected remaining DPD enzyme activity and can be applied to patients who are heterozygous carriers of a single *DPYD* variant. For homozygous *DPYD* variant allele carriers (two identical variants) and compound heterozygous *DPYD* variant allele carriers (two or more different variants), dosing guidelines are not yet available (or treatment with an alternative drug is advised), although safe treatment with low-dose fluoropyrimidines in these homozygous *DPYD* patients was demonstrated by a recent case series [21].

Patients who carry multiple variants (compound heterozygous) can carry the variants on a single allele (in *cis*) or on different alleles (in *trans*). In the first case, one functionally active allele remains, whereas in the latter case, both alleles are affected, which may result in a proportionally decreased enzyme activity (Figure 1). With currently used genotyping techniques, the allelic location of variants (phasing) cannot be determined. This uncertainty hampers adequate interpretation of the pharmacogenetic test result in compound heterozygous patients and makes it impossible to give an appropriate dose recommendation based on the genotype alone. Since it is likely that in the future, even more *DPYD* variants will be tested, the probability of finding compound heterozygous *DPYD* variant allele carriers will increase. The aims of this study are to examine diagnostic and therapeutic strategies for fluoropyrimidine treatment of patients carrying multiple *DPYD* variants and the frequency and phasing of variants of compound heterozygous *DPYD* patients in publicly available databases.

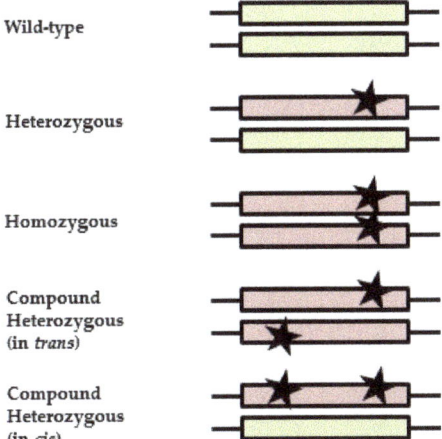

Figure 1. Illustration of zygosity and clinical interpretations. Black stars represent variants; boxes represent alleles. A wild-type patient carries no variants, resulting in normal-activity alleles (green). A heterozygous patient carries one variant, resulting in one reduced or inactive allele (red) and one active allele (green). A partly reduced enzyme activity is expected, since there is still one active allele left. For homozygous patients, both variants result in a reduced or inactive allele (red). Depending on the effect of the variants on the protein, a reduced or absent enzyme activity is expected. Compound heterozygous patients can carry variants on different alleles (in *trans*) or on one allele (in *cis*), resulting in differences in enzyme function, either like that of a heterozygous patient or a homozygous patient.

2. Materials and Methods

In this study, we present seven compounds heterozygous *DPYD* variant allele carriers as clinical cases. In addition, we have performed in silico research in publicly available databases.

2.1. Patients

Data and DNA from patient cases carrying multiple *DPYD* variants were collected. Patients were identified either after development of severe toxicity from fluoropyrimidine-containing therapy, by additional retrospective genotyping in a clinical trial (clinicaltrials.gov identifier NCT00838370, [13]), or prior to treatment in routine clinical care. The study was reviewed and approved by the institutional review board of the Leiden University Medical Centre (LUMC, G18.015). Patient data from the electronic medical records was handled following the codes of proper use and proper conduct in the self-regulatory codes of conduct [22]. Toxicity to fluoropyrimidine-containing therapy was graded by the treating physicians using the National Cancer Institute CTC-AE version 4.03 [23], and severe fluoropyrimidine-induced toxicity was defined as CTC-AE grade ≥ 3. In some cases, additional patient material to determine the phasing of the *DPYD* variants was collected. In these cases, additional patient consent was obtained.

2.2. Dihydropyrimidine Dehydrogenase Enzyme Activity Measurements

For all patients, DPD enzyme activity was determined. This could be either prior to treatment or retrospectively after the occurrence of severe toxicity. DPD enzyme activity measurement in peripheral blood mononuclear cells (PBMCs) [24,25] was used as a reference to assess DPD activity, and has been used previously to determine dosages in *DPYD* variant-carrying patients [21,26]. A validated method [27] was used, containing radiolabeled thymine as a substrate and consisting of high-performance liquid chromatography (HPLC) with online radioisotope detection using liquid scintillation counting. Normal values for healthy volunteers are 9.9 ± 2.8 nmol/(mg×h), for DPD-deficient patients are 4.8 ± 1.7 nmol/(mg×h), and reference values range from 5.9 to 14 nmol/(mg×h) [28]. Dose reductions based on DPD enzyme activity were performed in a one-to-one ratio, as was previously described by Henricks et al. [21]. Thereafter, toxicity-guided dosing was used.

2.3. Molecular Methods for Estimation of Phasing

In regard to the size of the *DPYD* gene, the location of the variants, and the material available (DNA, RNA) from the patients, three molecular methods to determine the phasing of the variants could be used in this study. In four patients, we could execute one or more of these methods. These methods are explained and illustrated in the supplementary material (Figure S1). Details on these techniques have been published elsewhere [29–31].

2.4. Frequencies of Compound Heterozygous DPYD Carriers

To investigate the incidence of compound heterozygous *DPYD* variant allele carriers (of the four genotyped *DPYD* variants), large databases were queried [32,33]. The incidence was calculated using minor allele frequencies (MAFs) of each variant identified in the databases separately. Since the determined variants are not in the same haplotype, it was assumed that the inheritance of these individual *DPYD* variants is independent. All genotypes from the databases were calculated to be in Hardy–Weinberg equilibrium, except for *DPYD*2A and c.1236G>A for the Exome Aggregation Consortium (ExAC, http://exac.broadinstitute.org/) [32] and Genome Aggregation Database (gnomAD, http://gnomad.broadinstitute.org/) [33] due to a slight overrepresentation of homozygous cases. The calculated frequencies were compared to frequencies from databases in which phasing could be determined.

Exome Aggregation Consortium and Genome Aggregation Database

Both the ExAC [32] and gnomAD [33] databases collect exome sequencing data and aggregate the data for public use. The ExAC dataset (v0.3.1) contains sequenced data of 60,706 unrelated individuals. The gnomAD dataset (v2.0) contains sequenced data of 123,136 exomes and 15,496 genomes from unrelated individuals. In ExAC, 2791 *DPYD* variants, and in gnomAD, 2190 *DPYD* variants were found. MAFs of *DPYD* variants from these databases reflect those of the population due to the large group size in the databases. Since both ExAC and gnomAD do not contain individual matched or phased data, it is not possible to search for compound heterozygous patients in these databases.

2.5. Phasing in Compound Heterozygous DPYD Carriers

Three databases were used to identify compound heterozygous *DPYD* variant allele carriers and determine the phasing, i.e., allelic location, of variants.

2.5.1. Genome of the Netherlands Datasets

The Genome of the Netherlands (GoNL, http://www.nlgenome.nl/) trio datasets contain information of related fathers, mothers, and children, and phasing information is therefore available. Datasets were previously processed and phased using trio-aware variant calling [34]. After the exclusion of children, phased variant call format (VCF) files for 496 subjects (fathers and mothers) were obtained from the GoNL repository. The toolset Bedtools (https://bedtools.readthedocs.io/en/latest/, v2) was used to extract all variants found in the *DPYD* locus (chr1:97,543,300–98,386,615). Next, for all individuals, the carrier status of *DPYD*2A, *DPYD*13, c.1236G>A, and c.2846A>T was examined. Individuals who carry at least one of the four actionable *DPYD* variants were identified, and using a custom Python [35] script, the phasing of variants was assessed for individuals with multiple variants.

2.5.2. 1000 Genomes Database

The 1000 Genomes Project (http://www.internationalgenome.org/) is the largest publicly available catalogue of human variation and genotyped phased data. It originally ran from 2008 until 2015, and thereafter it was maintained and expanded by the International Genome Sample Resource (IGSR) [36]. On 27 October 2016, phased data of the *DPYD* gene (chr1: 97,543,300–98,386,615) was downloaded from the 1000 Genomes ftp server (phase 3; GRCh37; chr1: 97,543,300–98,386,615) using Tabix (v1.1) [37]. The statistical program R (v3.2.5) [38] was used to select the genotypes at four *DPYD* risk alleles in unrelated individuals of Caucasian descent.

2.5.3. Exome Trios Leiden University Medical Centre Database

This diagnostic database of the clinical genetics department of LUMC contains 433 complete exome trios (father, mother, and child). The exome was enriched by the Agilent sureselect v5 kit and sequenced using various Illumina (San Diego, CA, USA) sequencers (Hiseq 2000, 2500, 4000, Nextseq). Carrier status of the abovementioned *DPYD* variants was established by querying the trio VCF files. We also investigated all samples with sufficient coverage of this region to obtain a reliable frequency estimate. In the case of trios, only parents were taken into account.

3. Results

3.1. Patient Cases and Clinical Implications

Details of the demographics and clinical characteristics of the seven cases are described in the supplementary material (patient cases). All patients received treatment with fluoropyrimidines and were identified as compound heterozygous *DPYD* variant allele carriers either prior to the start of treatment or retrospectively. Table 1 shows an overview of the cases. Table 2 shows all genotype and phenotype results. With additional genetic testing, phasing could be determined in four out of seven patients. In three patients, the variants were located in *trans*, and one patient carried the variants in *cis*. With the phasing information available, it is possible to calculate a dose recommendation using publicly available pharmacogenetic dosing guidelines [19,20]. For example, patient 1 carried *DPYD*2A and c.1236G>A in *trans*. The gene activity values range from inactive (0) to fully active (1). *DPYD*2A and c.1236G>A/HapB3 have values of 0 and 0.5, respectively. As this patient carries the variants in *trans*, each allele contains one variant and no fully functional allele remains. Therefore, the cumulated gene activity score (GAS) is 0.5. The GAS can be used to determine dose recommendations according to the genotype, as was previously described [12]. The GAS ranges from 0 to 2, and a score of 0.5 corresponds to a dose recommendation of 25%. The DPD enzyme activity of patient 1 was 0.9 nmol/(mg×h). This was divided by the mean of the reference value (9.9), which results in a theoretical DPD activity of 9%. For each patient for whom phasing details were known, the GAS was determined and compared to the theoretical DPD activity. Dose recommendations according to the GAS (genotype) and theoretical DPD activity (phenotype) were divergent in almost all cases, as shown in Table 2.

3.2. Preventing Toxicity

Three of the seven case patients were identified as carriers of one or more *DPYD* variants prior to the start of therapy. For one patient, the DPD enzyme activity was determined prior to the start of therapy. Based on their genotype or phenotype, these three patients received initially reduced fluoropyrimidine dosages of 50%. They experienced limited and reversible toxicity (CTC-AE grades 0–2). The dose of one patient was increased to 70% in the second treatment cycle, after which CTC-AE grade 3 toxicity occurred.

Four of the seven case patients received a full dose, since their genotype was unknown prior to the start of therapy. These patients all experienced severe toxicity (CTC-AE grades 3–5), and three of them were admitted to the hospital for 7–14 days. An overview of cases, including the toxicity, is shown in Table 3.

3.3. Frequencies of Compound Heterozygous DPYD Carriers without Phasing Information

The ExAC and gnomAD databases revealed an average MAF for *DPYD*2A*, *DPYD*13*, c.1236G>A, and c.2846A>T of 0.55%, 0.03%, 1.43%, and 0.27%, respectively. MAFs for ExAC and gnomAD separately are summarized in Table 4. The probability of identifying a compound heterozygous *DPYD* patient for two variants according to these databases was ≤ 0.008%, as was calculated using frequencies of combinations of *DPYD* variants. Results for each combination of *DPYD* variants are shown in Table 5. With several million fluoropyrimidine users each year, thousands of patients worldwide are compound heterozygous for a subset of these four *DPYD* variants.

3.4. Frequencies of Compound Heterozygous DPYD Carriers with Phasing Information

In the GoNL database, genetic data from 496 subjects (fathers and mothers only) was reviewed. One subject was found who carried two *DPYD* variants. This subject was a carrier of the *DPYD* c.1236G>A and *DPYD* c.2846A>T variants, both of which were located on a single allele (in *cis*). Based upon the data in GoNL, the probability of having compound heterozygosity of the four *DPYD* variants is <0.2%.

In the 1000 Genomes database, data of 2513 individuals were available. After the selection of unique, unrelated individuals, 407 individuals remained. One subject was found who carried two *DPYD* variants. This subject was a carrier of *DPYD* c.1236G>A and *DPYD* c.2846A>T, both of which were located on different alleles (in *trans*). Based upon the data in 1000 Genomes, the probability of having compound heterozygosity of the four *DPYD* variants is <0.3%.

In the LUMC clinical genetics database (exome trios LUMC), the analysis was restricted to the children, since this would allow phasing. None of the 433 children carried more than one *DPYD* variant, thus compound heterozygosity in this database is <0.2%.

Despite the low frequency, compound heterozygous patients were identified in all databases except the LUMC clinical genetics database. However, the low frequency did not allow to determine the probability of in *cis* or in *trans* phasing of variants in a patient.

Table 1. Characteristics of patient cases. Shown per patient are primary tumor, treatment, capecitabine dose, executed assays (genotype, dihydropyrimidine dehydrogenase (DPD) enzyme activity, and additional assays) information. Additional assays are droplet digital PCR, PacBio sequencing (Menlo Park, CA, USA), or an in-house developed technique. For the executed assays, it is shown whether these were executed prior to treatment (P) or retrospectively (R). *Abbreviations*: BC: breast cancer; CRC: colorectal cancer; CAP: capecitabine; RT: radiotherapy; OX: oxaliplatin; BEV: bevacizumab; bid: *bis in die*/twice a day.

Patient #	Primary Tumor	Treatment	Capecitabine Dose	Executed Assays
1	BC	CAP	1000 mg/m²/bid	Genotyping (R), DPD activity (R), in-house technique (R), droplet digital PCR (R)
2	BC	CAP	800 mg bid (50%)	Genotyping (P), DPD activity (R), in-house technique (R)
3	CRC	CAP + OX	900 mg bid (50%) [1]	Genotyping (P), DPD activity (P), PacBio (R)
4	BC	CAP	1500 mg bid	Genotyping (R), DPD activity (R²)
5	CRC	CAP + RT	800 mg bid (50%)	Genotyping (P + R³), DPD activity (R⁴), PacBio (R)
6	CRC	CAP + OX	1000 mg/m²/bid	Genotyping (R), DPD activity (R)
7	CRC	CAP + OX + BEV	1000 mg/m²/bid	Genotyping (R), DPD activity (R)

[1] Increased to 70% in the second cycle; [2] during hospital admission; [3] *DPYD*2A was prospectively identified, c.2846A>T was retrospectively identified; [4] during treatment.

Table 2. Dose advice for compound heterozygous *DPYD* variant allele carriers. Shown per patient are *DPYD* variants, GAS, retrospective DPWG dosing advice based on phasing, DPD enzyme activity, and percentage of DPD enzyme activity considered for dose advice. According to the DPWG guidelines [19], a gene activity score can be given to compound heterozygous patients when phasing is known. Fully functional/reduced functionality = gene activity score of 1.5; fully functional/inactive = gene activity score of 1; reduced functionality/reduced functionality = gene activity score of 1; reduced functionality/inactive = gene activity score of 0.5; inactive/inactive = gene activity score of 0. *Abbreviations*: DPD: dihydropyrimidine dehydrogenase; GAS: gene activity score; DPWG: Dutch Pharmacogenetic Working Group; X: could not be determined.

Patient #	DPYD Variants	Phasing	GAS [12]	DPWG Dose Advice (% of Regular Dose)	DPD Activity (nmol/(mg×h))	Percentage of DPD Activity [1]
1	DPYD*2A + c.1236G>A	in *trans*	0.5	25%	0.9	9%
2	DPYD*2A + c.2846A>T	in *trans*	0.5	25%	6.0	60%
3	c.1236G>A + c.2846A>T	in *trans*	1	50%	4.5	45%
4	DPYD*2A + c.2846A>T	unknown	X	X	0.11	1%
5	DPYD*2A + c.2846A>T	in *cis*	1	50%	7.2	72%
6	DPYD*2A + c.1236G>A	unknown	X	X	3.8	38%
7	DPYD*2A + c.1236G>A	unknown	X	X	1.6	16%

[1] The reference DPD activity ranges from 5.9–14 nmol/(mg×h) [28], and therefore the percentage of DPD activity can be calculated using the average of the reference (9.9 nmol/(mg×h)). This percentage could be used as a percentage of the regular dose.

Table 3. Toxicity profiles of compound heterozygous *DPYD* variant allele carriers. Shown per patient are *DPYD* variants, fluoropyrimidine dose as a percentage of the regular dose, and experienced toxicity with this dose. All patients retrospectively identified as *DPYD* variants carrier received full doses and experienced severe (CTC-AE ≥ 3) toxicity. All patients prospectively identified as *DPYD* variant(s) carrier received dose reductions and experienced a maximum of CTC-AE grade 2 toxicity with the initial dose. *Abbreviations*: CTC-AE: Common Terminology Criteria for Adverse Events v4.03.

Patient #	DPYD variants	Dose (% of Regular Dose)	Toxicity (Maximal CTC Grade)
1	DPYD*2A + c.1236G>A	100%	4
2	DPYD*2A + c.2846A>T	50%	1–2
3	c.1236G>A + c.2846A>T	50% → 70%	0 (on 50% dose) → 3 (on 70% dose)
4	DPYD*2A + c.2846A>T	100%	5
5	DPYD*2A + c.2846A>T	50%	0
6	DPYD*2A + c.1236G>A	100%	4
7	DPYD*2A + c.1236G>A	100%	3

Table 4. MAF per database. Three databases (GoNL, 1000 Genomes, and exome trios LUMC) containing phased data were checked for four *DPYD* variants. Two large online databases (ExAC and gnomAD) were checked to identify the MAFs of the individual *DPYD* variants. For each *DPYD* variant, the genotype distribution and MAF are shown. *Abbreviations*: MAF: minor allele frequency; HW: homozygous wild-type; HE: heterozygous carrier; HM: homozygous carrier; GoNL: Genome of the Netherlands; ExAC: Exome Aggregation Consortium; gnomAD: Genome Aggregation Database.

Variants	DPYD*2A (rs3918290)		DPYD*13 (rs55886062)		c.1236G>A (rs56038477)		c.2846A>T (rs67376798)	
Databases	HW/HE/HM	MAF	HW/HE/HM	MAF	HW/HE/HM	MAF	HW/HE/HM	MAF
GoNL	489/7/0	0.7%	494/2/0	0.2%	475/21/0	2.1%	490/6/0	0.6%
1000 Genomes	405/2/0	0.2%	406/1/0	0.1%	389/18/0	2.2%	403/4/0	0.5%
Exome Trios LUMC	946/15/0	0.8%	946/0/0	0.00%	946/46/0	2.3%	946/2/0	0.1%
ExAC	60,627/624/5	0.5%	60,320/42/0	0.03%	60,652/1808/27	1.5%	60,687/317/1	0.3%
gnomAD	138,489/1586/10	0.6%	138,166/83/0	0.03%	138,407/3841/39	1.4%	138,478/792/1	0.3%

Table 5. Calculated frequencies for compound heterozygous *DPYD* patients. Using the average MAFs of the ExAC and gnomAD databases (for *DPYD*2A*, *DPYD*13*, c.1236G>A, and c.2846A>T, these are 0.55%, 0.03%, 1.43%, and 0.27%, respectively), possible combinations for two out of four currently genotyped *DPYD* variants are shown. *Abbreviations:* MAF: minor allele frequency; ExAC: Exome Aggregation Consortium; gnomAD: Genome Aggregation Database.

Combination of *DPYD* Variants	Calculated Frequency
*DPYD*2A* + *DPYD*13*	0.0002%
*DPYD*2A* + c.1236G>A	0.008%
*DPYD*2A* + c.2846A>T	0.001%
*DPYD*13* + c.1236G>A	0.0005%
*DPYD*13* + c.2846A>T	0.0001%
c.1236G>A + c.2846A>T	0.004%

4. Discussion

Prospective genotyping of *DPYD* variants followed by individual dose adjustments is increasingly applied as the standard of care for patients starting fluoropyrimidine therapy. Standard dose reductions from CPIC and DPWG guidelines cannot be applied in patients who carry more than one *DPYD* variant, as the phasing of the variants is unknown. Despite the low population frequency of < 0.2%, the absolute number of identified compound heterozygous patients will increase as the number of genotyped patients increases and the panel of tested variants is expanded. To the best of our knowledge, this is the first study that describes a case series of compound heterozygous *DPYD* variant allele carriers and investigates diagnostic and therapeutic strategies for these patients.

Our study shows the clinical need for further information on the genotype, as four patients were identified as compound heterozygous carriers retrospectively and all of them experienced severe toxicity. These compound heterozygous *DPYD* variant allele carriers have an increased risk of developing severe fluoropyrimidine-induced toxicity if dosages are not adequately adjusted. Previously, compound heterozygous patients have been described with severe or even lethal side effects after fluoropyrimidine treatment [39,40]. Three patients in this study were prospectively identified as compound heterozygous carriers, received initial dose reductions, and developed only mild toxicities.

Out of the four patients for whom we were able to retrieve phasing information, three were in *trans* and one was in *cis* orientation. Data from publicly available databases also showed that both in *cis* and in *trans* orientations exist. However, the recently updated CPIC guidelines on *DPYD* assumes in *trans* phasing for compound heterozygous patients [20]. The DPWG guidelines do not mention phasing; however, the dosing recommendations of the DPWG use the GAS, a score based on the activity of individual alleles [19]. This implies the need for phasing information. The assumption of in *trans* phasing could result in the underdosing of patients with variants phased in *cis*, and thus exemplifies the need for the determination of the phasing of variants.

In this study, we looked at different diagnostic strategies to determine the phasing of *DPYD* variants in compound heterozygous patients. In four patients, the phasing of *DPYD* variants could be determined using one of three different molecular methods. These methods are in the early phases of development, not routinely available, quite expensive, and not always conclusive. For two of these techniques, patient RNA is used, which degrades quickly after the blood draw unless specifically designed blood tubes are used. Compound heterozygous patients are rare, yet here we describe seven patients heterozygous for multiple *DPYD* variants. A limitation of our study is that most patients were identified retrospectively and in different institutions. Because of this, not enough of or not the right material was available for analysis, thus not all genotyping techniques could be executed in each patient. For two samples, tests failed or produced inconclusive results. For this reason, a formal comparison of their suitability to identify phasing was not possible. However, of the three explored molecular methods, PacBio sequencing seems most promising. While phasing improved the prediction of DPD enzyme activity, patients with identical combinations of *DPYD* variants and identical phasing showed considerable differences in DPD enzyme activity, which could potentially limit the added value of the determination of the phasing of *DPYD* variants. However, larger numbers of compound heterozygous *DPYD* variant allele carriers would be necessary to draw a firm conclusion.

The measurement of DPD enzyme activity in PBMCs was used as a reference to assess DPD activity. The method is well-established, commonly available, and shows limited intra- and interpatient variability [27]. However, recently, differences in intrapatient variability in DPD enzyme activity related to circadian rhythm were shown [41], which can result in the under- or overestimation of DPD enzyme activity. In this study, we present one patient with extremely low DPD enzyme activity, which could possibly be influenced by the presence of severe neutropenia, as DPD activity is normally measured in mononuclear cells. Therefore, DPD enzyme activity can differ depending on the clinical condition of the patient and should thus be measured prior to treatment.

A major question is whether genotyping or phenotyping is the best method to determine DPD activity to guide fluoropyrimidine dosing in patients carrying multiple *DPYD* variants. Despite the low population frequency, we present seven patients carrying multiple *DPYD* variants, of which three received initially reduced fluoropyrimidine dosages. However, based on these data, it is not possible to determine if a dose recommendation based on phased genetic information or DPD enzyme activity measured in PBMCs is safer. In three out of four cases, differences were observed between the theoretically calculated DPD activity using genotyping or phenotyping. These differences would result in different dosing recommendations. For example, there is a considerable interpatient variability in DPD enzyme activity in carriers of the *DPYD* variant c.1236G>A/HapB3 [12]. Due to this variability, genetic dose recommendations are categorized (e.g., 25 or 50%) on the average of the phenotypes. This categorization could explain the observed dosing differences derived from genotyping and phenotyping. Other variants of *DPYD* currently not routinely tested for or variants in other genes, e.g., *MIR27A* [42], might also be involved in reducing DPD activity or explaining fluoropyrimidine-induced toxicity. DPD enzyme activity measurements are well-established, and additional molecular methods to resolve phasing are still in early phases of development. Therefore, in our opinion, the current therapeutic strategy for compound heterozygous *DPYD* variant allele carriers should be to determine initial dose reductions based on a DPD phenotyping test, for example, by measuring enzyme activity in PBMCs. Dosing could be adjusted by the treating physician in subsequent cycles based on observed severe toxicity (or lack thereof).

5. Conclusions

In conclusion, patients carrying multiple *DPYD* variants are at high risk of developing severe toxicity. Additional analyses are required to determine the correct dose of fluoropyrimidine treatment. In patients carrying multiple *DPYD* variants, we recommend that a DPD phenotyping assay be carried out to determine a safe starting dose. The dose could be titrated in subsequent cycles based on observed toxicity.

Supplementary Materials: The following are available online at http://www.mdpi.com/2073-4425/9/12/585/s1; Description of patient cases (1 to 7) and Figure S1 illustration of molecular methods.

Author Contributions: Conceptualization, C.A.T.C.L., H.G., H.-J.G. and J.J.S.; Data curation, C.A.T.C.L., L.M.H. and A.B.P.v.K.; Formal analysis, C.A.T.C.L., H.-J.G. and J.J.S.; Methodology, C.A.T.C.L., H.-J.G. and J.J.S.; Supervision, H.G., H.-J.G. and J.J.S.; Writing—original draft, C.A.T.C.L.; Writing—review & editing, L.M.H., A.B.P.v.K., R.H.J.M., J.H.M.S., H.G., H.-J.G. and J.J.S.

Funding: This research received no external funding.

Acknowledgments: The authors thank S.Y. Anvar, G.W.E. Santen, E.B. van den Akker and H. Mei for assistance with the databases; R.H.A.M. Vossen, E.J. de Meijer and R.J.H.M van der Straaten for execution of the molecular methods for estimation of phasing; and F.M. de Man for the collection of patient material and clinical data.

Conflicts of Interest: The authors declare no conflict of interest. C. Lunenburg was previously supported by an unrestricted grant from Roche Pharmaceuticals. There was no involvement in the study design, data collection, analysis, or interpretation of the data.

References

1. *Scrip's Cancer Chemotherapy Report*; Scrip world pharmaceutical news; PJB Publications Ltd.: London, UK, 2002.
2. Walko, C.M.; Lindley, C. Capecitabine: A review. *Clin. Ther.* **2005**, *27*, 23–44. [CrossRef] [PubMed]
3. Malet-Martino, M.; Martino, R. Clinical studies of three oral prodrugs of 5-fluorouracil (capecitabine, UFT, S-1): A review. *Oncologist* **2002**, *7*, 288–323. [CrossRef] [PubMed]
4. Rosmarin, D.; Palles, C.; Pagnamenta, A.; Kaur, K.; Pita, G.; Martin, M.; Domingo, E.; Jones, A.; Howarth, K.; Freeman-Mills, L.; et al. A candidate gene study of capecitabine-related toxicity in colorectal cancer identifies new toxicity variants at *DPYD* and a putative role for *ENOSF1* rather than *TYMS*. *Gut* **2015**, *64*, 111–120. [CrossRef]
5. Terrazzino, S.; Cargnin, S.; Del Re, M.; Danesi, R.; Canonico, P.L.; Genazzani, A.A. *DPYD* IVS14+1G>A and 2846A>T genotyping for the prediction of severe fluoropyrimidine-related toxicity: A meta-analysis. *Pharmacogenomics* **2013**, *14*, 1255–1272. [CrossRef]
6. Saltz, L.B.; Niedzwiecki, D.; Hollis, D.; Goldberg, R.M.; Hantel, A.; Thomas, J.P.; Fields, A.L.; Mayer, R.J. Irinotecan fluorouracil plus leucovorin is not superior to fluorouracil plus leucovorin alone as adjuvant treatment for stage III colon cancer: Results of CALGB 89803. *J. Clin. Oncol.* **2007**, *25*, 3456–3461. [CrossRef] [PubMed]
7. Van Kuilenburg, A.B. Dihydropyrimidine dehydrogenase and the efficacy and toxicity of 5-fluorouracil. *Eur. J. Cancer* **2004**, *40*, 939–950. [CrossRef] [PubMed]
8. Gonzalez, F.J.; Fernandez-Salguero, P. Diagnostic analysis, clinical importance and molecular basis of dihydropyrimidine dehydrogenase deficiency. *Trends Pharmacol. Sci.* **1995**, *16*, 325–327. [CrossRef]
9. Van Kuilenburg, A.B.; Meijer, J.; Maurer, D.; Dobritzsch, D.; Meinsma, R.; Los, M.; Knegt, L.C.; Zoetekouw, L.; Jansen, R.L.; Dezentje, V.; et al. Severe fluoropyrimidine toxicity due to novel and rare *DPYD* missense mutations, deletion and genomic amplification affecting DPD activity and mRNA splicing. *Biochim. Biophys. Acta* **2017**, *1863*, 721–730. [CrossRef]
10. Meulendijks, D.; Henricks, L.M.; van Kuilenburg, A.B.; Jacobs, B.A.; Aliev, A.; Rozeman, L.; Meijer, J.; Beijnen, J.H.; de Graaf, H.; Cats, A.; et al. Patients homozygous for *DPYD* c.1129-5923C>G/haplotype B3 have partial DPD deficiency and require a dose reduction when treated with fluoropyrimidines. *Cancer Chemother. Pharmacol.* **2016**, *78*, 875–880. [CrossRef]
11. Offer, S.M.; Fossum, C.C.; Wegner, N.J.; Stuflesser, A.J.; Butterfield, G.L.; Diasio, R.B. Comparative functional analysis of *DPYD* variants of potential clinical relevance to dihydropyrimidine dehydrogenase activity. *Cancer Res.* **2014**, *74*, 2545–2554. [CrossRef]
12. Henricks, L.M.; Lunenburg, C.A.; Meulendijks, D.; Gelderblom, H.; Cats, A.; Swen, J.J.; Schellens, J.H.; Guchelaar, H.J. Translating *DPYD* genotype into DPD phenotype: Using the *DPYD* gene activity score. *Pharmacogenomics* **2015**, *16*, 1277–1286. [CrossRef] [PubMed]
13. Deenen, M.J.; Meulendijks, D.; Cats, A.; Sechterberger, M.K.; Severens, J.L.; Boot, H.; Smits, P.H.; Rosing, H.; Mandigers, C.M.; Soesan, M.; et al. Upfront genotyping of *DPYD**2A to individualize fluoropyrimidine therapy: A safety and cost analysis. *J. Clin. Oncol.* **2016**, *34*, 227–234. [CrossRef] [PubMed]
14. Lunenburg, C.A.; van Staveren, M.C.; Gelderblom, H.; Guchelaar, H.J.; Swen, J.J. Evaluation of clinical implementation of prospective *DPYD* genotyping in 5-fluorouracil- or capecitabine-treated patients. *Pharmacogenomics* **2016**, *17*, 721–729. [CrossRef] [PubMed]
15. Henricks, L.M.; Lunenburg, C.; de Man, F.M.; Meulendijks, D.; Frederix, G.W.J.; Kienhuis, E.; Creemers, G.J.; Baars, A.; Dezentje, V.O.; Imholz, A.L.T.; et al. *DPYD* genotype-guided dose individualisation of fluoropyrimidine therapy in patients with cancer: A prospective safety analysis. *Lancet Oncol.* **2018**, *19*, 1459–1467. [CrossRef]
16. Lunenburg, C.A.; Henricks, L.M.; Guchelaar, H.J.; Swen, J.J.; Deenen, M.J.; Schellens, J.H.; Gelderblom, H. Prospective *DPYD* genotyping to reduce the risk of fluoropyrimidine-induced severe toxicity: Ready for prime time. *Eur. J. Cancer* **2016**, *54*, 40–48. [CrossRef] [PubMed]
17. Meulendijks, D.; Henricks, L.M.; Sonke, G.S.; Deenen, M.J.; Froehlich, T.K.; Amstutz, U.; Largiader, C.R.; Jennings, B.A.; Marinaki, A.M.; Sanderson, J.D.; et al. Clinical relevance of *DPYD* variants c.1679T>G, c.1236G>A/HapB3, and c.1601G>A as predictors of severe fluoropyrimidine-associated toxicity: A systematic review and meta-analysis of individual patient data. *Lancet Oncol.* **2015**, *16*, 1639–1650. [CrossRef]

18. Result Survey Screening for DPD Deficiency. *Medische Oncologie*. October 2016. Available online: https://www.nvmo.org/magazine/ (accessed on 1 November 2016).
19. KNMP. Royal Dutch Society for the Advancement of Pharmacy. Fluorouracil/Capecitabine DPD Gene Activity Score and Guidelines. Available online: https://kennisbank.knmp.nl/article/farmacogenetica/2552-4893-4894.html (accessed on 5 May 2017).
20. Amstutz, U.; Henricks, L.M.; Offer, S.M.; Barbarino, J.; Schellens, J.H.M.; Swen, J.J.; Klein, T.E.; McLeod, H.L.; Caudle, K.E.; Diasio, R.B.; et al. Clinical pharmacogenetics implementation consortium (CPIC) guideline for dihydropyrimidine dehydrogenase genotype and fluoropyrimidine dosing: 2017 update. *Clin. Pharmacol. Ther.* **2018**, *103*, 210–216. [CrossRef]
21. Henricks, L.M.; Kienhuis, E.; de Man, F.M.; van der Veldt, A.A.M.; Hamberg, P.; van Kuilenburg, A.B.P.; van Schaik, R.H.N.; Lunenburg, C.A.T.C.; Guchelaar, H.J.; Schellens, J.H.M.; et al. Treatment algorithm for homozygous or compound heterozygous *DPYD* variant allele carriers with low dose capecitabine. *JCO Precis. Oncol.* **2017**, *1*, 1–10, Published online October 6. [CrossRef]
22. Federa. Available online: federa.org (accessed on 9 September 2017).
23. National Cancer Institute: Common Terminology Criteria for Adverse Events v4.03. Available online: https://evs.nci.nih.gov/ftp1/CTCAE/CTCAE_4.03_2010-06-14_QuickReference_8.5x11.pdf (accessed on 9 September 2017).
24. Meulendijks, D.; Cats, A.; Beijnen, J.H.; Schellens, J.H. Improving safety of fluoropyrimidine chemotherapy by individualizing treatment based on dihydropyrimidine dehydrogenase activity—Ready for clinical practice? *Cancer Treat. Rev.* **2016**, *50*, 23–34. [CrossRef]
25. Van Staveren, M.C.; van Kuilenburg, A.B.; Guchelaar, H.J.; Meijer, J.; Punt, C.J.; de Jong, R.S.; Gelderblom, H.; Maring, J.G. Evaluation of an oral uracil loading test to identify DPD-deficient patients using a limited sampling strategy. *Br. J. Clin. Pharmacol.* **2016**, *81*, 553–561. [CrossRef]
26. Henricks, L.M.; Siemerink, E.J.M.; Rosing, H.; Meijer, J.; Goorden, S.M.I.; Polstra, A.M.; Zoetekouw, L.; Cats, A.; Schellens, J.H.M.; van Kuilenburg, A.B.P. Capecitabine-based treatment of a patient with a novel *DPYD* genotype and complete dihydropyrimidine dehydrogenase deficiency. *Int. J. Cancer* **2018**, *142*, 424–430. [CrossRef]
27. Van Kuilenburg, A.B.; Van Lenthe, H.; Tromp, A.; Veltman, P.C.; Van Gennip, A.H. Pitfalls in the diagnosis of patients with a partial dihydropyrimidine dehydrogenase deficiency. *Clin. Chem.* **2000**, *46*, 9–17. [PubMed]
28. Van Kuilenburg, A.B.; Meinsma, R.; Zoetekouw, L.; Van Gennip, A.H. Increased risk of grade IV neutropenia after administration of 5-fluorouracil due to a dihydropyrimidine dehydrogenase deficiency: High prevalence of the IVS14+1g>a mutation. *Int. J. Cancer* **2002**, *101*, 253–258. [CrossRef]
29. Regan, J.F.; Kamitaki, N.; Legler, T.; Cooper, S.; Klitgord, N.; Karlin-Neumann, G.; Wong, C.; Hodges, S.; Koehler, R.; Tzonev, S.; et al. A rapid molecular approach for chromosomal phasing. *PLoS ONE* **2015**, *10*, e0118270. [CrossRef] [PubMed]
30. Buermans, H.P.; Vossen, R.H.; Anvar, S.Y.; Allard, W.G.; Guchelaar, H.J.; White, S.J.; den Dunnen, J.T.; Swen, J.J.; van der Straaten, T. flexible and scalable full-length CYP2D6 long amplicon PacBio sequencing. *Hum. Mutat.* **2017**, *38*, 310–316. [CrossRef]
31. Van der Straaten, T.; Swen, J.; Baak-Pablo, R.; Guchelaar, H.J. Use of plasmid-derived external quality control samples in pharmacogenetic testing. *Pharmacogenomics* **2008**, *9*, 1261–1266. [CrossRef] [PubMed]
32. ExAC. Exome Aggregation Consortium. ExAC Browser (Beta). Available online: http://exac.broadinstitute.org/ (accessed on 13 December 2017).
33. gnomAD. genome Aggregation Database. gnomAD browser (Beta). Available online: http://gnomad.broadinstitute.org/ (accessed on 14 July 2017).
34. Francioli, L.; Menelaou, A.; Pulit, S.; van Dijk, F.; Palamara, P.; Elbers, C.; Neerincx, P.; Ye, K.; Guryev, V.; Kloosterman, W.; et al. Genome of The Netherlands Consortium. Whole-genome sequence variation, population structure and demographic history of the Dutch population. *Nat. Genet.* **2014**, *46*, 818–825. [CrossRef] [PubMed]
35. Python. Python Software Foundation©. Available online: https://www.python.org/ (accessed on 9 September 2017).
36. IGSR. The International Genome Sample Resource. Available online: http://www.internationalgenome.org/ (accessed on 29 June 2017).

37. Li, H. Tabix: Fast retrieval of sequence features from generic TAB-delimited files. *Bioinformatics* **2011**, *27*, 718–719. [CrossRef] [PubMed]
38. R Core Team. R: A Language and Environment for Statistical Computing 2018. Available online: https://www.R-project.org. (accessed on 9 September 2017).
39. Toffoli, G.; Giodini, L.; Buonadonna, A.; Berretta, M.; De, P.A.; Scalone, S.; Miolo, G.; Mini, E.; Nobili, S.; Lonardi, S.; et al. Clinical validity of a *DPYD*-based pharmacogenetic test to predict severe toxicity to fluoropyrimidines. *Int. J. Cancer* **2015**, *137*, 2971–2980. [CrossRef] [PubMed]
40. Johnson, M.R.; Wang, K.; Diasio, R.B. Profound dihydropyrimidine dehydrogenase deficiency resulting from a novel compound heterozygote genotype. *Clin. Cancer Res.* **2002**, *8*, 768–774.
41. Jacobs, B.A.; Deenen, M.J.; Pluim, D.; van Hasselt, J.G.; Krahenbuhl, M.D.; van Geel, R.M.; de Vries, N.; Rosing, H.; Meulendijks, D.; Burylo, A.M.; et al. Pronounced between-subject and circadian variability in thymidylate synthase and dihydropyrimidine dehydrogenase enzyme activity in human volunteers. *Br. J. Clin. Pharmacol.* **2016**, *82*, 706–716. [CrossRef] [PubMed]
42. Meulendijks, D.; Henricks, L.M.; Amstutz, U.; Froehlich, T.K.; Largiader, C.R.; Beijnen, J.H.; de Boer, A.; Deenen, M.J.; Cats, A.; Schellens, J.H. Rs895819 in *MIR27A* improves the predictive value of *DPYD* variants to identify patients at risk of severe fluoropyrimidine-associated toxicity. *Int. J. Cancer* **2016**, *138*, 2752–2761. [CrossRef] [PubMed]

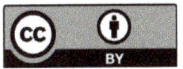

© 2018 by the authors. Licensee MDPI, Basel, Switzerland. This article is an open access article distributed under the terms and conditions of the Creative Commons Attribution (CC BY) license (http://creativecommons.org/licenses/by/4.0/).

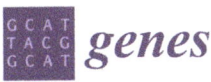

Article

FARMAPRICE: A Pharmacogenetic Clinical Decision Support System for Precise and Cost-Effective Therapy

Rossana Roncato [1], Lisa Dal Cin [1], Silvia Mezzalira [1], Francesco Comello [1], Elena De Mattia [1], Alessia Bignucolo [1], Lorenzo Giollo [2], Simone D'Errico [2], Antonio Gulotta [2], Luca Emili [3], Vincenzo Carbone [3], Michela Guardascione [1], Luisa Foltran [4], Giuseppe Toffoli [1,*] and Erika Cecchin [1,*]

1. Clinical and Experimental Pharmacology, Centro di Riferimento Oncologico di Aviano (CRO) IRCCS, 33081 Aviano, Italy; rroncato@cro.it (R.R.); lisa.dalcin@cro.it (L.D.C.); silvia.mezzalira@cro.it (S.M.); francesco.comello@cro.it (F.C.); edemattia@cro.it (E.D.M.); alessia.bignucolo@cro.it (A.B.); michela.guardascione@cro.it (M.G.)
2. GPI, Società per Azioni (SpA), 38123 Trento, Italy; lorenzo.giollo@gpi.it (L.G.); simone.derrico@gpi.it (S.D.); antonio.gulotta@gpi.it (A.G.)
3. InSilicoTrials Technologies società a responsabilità limitata (s.r.l.), 34148 Trieste, Italy; luca.emili@insilicotrials.com (L.E.); vincenzo.carbone@insilicotrials.com (V.C.)
4. Department of Medical Oncology, Centro di Riferimento Oncologico di Aviano (CRO), IRCSS, 33081 Aviano, Italy; luisa.foltran@cro.it
* Correspondence: gtoffoli@cro.it (G.T.); ececchin@cro.it (E.C.); Tel.: +39-0434-659-612 (G.T.); +39-0434-659-667 (E.C.)

Received: 28 February 2019; Accepted: 1 April 2019; Published: 4 April 2019

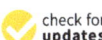

Abstract: Pharmacogenetic (PGx) guidelines for the precise dosing and selection of drugs remain poorly implemented in current clinical practice. Among the barriers to the implementation process is the lack of clinical decision support system (CDSS) tools to aid health providers in managing PGx information in the clinical context. The present study aimed to describe the first Italian endeavor to develop a PGx CDSS, called FARMAPRICE. FARMAPRICE prototype was conceived for integration of patient molecular data into the clinical prescription process in the Italian Centro di Riferimento Oncologico (CRO)-Aviano Hospital. It was developed through a coordinated partnership between two high-tech companies active in the computerization of the Italian healthcare system. Introducing FARMAPRICE into the clinical setting can aid physicians in prescribing the most efficacious and cost-effective pharmacological therapy available.

Keywords: CDSS; pharmacogenetics; implementation

1. Introduction

The response to drugs is highly variable among individuals. Indeed, genetic variants are estimated to affect between 20–95% of the response variability, depending on the drug [1]. Germline genetic variants can influence drug Adsorption, Distribution, Metabolism, and Elimination (ADME) and they can be responsible for reduced drug efficacy or increased toxicity. Patients might benefit from using pharmacogenetics (PGx) to inform treatment decisions regarding drug selection and dosing. The PGx approach has the potential of improving drug efficacy and/or avoiding unwanted side effects; these improvements could lead to better treatment adherence and outcomes [2]. An inherently personalized approach to medicine could provide non-negligible offsets to Healthcare system costs [3,4].

PGx guidelines for drug dosing have become available for a wide range of medications associated with gene-drug interactions that could potentially be clinically actionable. To date, over 160 medications, ranging from heart disease medications to psychiatric drugs, currently have PGx labeling registered with the US Food and Drug Administration (FDA) [5]. The publicly available online knowledge base, PharmGKB [6], is an interactive tool that collects PGx recommendations. It includes PGx-based drug dosing guidelines established by the Clinical Pharmacogenetics Implementation Consortium (CPIC), the Royal Dutch Association for the Advancement of Pharmacy—Pharmacogenetics Working Group (DPWG), the Canadian Pharmacogenomics Network for Drug Safety (CPNDS) and other professional societies.

PGx tests have been used in the past, but mainly as a reactive approach to an aberrant clinical outcome in individual patients. Physicians typically ordered PGx tests on an "as needed" basis, after the occurrence of unexpected severe toxicity or a lack of response. Currently, the use of PGx as a tool for evidence-based medication management is gaining acceptance among many healthcare providers. PGx tests can be used to predict drug efficacy and side effects in individual patients. Consequently, PGx testing has moved to the pre-therapeutic setting, where the test is typically ordered at the first prescription of a drug that is associated with a PGx guideline.

Despite a recent survey, which showed that 97.6% of clinicians agreed that genetic variations might influence drug response, only 12.9% of clinicians had ordered a PGx test during the prior six months. In fact, translating PGx knowledge into clinical practice has been slow and hindered by many barriers that have prevented its large-scale implementation. Apart from the established statistical associations between PGxs and drug therapy outcomes (clinical validity), large scale implementation of PGx translation requires evidence of clinical-utility and cost-effectiveness. Moreover, that evidence will likely result in favorable reimbursement decisions from payers [7]. Additionally, to aid the implementation of PGx in clinical practice, we need to set up a straightforward workflow from the test prescription to the application of the guidelines, combined with appropriate training and education programs about the clinical use of PGx for healthcare practitioners [8].

The poor application of PGx in the clinical routine is related to the need for a "physician-friendly" electronic "educational resource" that aids clinicians in managing PGx results during routine clinical practice [9]. The implementation of a point-of-care electronic clinical decision support system (CDSS) is urgently needed to guide drug prescriptions in a community-based practice setting [10].

In recent years, a growing body of literature has been produced in developing and implementing PGx CDSSs for improving patient care. A PGx CDSS is a critical tool that can address some of the barriers to implementing PGx guidelines into the clinical routine. They are computer-based systems intended to improve medical decision-making at the point-of-care by supporting physicians in decisions regarding prescriptions. The CDSS infrastructure was designed to store the patient's genomic data and create filtered PGx information, such as pop-up alerts, to inform physicians and other healthcare providers when a gene-drug interaction is available for a specific patient [11]. Thus, this information technology (IT) tool can translate genetic information into practical therapeutic recommendations. It can be used to customize, as much as possible, pharmacological treatments, in terms of drug selection and dosing. The dynamic nature of PGx guidelines warrants long-term maintenance and continuous updating of the PGx CDSS, as new evidence becomes available. To that end, PGx CDSS tools must be fully scalable and sustainable in an automated way [12].

With the aim of providing clinicians with an IT infrastructure (CDSS) for the automated management of patient molecular data, which could be translated into specific prescription indications the FARMAPRICE partnership was created. The partnership comprises the Clinical and Experimental Pharmacology unit of the Centro di Riferimento Oncologico (CRO)-Aviano Hospital and two high-tech companies, InSilicoTrials Technologies, Trieste, Italy, and GPI company, Trento, Italy, which are active in developing solutions for the healthcare system. They put forth a coordinated effort to bring together scientific, clinical and technological expertise in the PGx field. In 2017, the FARMAPRICE partnership proposed a project that was financed by POR FESR 2014–2020, which aimed to promote innovation in the drug prescription process by implementing the preemptive PGx approach in Italy.

The present article aimed to describe the Italian project, FARMAPRICE, a CDSS designed for integration into the clinical prescription process in the Italian CRO-Aviano Hospital.

2. Materials and Methods

FARMAPRICE CDSS was designed to aid clinicians in prescribing the most efficacious and cost-effective pharmacological therapy available by providing support for prescribing drugs within available PGx guidelines. Prescribing physicians can interrogate the FARMAPRICE platform to get specific dosing recommendation. To that end, the FARMAPRICE platform queries two repositories: The first is the patient's complete genetic data; the second is the list of all PGx guidelines based on validated gene-drug interactions (Figure 1).

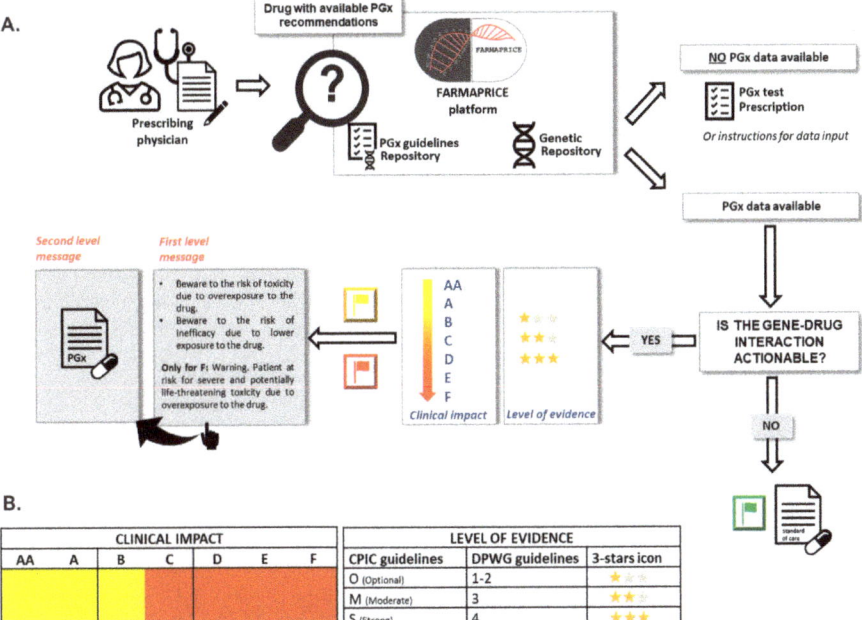

Figure 1. FARMAPRICE platform workflow. (**A**) The prescribing physician interrogates FARMAPRICE platform to discover if the drug to be prescribed presents validated gene-drug interactions and if that specific patient has a potentially clinically actionable genotype. In the negative case instructions are given for a pharmacogenetic (PGx) test prescription. In the affirmative case, a PGx-based recommendation integrated with its level of evidence and clinical impact will be provided. This will allow prescribers to weigh the strength of evidence available and to decide whether to follow the recommendation or not. A PGx-based recommendation will be first delivered as a "first level message" briefly describing the involved risk (inefficacy or toxicity) for that specific patient at standard dosage. A "second level message" (complete PGx-based drug selection or dosing recommendation) is displayed by clicking on "first level message". (**B**) Clinical impact of a specific gene-drug interaction is delivered with a different colors flag icon basing on Swen et al. [13]. Correspondence between rating from AA to F and the color code is here defined. Conversely, the level of evidence will be delivered as a three-star icon basing on both Clinical Pharmacogenetics Implementation Consortium (CPIC) and Royal Dutch Association for the Advancement of Pharmacy—Pharmacogenetics Working Group (DPWG) latest guidelines available for that gene-drug interaction as herein described.

The development of the project was divided into three phases: First, the selection of actionable gene-drug pairs to be integrated into the CDSS; second, the development of a CDSS prototype; and third, an evaluation of the IT platform prototype in a medical setting.

2.1. First Phase: The Selection of Actionable Gene-Drug Pairs to be Integrated into the CDSS

Between January and June 2018, the PGx team of the Experimental and Clinical Pharmacology Unit of CRO-Aviano elaborated a list of gene-drug interactions based on the most recent PGx guidelines [6].

In the first phase of the project, the PharmGKB website was consulted to obtain the most complete, up-to-date list of all available PGx guidelines. The PharmGKB summarizes guidelines from the two most widely recognized consortia, CPIC and DPWG. Although these consortia are currently working on harmonizing their clinical recommendations, controversial information might arise from different guidelines, which could generate uncertainty in treatment decisions. Within the FARMAPRICE development project, the PGx-based recommendations provided by the CPIC and DPWG consortia were merged into a unique therapeutic recommendation. In cases of discrepancies, the software provides prescribing physicians with the most restrictive/conservative recommendation, to ensure patient safety, and it adds the following statement: "Further modification of the therapy is advised, based on the patient's individual response".

Gene-drug pairs to be integrated were selected based on their actionability and on the availability of the drug in Italy. The genetic variants of these pharmacogenes were selected based on the most recent scientific publications and the level of evidence on the functional effect of the genetic variant on the encoded protein, according to the most updated CPIC guidelines [14]. These genetic variants were classified according to their functional impact. Then, they were combined to obtain all possible genotypes and diplotypes that could be linked to a specific therapeutic recommendation, consistent with published guidelines [15].

2.2. Second Phase: Development of the FARMAPRICE Prototype

A series of synoptic tables was created that linked genotypes to phenotypes and therapeutic recommendations for each selected drug. These tables were forwarded to IT developers for the configuration of the CDSS prototype. The IT tools for collecting medical-molecular data were configured together with corresponding protocols for the acquisition and integration of molecular data in a standardized form. To guarantee greater longevity, open source solutions were implemented: The application was developed using Protected Health Information (PHI) Technology, an open-source framework based on Eclipse IDE (Integrated Development Environment). It provides tools and components to design eHealth applications (named PHI Solutions) to be executed in a runtime environment independent from the underlying operating system. It adopts Model Driven Architecture (MDA) and Business Processes Management (BPM) tools combined with Service Oriented Architecture (SOA), completely based on the latest open standards (HL7, IHE, DICOM, XDS).

These elements assure the longest lifetime of the applications and back the whole diagnostic, therapeutic and processes. This choice guarantees a high level of interoperability, in view of potential integration into systems of production and in complex environments, such as hospital information systems, including the EHR [16].

2.3. Third Phase: FARMAPRICE User Experience

Ideally, the genetic reports and the service provided should be formatted and focused, based on feedback from clinicians. Maximizing the effectiveness of the alerts will aid in the integration of CDSSs and their adoption by practitioners [17]. The IT companies involved in FARMAPRICE development carried out a study to determine the software requirements for the most effective user experience on: (i) Platform usability, (ii) functional specifications and content requirements, (iii) information architecture, and (iv) Information design, interface design, and navigation.

Software requirements were gathered by the project partners to collect, analyze and document the System Requirements Specification. The approach adopted was not the usual waterfall model where software development follows a linear succession of steps to the final product. A prototypal approach was implemented, instead. The development of a prototype with a minimum set of functionalities made the formalization of the requirements easier and the adaptation to the users' real needs through consecutive approximation. The partners carried out a study to determine the best software Graphical User Interface (GUI) using the designing tools of the User Experience (UX). Users were separated into two classes of archetypical users (so called personas) who represent the needs of a larger group of users, i.e., "clinicians" and "researchers". The observation of these two classes was realized considering the environment in which a persona operates, which tools it uses, its background information, and the behavior working patterns. As a result, the study output gives back slightly different users' interactions with the software that will be considered in further implementations. The use of REST (Representational State Transfer) services ensures the separation between the application back-end and front-end. Process execution, information classes and the persistence management (permanent data storage) are then unlinked by the front-end that can be migrated to other frameworks (Angular JS, React etc.) with no impact on the application business logic.

The study outcome indicated the necessity of two different interfaces and two different sets of data access and access privileges, due to privacy concerns. About the latter, "clinicians" have data access to all the information (i.e., they can see all the data without modification of genomic data), while "researchers" have data access constraints to patient personal data, but have access privileges to modify all genetic information (i.e., they cannot see who the patient is, but can update/modify the data, the PGx guidelines, etc.). The "clinicians" GUI is oriented to the clinical aspects, similarly to an EHR presenting the evidence-based therapeutic recommendations, together with the actual clinical impact; the "researchers" GUI is designed for the collection, modification, integration of the background information.

3. Results

3.1. First Phase: The Selection of Actionable Gene-Drug Pairs to be Integrated into the CDSS

The selection process of gene-drug pairs based on both their actionability and availability of the drug in Italy resulted in the inclusion of 46 drugs in the final selection. FARMAPRICE drugs span several pharmacological classes, including anti-neoplastic agents, anti-viral agents, anti-coagulant agents, oral contraceptives, analgesics, anti-emetics, immunosuppressives, anti-epileptics, anti-arrhythmics, anti-gout drugs, anti-depressants (SSRI, TCA and other), psychostimulants, anti-psychotics, anti-hypertensive drugs, drugs for cystic fibrosis treatment, cholesterol-lowering drugs, and anti-fungals (Table 1). Among the pharmacogenes that impacted the outcome of the identified drugs, 14 were included in the final selection. This selection process identified 374 variants with documented impact on gene transcription.

Table 1. Drugs included in FARMAPRICE clinical decision support system (CDSS).

Drug Classification	Drugs
Analgesics	Codeine, Tramadol
Anti-arrhythmics	Propafenone, Flecainide
Anti-coagulant agents	Acenocoumarol, Phenprocoumon, Clopidrogel, Warfarin
Antidepressant	Venlafaxine
Antidepressant (SSRI)	Citalopram, Escitalopram, Sertraline, Paroxetine
Anti-depressants (TCA)	Amitriptyline, Clomipramine, Nortriptyline, Trimipramine
Anti-emetics	Ondasetron, Tropisetron
Anti-epileptics	Carbamazepine, Phenytoin, Oxacarbamazepine
Anti-fungals	Voriconazole
Anti-gout drugs	Allopurinol, Rasburicase

Table 1. *Cont.*

Drug Classification	Drugs
Anti-hypertensive drugs	Metoprolol
Anti-neoplastic agents	5-Fluorouracil, Capecitabine, Irinotecan, Tamoxifen, Tioguanine, Mercaptopurine, Azathioprine
Anti-psychotics	Aripiprazole, Haloperidol, Zuclopenthixol
Anti-viral agents	Abacavir, Atazanavir, Ribavirin, PEG-IFN
Cholesterol-lowering drugs	Atorvastatin, Simvastatin
Cystic fibrosis treatment	Ivacaftor
Immunosuppressives	Tacrolimus
Oral contraceptives	Hormonal contraceptives for systemic use
Psychostimulants	Atomoxetine

3.2. Second Phase: Development of the FARMAPRICE Prototype

FARMAPRICE was developed as an active PGx CDSS functional prototype integrated with PGx guidelines and patient genetic information in a web service platform. It was considered that the Italian health care system is currently lacking a common EHR platform among its different regions, thus resulting in a fragmented healthcare delivery system with limited EHR interoperability. Since sharing healthcare data among different providers is hampered, FARMAPRICE was conceived as a stand-alone system that could be eventually integrated into the EHR system. Specific requirements were then to guarantee a correct exchange of data, in particular the checking of data entry (in support of the researchers and the clinicians to eliminate any input errors), the certification of the prescription algorithm (avoiding the risk of incurring possible modifications), and the verification of the output data (to have indications for further improvement of the effectiveness of the guidelines underlying the system itself). Specifically, the solution has been designed as a web application, implemented using open-source components and technologies: The integration with an EHR can be reached through integration profiles that manage HL7 input/output messages. It is designed to be a module: It defines and enforce logical boundaries, it is pluggable with another module that expects its interface, and it is a single unit to be easily deployed, overcoming fragmentation issues.

The prototype is structured into four principal parts. The section "Patients" provides the prescribing physician access to the patient's genetic data (genetic data repository). Moreover, in this section, the prescriber can configure a new patient record and input the relevant genetic data. In the section "Prescription", the clinician can interrogate the system to obtain a specific recommendation for a selected patient that requires a new drug prescription. An alphabetically ordered drug list will pop-up. Once a new drug prescription is selected, the dosing recommendation will be provided, based on the patient's genetic profile. When relevant genetic data are missing, the system will request input of additional information to ensure the correct drug recommendation is provided. In addition, the user can track a patient's clinical history to obtain information about all the drugs previously prescribed through FARMAPRICE. Other sections (e.g., "File configuration" and "Drug configuration") are reserved for developers and researchers that update the FARMAPRICE CDSS with the latest PGx guidelines.

Due to the security risks associated with storing large quantities of personal data, specifically genetic data, the CDSS prototype was implemented on a "research and development" project setting, meaning that all the genetic data were handled anonymously. For future developments, an electronic register has been designed for the safe storage and management of acquired genetic data, and for qualitative-quantitative analysis, aiming to enlarge the register with new data deriving from other hospital structures present in the region. The OpenClinica technology (OpenClinica, LLC, Waltham, MA, USA), representing the first open source clinical trial software in the world for the management of clinical data (CDM) of Electronic Data Capture (EDC), was chosen for the underlying electronic database. The underlying technologies of the OpenClinica web application are: Java as a programming language, Spring Framework as an application framework and PostgreSQL as a report database.

The early modular design was prepared for integration with security technologies on the cloud, such as Microsoft Azure, to benefit from safety and compliance in the healthcare field with the latest standards of anonymization, security, and data maintenance as required by the European Medicine Agency (EMA) and the Food and Drug Administration (FDA) USA.

FARMAPRICE employs both types of alert messages typically used by CDSS: "Pre-test" and "Post-test" alerts. Pre-test alerts can be useful for reminding clinicians when a PGx test is necessary to ensure that a specific drug is safe for the patient. When prescribing a medication that is affected by a PGx guideline, the alert informs the clinician that the patient record lacks genotyping results. Conversely, a post-test alert appears when the PGx test results are available. This alert informs the prescribing physician that the patient has an actionable genotype and recommends a corresponding therapy [18]. This alert includes patient-specific dosing recommendations and highlights the strength of supporting evidence.

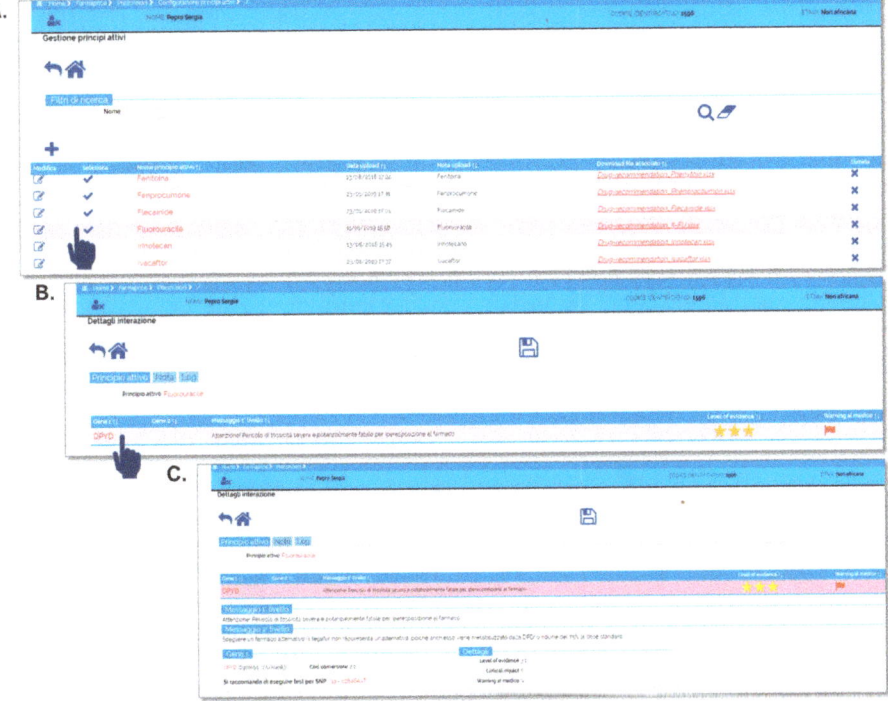

Figure 2. Demo prescription using FARMAPRICE tool. (**A**) the physician prescribes 5-fluorouracil to a patient who is DihydroPYrimidine-Dehydrogenase (*DPYD*) poor metabolizer. (**B**) This action triggers a pop-up with a first level message. (**C**) This in turn can trigger the real PGx-based recommendation of drug selection or dosage by clicking directly on the first level message.

Post-test alerts consist of two levels of messages. At the time a drug is ordered, a pop-up alert (first level message) appears when the patient has an actionable genotype listed in the PGx results repository. This first level message is a standardized text that describes the expected clinical effect of a specific genotype-drug interaction. This text was designed to be concise, and it includes the most important information needed for a prescription. Next to the first level text message, FARMAPRICE places stars and flags to indicate the *level of evidence* and the *clinical impact*, respectively, of the proposed dosing guideline. The *level of evidence* refers to the strength of the literature-based evidence that links the genotype to the phenotype. FARMAPRICE indicates the level of evidence with one to three stars to indicate the lowest to highest levels of evidence, respectively. The *clinical impact* is related to the clinical relevance of the potential adverse drug event. The clinical impact is indicated with colored flags: Yellow for low clinical impact (scored AA to C in the DPWG guidelines); red for high clinical impact (D to F in the DPWG guidelines [13]); and green for no clinical impact. Thus, a green flag combined with the first level message, "no recommendation, start with the standard dosage", indicates that no actionable genotype-drug interaction is available. For red and yellow flags, the prescribing physician can click on the first-level message to activate a hypertext link that will redirect to a second-level message. This message gives a recommendation on drug dosing and alternate drug selection. This second level message contains a more extensive text explanation, with details on the recommended changes in drug dosing and selection (Figure 2).

3.3. Third Phase: FARMAPRICE User Experience

Once the prototype was ready, the graphical interface was accurately reviewed and modified according to the medical doctors feed-back. The software GUI was implemented using PHI Technology GUI Designer which provides web-based user interfaces created on the underlying processes. This capability to render a GUI model is owed to the modeling framework of Eclipse, combined with the templating framework and guarantee a framework based on the logical processes of the software user, to consider all the crucial information. Yet this does not ensure the intuitiveness of the UI: Icons symbolize common actions which are consistent for homogeneous groups of users (i.e., "clinicians" and "researchers"). The feedback provided by the users led to the selection of an alternative set of icons understandable to the CDSS users, namely "clinicians" and "researchers". Warning messages were also implemented to allow prescribers to better weigh the strength of evidence available and decide whether to follow the recommendation or not [2]. The FARMAPRICE prototype is currently in experimental use by the medical oncologists of the Medical Oncology Department of the CRO-Aviano Hospital. These physicians have agreed to provide feed-back on their user experience, which will inform the developers on ways to optimize the software graphical interface and its operative performance.

4. Discussion

The preemptive PGx approach is typically used only for single gene-drug pairs with a relevant clinical impact, as is the case for highly toxic drugs, such as capecitabine, 5-fluorouracil, or 6-mercaptopurine. Preferably, in the future, this type of preemptive testing will be integrated into clinical practice. In that context, patients could be screened for drug-related genes in anticipation of future prescription events, consistent with the lifetime value of PGx testing. Then, in decisions regarding prescriptions, PGx results will be considered an inherent patient characteristic, like age, weight, renal function, and allergy status. Indeed, physicians are in a front-line position to handle the potential volume of such information by reviewing, interpreting, and delivering PGx test results and providing follow-up to the patient. Moreover, in future, the PGx knowledge base is likely to increase with the discovery of new gene-drug interactions, as next generation sequencing (NGS) continues to advance. In this study we have presented the results of an Italian coordinated effort to develop a CDSS tool, FARMAPRICE, that could help the PGx implementation in the current clinical practice.

Many initiatives both in Europe and the United States are and have been trying to address this hurdle. The main research networks involved in the integration of genetic data into the EHR are the Electronic Medical Records and Genomics Network (eMERGE) and the Implementing Genomics in Practice (IGNITE) [19]. The eMERGE network was formed by a partnership between eMERGE and the Pharmacogenomics Research Network (PGRN), which involves ten US sites. One of its main goals is to integrate clinically validated PGx genotypes into the EHR and associated CDSSs and to assess the process and clinical outcomes of implementation [20]. A few medical institutions have pilot projects that have surpassed "reactive genotyping" to include "preemptive genotyping". For example, the Mayo Clinic, with the RIGHT project, the Icahn School of Medicine at Mount Sinai, with CLIPMERGE, and Vanderbilt University Medical Center (VUMC), with PREDICT. These projects aim to drive point-of-care CDSSs with the integration of clinically actionable PGx variants into the EHR [21–23].

The Mayo clinic Biobank enrolled 1013 participants within 3 years into the "Right Drug, Right Dose, Right Time" project. The study aimed at optimizing preemptive genotyping in patients with a high probability of initiating statin therapy during the study period. One result of that study was the integration of PGx results into the EHR and the development of a point-of-care CDSS, including: (i) Pre-test and post-test alerts; and (ii) a CDSS integrated with additional PGx educational support links to aid clinicians. In addition, the Mayo Clinic developed a long-term maintenance strategy, with a CDSS that could automatically update itself with newly discovered gene-drug interactions. Moreover, that CDSS could automatically send an email to the technical team when an unreadable result occurred [11,19,21,24,25].

A member of the eMERGE network, the CLIPMERGE PGx program at Mount Sinai Medical Center, developed an active CDSS that delivered post-PGx-test alerts to clinicians at the point-of-care. That project aimed to implement the use of PGx testing by integrating it in CDSS and EHR using a DNA biobank-derived cohort (*BioMe*). Initially, 1500 pilot participants were recruited and preemptively genotyped for known variants associated with the use of warfarin, clopidogrel, simvastatin, and several types of antidepressants [22,25,26].

As mentioned previously, another relevant network involved in the integration of patient genetic data into clinical care is the IGNITE network. This network includes six US sites, and of these, three deal with PGx implementation: The University of Florida's Personalized Medicine Program; Indiana University's INGENIOUS program; and Vanderbilt University's I3P program [27]. Other initial efforts that aim to implement PGx in clinical care include Cleveland Clinic's Personalized Medication Program, St. Jude Children's Research Hospital's PG4KDS program, the University of Chicago's 1200 Patient Project, and the University of Maryland's Personalized Anti-Platelet Pharmacogenetics Program [18,28–30]. In Europe the PREemptive Pharmacogenomic testing for prevention of Adverse drug Reactions (PREPARE) clinical trial was conducted within the European Ubiquitous Pharmacogenomics (U-PGx) project [26,31]. They selected a panel of 50 variants in 13 pharmacogenes. This project put together different implementation sites in different European countries, with widely varying health care systems. In this context a spectrum of complementary CDSS solutions was developed, with the unique implementation experience of a portable CDSS, the "Safety-Code card".

For many years, genotyping was limited by the single-gene approach. The recent introduction of genotyping array technologies in the clinical practice made it possible to simultaneously evaluate several relevant pharmacogenes [32]. This technological approach has led to high-quality and economically affordable results. Indeed, the genotyping method for preemptive testing that has been adopted by ongoing implementation programs is mainly based on the use of array genotyping platforms [33]. These platforms offer robust interpretations of the results, and they are well-suited to automation, where PGx results are automatically uploaded into a structured IT system. The most suitable genotyping approach should be selected from the currently available commercial and custom panels. This selection is guided by features of feasibility and cost-effectiveness, such as: The turnaround time from isolated DNA to genotype; the instrumental and technical equipment of the laboratory involved in generating the genotype; the potential number of samples per array; the cost of the array; and the content and potential flexibility of the array [34].

A CDSS can be designed as an active or passive system. In the passive (or asynchronous) CDSS, the information is available only when the clinician specifically requests it, and it is reported as a static warning note. In contrast, the active (or synchronous) CDSS processes information and interacts with clinical data by following rules and issuing alerts [12,24]. Indeed, FARMAPRICE can be interrogated by healthcare providers at the point-of-care by accessing the web-based platform to determine whether a specific drug has a potentially clinically actionable gene-drug interaction. Rules will predict phenotype-predicted genotype and interactive alerts will be triggered both when a high-risk drug is prescribed and when a specific PGx result should be obtained before prescribing the intended drug.

PGx CDSSs are typically developed as stand-alone systems that function autonomously as a web service or a mobile application, rather than being integrated into the existing local hospital infrastructure. However, because PGx results are relevant throughout a patient's life, ideally, they should be stored in a time-independent manner to ensure accessibility to future providers [12]. Currently, the long-term availability of PGx results at the point-of-care can only be guaranteed by a CDSS that is embedded into an Electronic Health Record (EHR) [35]. With this method, PGx results can be shared among different healthcare providers (pharmacists, general practitioners, specialists), and they can be used at different stages of the clinical workflow to guide clinical decision-making processes [19]. However, linking the EHR to the CDSS is challenging; thus, it is not yet a common practice. Caraballo et al pointed out that modern EHRs have not been designed for long-term storage of genetic data. Due to the lack of a specific repository, to date, PGx data have been stored in EHRs on either a "problem list" or an "allergy list", which provides time-independent documentation of possible gene-drug interactions. Other issues that make it challenging to incorporate PGx results into the EHR are the increasing amount of genetic data and the unstandardized formats of available data, which makes them difficult to share in a multi-center setting [19,24]. The Italian health care system is currently lacking a common EHR platform among its different regions. This lack has resulted in a fragmented healthcare delivery system with limited EHR interoperability. Thus, sharing healthcare data among different providers is hampered. Consequently, FARMAPRICE was conceived as a stand-alone system that could be eventually integrated into the EHR system.

Indeed, successful implementation of a CDSS is not only related to its clinical utility in terms of improving treatment safety and efficacy, but also to its perceived feasibility and usability by the prescribing physicians. When looking at the software requirements for the most effective user experience, clinicians considered that excess alerts (e.g., not relevant or repeated alerts, a phenomenon termed "alert fatigue") could put a strain on the clinician's workload, and this could have adverse effects on patient care [36]. In the evaluation of FARMAPRICE prototype, a user-friendly design was sought and designed to ensure that the interruptions would not overload busy clinicians [24]. The user experience is now in the experimental evaluation phase by prescribing physicians in the CRO-Aviano hospital.

It must be further considered that, in the first place, the use of this kind of tool is primarily related to the health practitioners personal motivation and of their awareness of the opportunity to use PGx in their everyday routine. Other implementation experiences have demonstrated that although physicians may perceive the benefit of using PGx, the lack of formal training about PGx, together with concerns regarding feasibility, clinical utility, and integration in the clinical workflow have been reported by physicians as the major barriers to a more routine use of PGx [8]. It must be not forgotten that education is a crucial step for implementing PGx into the clinic. Educational and training programs must be offered to health practitioners in an interprofessional context to drive interest and continuous learning about PGx, to allow a critical and conscious use of PGx in the clinical practice also with the aid of innovative IT tools, such as FARMAPRICE.

5. Conclusions

Patients and healthcare providers are important stakeholders in the implementation of PGx. Among the provider-perceived barriers to adopting this information are inadequate knowledge about PGx, the lack of clear guidelines for many drugs, and the absence of convincing cost-effectiveness data to support PGx clinical utility. In addition, an emerging barrier to the PGx clinical implementation process is the lack of user-friendly tools to integrate genetic information and their interpretation into the clinical prescription workflow.

Health-related ITs, such as the CDSS, are designed to support clinicians in the decision-making process; to address the growing information pool, which overloads clinicians; and to provide a platform for incorporating evidence-based knowledge into care delivery. An Italian consortium has been set up to create FARMAPRICE, a CDSS designed to be used in the clinical setting to facilitate the use of PGx in the drug prescription process in Italy. A prototype has been created and is ready to be presented to clinicians for use in their routine practice. It is likely that, in the next few years, pre-treatment patient genotyping will become a more common clinical practice, and FARMAPRICE will represent a user-friendly, stand-alone system that can be integrated into every clinical context to manage genetic data and optimize patient treatments.

Author Contributions: Conceptualization: E.C., G.T., L.G., and L.E.; methodology: E.C., R.R., L.D.C., S.M., and F.C.; software: V.C., and E.D.S.; validation: M.G., E.D.M., A.B., L.F., and F.C.; original manuscript draft preparation: E.C., R.R., L.D.C., S.M., F.C., and E.D.M.; funding acquisition: E.C., L.G., L.E.

Funding: This research was funded by POR FESR 2014-2020 Friuli Venezia Giulia Attivita 1.3.b. Deliberazione della Giunta Regionale 849/2016 (FARMAPRICE) (EC).

Conflicts of Interest: The authors declare no conflict of interest. The funders played no role in the design of the study; in the collection, analyses, or interpretation of data; in writing the manuscript, or in the decision to publish the results.

References

1. Arwood, M.J.; Chumnumwat, S.; Cavallari, L.H.; Nutescu, E.A.; Duarte, J.D. Implementing Pharmacogenomics at Your Institution: Establishment and Overcoming Implementation Challenges. *Clin. Trans. Sci.* **2016**, *9*, 233–245. [CrossRef]
2. Mukerjee, G.; Huston, A.; Kabakchiev, B.; Piquette-Miller, M.; van Schaik, R.; Dorfman, R. User considerations in assessing pharmacogenomic tests and their clinical support tools. *Genom. Med.* **2018**, *3*, 26. [CrossRef]
3. Roncato, R.; Cecchin, E.; Montico, M.; De Mattia, E.; Giodini, L.; Buonadonna, A.; Solfrini, V.; Innocenti, F.; Toffoli, G. Cost Evaluation of Irinotecan-Related Toxicities Associated With the UGT1A1*28 Patient Genotype. *Clin. Pharmacol. Ther.* **2017**, *102*, 123–130. [CrossRef] [PubMed]
4. Toffoli, G.; Innocenti, F.; Polesel, J.; De Mattia, E.; Sartor, F.; Dalle Fratte, C.; Ecca, F.; Dreussi, E.; Palazzari, E.; Guardascione, M.; et al. The Genotype for DPYD Risk Variants in Patients With Colorectal Cancer and the Related Toxicity Management Costs in Clinical Practice. *Clin. Pharmacol. Ther.* **2019**, *105*, 994–1002. [CrossRef] [PubMed]
5. US Food and Drug Administration Home Page. Available online: https://www.fda.gov/ (accessed on 11 February 2019).
6. PharmGKB. Available online: https://www.pharmgkb.org/ (accessed on 14 February 2019).
7. Janssens, A.C.J.W.; Deverka, P.A. Useless until proven effective: The clinical utility of preemptive pharmacogenetic testing. *Clin. Pharmacol. Ther.* **2014**, *96*, 652–654. [CrossRef] [PubMed]
8. Borden, B.A.; Galecki, P.; Wellmann, R.; Danahey, K.; Lee, S.M.; Patrick-Miller, L.; Sorrentino, M.J.; Nanda, R.; Koyner, J.L.; Polonsky, T.S.; et al. Assessment of provider-perceived barriers to clinical use of pharmacogenomics during participation in an institutional implementation study. *Pharmacogenet. Genom.* **2019**, *29*, 31–38. [CrossRef] [PubMed]
9. Johansen Taber, K.A.; Dickinson, B.D. Pharmacogenomic knowledge gaps and educational resource needs among physicians in selected specialties. *Pharmgenom. Pers. Med.* **2014**, *7*, 145–162. [CrossRef] [PubMed]
10. Relling, M.V.; Evans, W.E. Pharmacogenomics in the clinic. *Nature* **2015**, *526*, 343–350. [CrossRef] [PubMed]
11. Hinderer, M.; Boeker, M.; Wagner, S.A.; Lablans, M.; Newe, S.; Hülsemann, J.L.; Neumaier, M.; Binder, H.; Renz, H.; Acker, T.; et al. Integrating clinical decision support systems for pharmacogenomic testing into clinical routine—A scoping review of designs of user-system interactions in recent system development. *BMC Med. Inform. Decis. Mak.* **2017**, *17*, 81. [CrossRef]
12. Hicks, J.K.; Dunnenberger, H.M.; Gumpper, K.F.; Haidar, C.E.; Hoffman, J.M. Integrating pharmacogenomics into electronic health records with clinical decision support. *Am. J. Health Syst. Pharm.* **2016**, *73*, 1967–1976. [CrossRef]
13. Swen, J.J.; Nijenhuis, M.; de Boer, A.; Grandia, L.; Maitland-van der Zee, A.H.; Mulder, H.; Rongen, G.A.P.J.M.; van Schaik, R.H.N.; Schalekamp, T.; Touw, D.J.; et al. Pharmacogenetics: From bench to byte—An update of guidelines. *Clin. Pharmacol. Ther.* **2011**, *89*, 662–673. [CrossRef] [PubMed]

14. Kalman, L.V.; Agúndez, J.; Appell, M.L.; Black, J.L.; Bell, G.C.; Boukouvala, S.; Bruckner, C.; Bruford, E.; Caudle, K.; Coulthard, S.A.; et al. Pharmacogenetic allele nomenclature: International workgroup recommendations for test result reporting. *Clin. Pharmacol. Ther.* **2016**, *99*, 172–185. [CrossRef] [PubMed]
15. Caudle, K.E.; Dunnenberger, H.M.; Freimuth, R.R.; Peterson, J.F.; Burlison, J.D.; Whirl-Carrillo, M.; Scott, S.A.; Rehm, H.L.; Williams, M.S.; Klein, T.E.; et al. Standardizing terms for clinical pharmacogenetic test results: Consensus terms from the Clinical Pharmacogenetics Implementation Consortium (CPIC). *Genet. Med.* **2017**, *19*, 215–223. [CrossRef] [PubMed]
16. PHI Technology White Paper. Available online: http://wiki.hl7.org/index.php?title=PHI_TECHNOLOGY_white_paper (accessed on 4 April 2019).
17. Lazaridis, K.N. PACE Forward-Making Pharmacogenomics Testing Available for Real-Life Clinical Utility. *Clin. Pharmacol. Ther.* **2019**, *105*, 42–44. [CrossRef] [PubMed]
18. Hicks, J.K.; Stowe, D.; Willner, M.A.; Wai, M.; Daly, T.; Gordon, S.M.; Lashner, B.A.; Parikh, S.; White, R.; Teng, K.; et al. Implementation of Clinical Pharmacogenomics within a Large Health System: From Electronic Health Record Decision Support to Consultation Services. *Pharmacotherapy* **2016**, *36*, 940–948. [CrossRef]
19. Caraballo, P.J.; Bielinski, S.J.; Sauver, J.S.; Weinshilboum, R.M. Electronic Medical Record-Integrated Pharmacogenomics and Related Clinical Decision Support Concepts. *Clin. Pharmacol. Ther.* **2017**, *102*, 254–264. [CrossRef] [PubMed]
20. Rasmussen-Torvik, L.J.; Stallings, S.C.; Gordon, A.S.; Almoguera, B.; Basford, M.A.; Bielinski, S.J.; Brautbar, A.; Brilliant, M.H.; Carrell, D.S.; Connolly, J.J.; et al. Design and anticipated outcomes of the eMERGE-PGx project: A multicenter pilot for preemptive pharmacogenomics in electronic health record systems. *Clin. Pharmacol. Ther.* **2014**, *96*, 482–489. [CrossRef]
21. Bielinski, S.J.; Olson, J.E.; Pathak, J.; Weinshilboum, R.M.; Wang, L.; Lyke, K.J.; Ryu, E.; Targonski, P.V.; Van Norstrand, M.D.; Hathcock, M.A.; et al. Preemptive genotyping for personalized medicine: Design of the right drug, right dose, right time-using genomic data to individualize treatment protocol. *Mayo Clin. Proc.* **2014**, *89*, 25–33. [CrossRef]
22. Gottesman, O.; Scott, S.A.; Ellis, S.B.; Overby, C.L.; Ludtke, A.; Hulot, J.-S.; Hall, J.; Chatani, K.; Myers, K.; Kannry, J.L.; et al. The CLIPMERGE PGx Program: Clinical implementation of personalized medicine through electronic health records and genomics-pharmacogenomics. *Clin. Pharmacol. Ther.* **2013**, *94*, 214–217. [CrossRef] [PubMed]
23. Pulley, J.M.; Denny, J.C.; Peterson, J.F.; Bernard, G.R.; Vnencak-Jones, C.L.; Ramirez, A.H.; Delaney, J.T.; Bowton, E.; Brothers, K.; Johnson, K.; et al. Operational implementation of prospective genotyping for personalized medicine: The design of the Vanderbilt PREDICT project. *Clin. Pharmacol. Ther.* **2012**, *92*, 87–95. [CrossRef] [PubMed]
24. Caraballo, P.J.; Hodge, L.S.; Bielinski, S.J.; Stewart, A.K.; Farrugia, G.; Schultz, C.G.; Rohrer-Vitek, C.R.; Olson, J.E.; St Sauver, J.L.; Roger, V.L.; et al. Multidisciplinary model to implement pharmacogenomics at the point of care. *Genet. Med.* **2017**, *19*, 421–429. [CrossRef] [PubMed]
25. Dunnenberger, H.M.; Crews, K.R.; Hoffman, J.M.; Caudle, K.E.; Broeckel, U.; Howard, S.C.; Hunkler, R.J.; Klein, T.E.; Evans, W.E.; Relling, M.V. Preemptive clinical pharmacogenetics implementation: Current programs in five US medical centers. *Annu. Rev. Pharmacol. Toxicol.* **2015**, *55*, 89–106. [CrossRef]
26. Van der Wouden, C.H.; Cambon-Thomsen, A.; Cecchin, E.; Cheung, K.C.; Dávila-Fajardo, C.L.; Deneer, V.H.; Dolžan, V.; Ingelman-Sundberg, M.; Jónsson, S.; Karlsson, M.O.; et al. Implementing Pharmacogenomics in Europe: Design and Implementation Strategy of the Ubiquitous Pharmacogenomics Consortium. *Clin. Pharmacol. Ther.* **2017**, *101*, 341–358. [CrossRef] [PubMed]
27. Weitzel, K.W.; Alexander, M.; Bernhardt, B.A.; Calman, N.; Carey, D.J.; Cavallari, L.H.; Field, J.R.; Hauser, D.; Junkins, H.A.; Levin, P.A.; et al. The IGNITE network: A model for genomic medicine implementation and research. *BMC Med. Genom.* **2016**, *9*, 1. [CrossRef]
28. Hoffman, J.M.; Haidar, C.E.; Wilkinson, M.R.; Crews, K.R.; Baker, D.K.; Kornegay, N.M.; Yang, W.; Pui, C.-H.; Reiss, U.M.; Gaur, A.H.; et al. PG4KDS: A Model for the Clinical Implementation of Pre-emptive Pharmacogenetics. *Am. J. Med. Genet. Semin. Med. Genet.* **2014**, *166C*, 45–55. [CrossRef]
29. O'Donnell, P.H.; Danahey, K.; Jacobs, M.; Wadhwa, N.R.; Yuen, S.; Bush, A.; Sacro, Y.; Sorrentino, M.J.; Siegler, M.; Harper, W.; et al. Adoption of a clinical pharmacogenomics implementation program during outpatient care—Initial results of the University of Chicago "1200 Patients Project". *Am. J. Med. Genet. Semin. Med. Genet.* **2014**, *166C*, 68–75. [CrossRef] [PubMed]

30. Shuldiner, A.R.; Palmer, K.; Pakyz, R.E.; Alestock, T.D.; Maloney, K.A.; O'Neill, C.; Bhatty, S.; Schub, J.; Overby, C.L.; Horenstein, R.B.; et al. Implementation of Pharmacogenetics: The University of Maryland Personalized Anti-Platelet Pharmacogenetics Program. *Am. J. Med. Genet. Semin. Med. Genet.* **2014**, *166C*, 76–84. [CrossRef]
31. Cecchin, E.; Roncato, R.; Guchelaar, H.J.; Toffoli, G. Ubiquitous Pharmacogenomics Consortium Ubiquitous Pharmacogenomics (U-PGx): The Time for Implementation is Now. An Horizon2020 Program to Drive Pharmacogenomics into Clinical Practice. *Curr. Pharm. Biotechnol.* **2017**, *18*, 204–209. [CrossRef] [PubMed]
32. Di Francia, R.; Frigeri, F.; Berretta, M.; Cecchin, E.; Orlando, C.; Pinto, A.; Pinzani, P. Decision criteria for rational selection of homogeneous genotyping platforms for pharmacogenomics testing in clinical diagnostics. *Clin. Chem. Lab. Med.* **2010**, *48*, 447–459. [CrossRef]
33. Dunnenberger, H.M.; Biszewski, M.; Bell, G.C.; Sereika, A.; May, H.; Johnson, S.G.; Hulick, P.J.; Khandekar, J. Implementation of a multidisciplinary pharmacogenomics clinic in a community health system. *Am. J. Health Syst. Pharm.* **2016**, *73*, 1956–1966. [CrossRef]
34. Johnson, J.; Burkley, B.; Langaee, T.; Clare-Salzler, M.; Klein, T.; Altman, R. Implementing Personalized Medicine: Development of a Cost-Effective Customized Pharmacogenetics Genotyping Array. *Clin. Pharmacol. Ther.* **2012**, *92*, 437–439. [CrossRef] [PubMed]
35. Swen, J.J.; Nijenhuis, M.; van Rhenen, M.; de Boer-Veger, N.J.; Buunk, A.-M.; Houwink, E.J.F.; Mulder, H.; Rongen, G.A.; van Schaik, R.H.N.; van der Weide, J.; et al. Pharmacogenetic Information in Clinical Guidelines: The European Perspective. *Clin. Pharmacol. Ther.* **2018**, *103*, 795–801. [CrossRef] [PubMed]
36. McCoy, A.B.; Thomas, E.J.; Krousel-Wood, M.; Sittig, D.F. Clinical decision support alert appropriateness: A review and proposal for improvement. *Ochsner. J.* **2014**, *14*, 195–202. [PubMed]

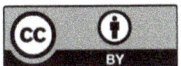

© 2019 by the authors. Licensee MDPI, Basel, Switzerland. This article is an open access article distributed under the terms and conditions of the Creative Commons Attribution (CC BY) license (http://creativecommons.org/licenses/by/4.0/).

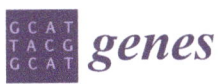

Article

Pharmacist-Initiated Pre-Emptive Pharmacogenetic Panel Testing with Clinical Decision Support in Primary Care: Record of PGx Results and Real-World Impact

Cathelijne H. van der Wouden [1,2], Paul C. D. Bank [1,2], Kübra Özokcu [3], Jesse J. Swen [1,2] and Henk-Jan Guchelaar [1,2,*]

1 Department of Clinical Pharmacy and Toxicology, Leiden University Medical Center, 2333 ZA Leiden, The Netherlands; j.j.swen@lumc.nl (J.J.S.)
2 Leiden Network for Personalised Therapeutics, 2333 ZA Leiden, The Netherlands
3 Division of Pharmacoepidemiology and Clinical Pharmacology, Utrecht Institute for Pharmaceutical Sciences (UIPS), Utrecht University, 3584 CG Utrecht, The Netherlands; K.Ozokcu@students.uu.nl
* Correspondence: H.J.Guchelaar@lumc.nl; Tel.: +31-(0)71-526-2790

Received: 29 March 2019; Accepted: 8 May 2019; Published: 29 May 2019

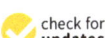

Abstract: Logistics and (cost-)effectiveness of pharmacogenetic (PGx)-testing may be optimized when delivered through a pre-emptive panel-based approach, within a clinical decision support system (CDSS). Here, clinical recommendations are automatically deployed by the CDSS when a drug-gene interaction (DGI) is encountered. However, this requires record of PGx-panel results in the electronic medical record (EMR). Several studies indicate promising clinical utility of panel-based PGx-testing in polypharmacy and psychiatry, but is undetermined in primary care. Therefore, we aim to quantify both the feasibility and the real-world impact of this approach in primary care. Within a prospective pilot study, community pharmacists were provided the opportunity to request a panel of eight pharmacogenes to guide drug dispensing within a CDSS for 200 primary care patients. In this side-study, this cohort was cross-sectionally followed-up after a mean of 2.5-years. PGx-panel results were successfully recorded in 96% and 68% of pharmacist and general practitioner (GP) EMRs, respectively. This enabled 97% of patients to (re)use PGx-panel results for at least one, and 33% for up to four newly initiated prescriptions with possible DGIs. A total of 24.2% of these prescriptions had actionable DGIs, requiring pharmacotherapy adjustment. Healthcare utilization seemed not to vary among those who did and did not encounter a DGI. Pre-emptive panel-based PGx-testing is feasible and real-world impact is substantial in primary care.

Keywords: pre-emptive; pharmacogenetics; panel

1. Introduction

An individual's response to a drug can be predicted by their pharmacogenetic (PGx) profile [1,2]. Incorporation of an individual's PGx profile into drug prescribing promises a safer, more effective and thereby more cost-effective drug treatment [3,4]. Several randomized controlled trials (RCTs) demonstrate the clinical utility of pre-emptive single gene tests to guide dosing [5–7], and drug selection [8], for individual drug-gene interactions. These studies are perceived as a proof-of-concept supporting the clinical utility of pre-emptive PGx testing, and may therefore also be applied to other drug-gene interactions, for which evidence of the same rigour may lack [9,10]. The Dutch Pharmacogenetics Working Group (DPWG) was established in 2005 to devise clinical guidelines for individual drug-gene interactions based on a systematic review of literature [11,12]. These guidelines provide clinicians with recommendations on how to manage drug-gene interactions. To date, the DPWG has developed guidelines for 97 drug-gene interactions, of which 54 are actionable drug-gene interactions, many of which are encountered principally in primary care. In parallel, the Clinical Pharmacogenetics Implementation Consortium (CPIC) has also devised guidelines for more than 40 drugs [13]. The DPWG and CPIC guidelines have ongoing efforts to harmonize the two [14]. In the Netherlands, the DPWG guidelines are incorporated into a nationwide clinical decision support system, called the "G-standaard", providing pharmacists and general practitioners (GPs) with relevant clinical recommendations at the point of care when an actionable drug-gene interaction is encountered.

Significant debate persists regarding the optimal approach for implementing PGx testing in clinical care; where some support using a pre-therapeutic single gene approach and others a pre-emptive panel-based approach [15]. The pre-therapeutic single gene approach has several drawbacks. In this one-at-a-time strategy, an individual gene is tested in response to a first prescription of an interacting target drug. If, however, patients receive prescriptions for multiple interacting target drugs over time, they may require testing for multiple single genes. Here, pharmacotherapy may be delayed in awaiting the PGx results. Furthermore, the costs of single gene testing may be allocated a multitude of times, while the marginal cost of testing and interpreting additional pharmacogenes simultaneously is near-zero [16,17]. These logistical and cost-effectiveness issues may be overcome and optimized when delivering PGx in a panel-based approach [18]. Here, a panel of variants within multiple genes, which are associated with drug response, are tested and saved for later use in preparation of future prescriptions [15]. In this way, the panel-results can be reused over time, as multiple drugs which interact with multiple variants are prescribed [19]. When an interacting target drug is prescribed, the corresponding PGx guideline can be deployed by the clinical decision support system at the point of care, thereby providing clinicians with the necessary information to guide prescribing by PGx, without any delay. Alternatively, a combination of the two strategies may be the optimal approach for delivering PGx. Here, a panel test is ordered reactively in response to an incident prescription and is saved in the electronic medical record (EMR) for pre-emptive use in future prescriptions. However, in order for the clinical decision support system to be enabled, it is crucial that the PGx results are recorded and preserved in the EMR. If this fails, a potential drug-gene interaction may go unnoticed. As a result, the added value of testing multiple genes is lost. A recent study showed that PGx results for *CYP2D6* were sparsely recorded; only 3.1% and 5.9% of reported PGx results were recorded in EMRs by general practitioners (GPs) and pharmacists, respectively, within a mean follow-up of 862 days [20]. This indicates that correct record of PGx results in the EMR may be a remaining barrier preventing the realization of panel-based testing. However, this is yet undetermined when reporting the results for multiple genes simultaneously. Therefore, we sought to investigate whether pharmacists and GPs are able to record PGx panel testing results within their EMR, in order to enable life-long use of PGx results through a clinical decision support system.

Another barrier preventing implementation of panel-based PGx testing is the lack of evidence demonstrating its clinical utility. Although there is a firm evidence base supporting the clinical utility of pre-emptive single gene PGx testing, evidence of similar quality supporting a panel-based approach is lacking [21]. Even so, several smaller studies report promising results indicating that pre-emptive panel-based PGx guided prescribing is indeed (cost-)effective in preventing adverse drug reactions among polypharmacy and psychiatry patients. However, this is yet to be determined within primary care [22–27]. Alternatively, the clinical impact of population-wide panel-based testing has previously been modelled by using Medicare prescription data; indicating half of patients above 65 will use at least one of the drugs for which PGx guidelines are available during a four year period, and one fourth to one third, will use two or more of these drugs [28]. Another study showed that more than 60% of the population would benefit from PGx guided prescribing within a 5-year period [19]. However, the clinical impact is yet undetermined in a real-world setting. This may differ from modelled estimations since the patients selected by pharmacists to receive panel testing may differ from those included in prescription datasets. Therefore, we aim to quantify the potential real-world impact of implementation of PGx panel in a clinical decision support system within a side-study of the Implementation of Pharmacogenetics into Primary care Project (IP3 study). In this side-study, the primary outcome is the frequency at which patients receive newly initiated prescriptions, with possible drug-gene interactions, for which PGx results are available in the EMR. To explore which target groups may benefit most from panel testing, we aim to investigate which patient sub-groups may more frequently initiate newly prescribed drugs within follow-up. Secondary outcomes include their downstream impact on healthcare utilization. Firstly, we hypothesize that patients who encounter an actionable drug-gene interaction and adhered to the DPWG guidelines will have a similar healthcare utilization compared to those who did not encounter an actionable drug-gene interaction. Secondly, we hypothesize that patients who encounter an actionable drug-gene interaction, but did not adhere to the DPWG guidelines, have a higher healthcare utilization compared to those who did not encounter an actionable drug-gene interaction.

2. Materials and Methods

2.1. Study Design, Participants

We performed a cross-sectional follow-up of The Implementation of Pharmacogenetics into Primary care Project (IP3 study) cohort, as a side-study. The IP3 study is a prospective multicenter observational pilot study with the objective to test the feasibility of pharmacist-initiated pharmacogenetics testing within a clinical decision support system in primary care. The study design, rationale and main study findings have previously been described elsewhere [29]. In brief, community pharmacies in the vicinity of Leiden, The Netherlands, were invited to participate in the study. Pharmacists who agreed on participation were provided with the opportunity to request free PGx tests for a panel of 40 variants in eight pharmacogenes (see Supplementary Table S1), to guide drug dispensing based on the DPWG guidelines, for a maximum of 200 patients. The genes selected to be tested were based on genes for which DPWG guidelines are available and which are either included in the Affymetrix Drug Metabolizing and Transporters (DMET) array (*CYP2C9, CYP2C19, CYP2D6, CYP3A5, SLCO1B1, TPMT* and *VKORC1*) or determined in clinical care (*DPYD*). This panel can be used in combination with the DPWG guidelines to guide drug prescribing for 41 drugs. Here, a combination of reactive and pre-emptive panel testing is implemented. A PGx panel is ordered reactively in response to an incident prescription and is saved in the EMR for pre-emptive use is future prescriptions. Adult patients receiving a first prescription (defined as no prescription for the first drug within the preceding 12 months) for at least 28 days for one of 10 drugs (amitriptyline, atomoxetine, atorvastatin, (es)citalopram, clomipramine, doxepin, nortriptyline, simvastatin or venlafaxine) in routine care were eligible. Additional in- and exclusion criteria are reported elsewhere [29]. After identification of the patients through automated queries, the participating pharmacists manually checked whether patients fulfilled the in- and exclusion criteria. Finally, patients not recruited within 14 days after dispensing the first prescription were excluded. When patients were eligible, pharmacists were able to select these patients for ordering a PGx panel. The panel test result could be used reactively for the drug of enrolment and pre-emptively for future prescriptions of 41 drugs with potential drug-gene interactions.

2.2. Healthcare Setting

In the Dutch healthcare system, patients are typically listed with one GP and one pharmacy. The GP plays a gatekeeping role in the provision of healthcare. The GP is consulted for all initial healthcare problems and may refer to specialized care when appropriate. Typically, GPs maintain EMRs for their patients and contain prescription history, lab results, correspondence with specialized physicians and reports regarding ER (emergency room) visits and hospitalizations. In parallel, pharmacists maintain a separate EMR containing dispensing history, relevant contra-indications and drug allergies and are used for medication surveillance at drug dispensing.

In routine care, PGx testing is predominantly performed within hospital pharmacy or clinical chemistry laboratories. Hospitals additionally maintain a separate EMR for registered patients. Generated PGx results are typically recorded in the hospital's EMR and are communicated with requesting pharmacists of physicians in primary care by paper or electronic reports.

2.3. Ethics Approval

All subjects gave their written informed consent for enrolment before they participated in the study. The study was conducted in accordance with the Declaration of Helsinki, and the protocol was approved by the Ethics Committee of Leiden University Medical Center (LUMC) (P14.081). Patients provided informed consent for data collection regarding their medication and related outcomes from both pharmacy and GP EMRs within 3 years of enrolment.

2.4. DNA Collection, Isolation, Extraction and Genotyping

After providing signed informed consent, pharmacists collected a 2mL saliva sample from participating patients using the Oragene DNA OG-250 (DNA Genotek Inc). The samples were transported to the PGx laboratory in Leiden University Medical Center by research staff or mail. DNA was extracted in accordance to Oragene DNA OG-250 isolation procedure, where a solution volume of 100µL, instead of 200 µL, was used. The DNA concentration was quantified in each sample with NanoDropPhotometer (Thermo Fisher Scientific), and DNA quality was assessed with the use of the 260 nm/280 nm absorbance ratio. Genotypes of *CYP2C9, CYP2C19, CYP2D6, CYP3A5, DPYD, SLCO1B1, TPMT* and *VKORC1* were determined using the Drug Metabolizing and Transporters (DMET) Plus Array (Affymetrix, Santa Clara, CA). *CYP2D6* copy number variants were detected with qPCR (Thermo Fisher Scientific, Massachusetts, USA). The DMET array was supplemented with the *DPYD* 1236G>A and 2846A>T variants which were routinely tested in clinic at the LUMC. Validation of the assays is described elsewhere [29].

2.5. Translation of Genotype to Phenotype and Return of Results

Genotypes for the eight pharmacogenes were translated into predicted phenotypes using the DPWG guidelines. A paper report holding the genotypes, predicted phenotypes and the DPWG therapeutic recommendation for the drug of enrollment was devised and sent to the patients' general practitioner (GP) and pharmacist by mail and/or fax (see Supplementary Figure S1 for an example report). The report held the request to record the entire PGx profile in the EMR to enable the clinical decision support system when drug-gene interaction is encountered during drug prescribing or dispensing (see Figure 1). Predicted phenotypes must be recorded in the EMR in a contra-indication format to enable deployment of the relevant guideline through the clinical decision support system. Even if patients are predicted to be extensive metabolizers (EM), we recommend that they still be recorded as contra-indications to record the performance of this test. However, pharmacy EMRs can hold a maximum of 10 contra-indications. It is important to note that the pilot study is initiated through the pharmacists and therefore the GPs who receive the paper report may have had no prior knowledge about the existence of the IP3 pilot study.

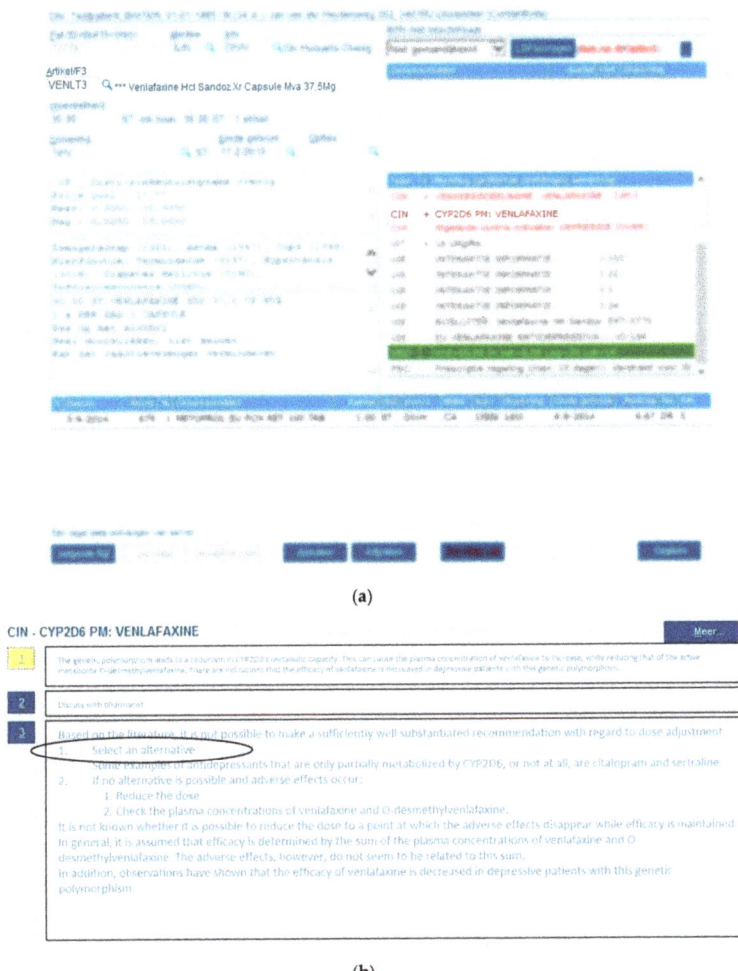

Figure 1. Clinical decision support during drug dispensing. A patient who is *CYP2D6* PM (as noted in the electronic medical record (EMR) as contra-indication, as indicated by "CIN" (contra-indication) receives a prescription for venlafaxine (**a**) which triggers a pop-up with the relevant Dutch Pharmacogenetics Working Group (DPWG) recommendation directing selection of alternative drug (**b**).

2.6. Healthcare Provider Incorporation of PGx Results in Drug Prescribing and Dispensing

When an actionable drug-gene interaction is encountered, the DPWG guideline directs adjustment of drug, dose or vigilance of pharmacotherapy to avoid potential adverse drug reactions or lack of efficacy. However, pharmacists are free to choose whether to adhere to the DPWG guidelines. In The Netherlands, and within the IP3 study, pharmacists must discuss pharmacotherapy alteration, resulting from medication surveillance, with the prescribing physicians before the prescription can be altered.

2.7. Groups for Analysis

Patients have been stratified into three groups for comparison (see Table 1): 1) those who did not encounter an actionable drug-gene interaction for the drug of enrolment, 2) those who encountered an actionable drug-gene interaction for the drug of enrolment and whose health care providers chose to adhere to the DPWG guideline, and 3) those who encountered an actionable drug-gene interaction for the drug of enrolment and whose health care providers chose not to adhere to the DPWG guideline.

2.8. Outcomes and Analyses

In this side-study, the primary outcome for quantifying the feasibility of the panel-based approach is whether the PGx panel results were recorded as a contra-indication in both the GP and pharmacist EMRs at the time of follow-up.

In this side-study, the primary outcome for quantifying the real-world impact of the panel-based approach is the number of newly initiated drugs for which potential drug-gene interactions are encountered, since enrolment, and whether these interactions are actionable. A potential drug-gene interaction is encountered when a patient, regardless of their phenotype (e.g., *CYP2D6* PM, IM or EM), receives a new prescription for a drug for which an actionable DPWG guideline is available and the interacting gene was included in the IP3 panel (e.g., metoprolol-*CYP2D6* guideline). A potential drug-gene interaction becomes an actionable when the patient's predicted phenotype directs adjustment of pharmacotherapy, based on the relevant DPWG guideline (e.g., patient is *CYP2D6* PM and initiates metoprolol). See Supplementary Table S2 for a list of drugs for which actionable DPWG guidelines are available and IP3 panel results can be used to identify potential and actionable drug-gene interactions. To explore which target group may benefit most from panel testing, we investigate whether baseline demographic variables (gender, age, BMI, number of comorbidities and number of comedications) are associated with an increasing number of prescribed drugs with potential drug-gene interactions within follow-up by using univariate negative binomial regression. The secondary outcome is healthcare utilization as a result of pre-specified drug-gene interaction associated adverse drug reactions within 12 weeks of enrolment. This is a composite endpoint of GP consults (in person, by phone or by e-mail), emergency department (ED) visits, and hospitalizations. These drug-gene interactions associated adverse drug reactions were defined before data collection was initiated and are based on the literature underlying the DPWG guidelines. For example, if a patient enrolled on simvastatin with a *SLCO1B1* TC genotype consults their GP regarding muscle pain symptoms within 12 weeks of initiation, this is considered a drug-gene interaction associated adverse drug reactions since *SLCO1B1* TC and CC carriers are at higher risk for statin-induced myopathy [30]. See Supplementary Table S3 for an overview of pre-specified drug-gene interaction associated adverse drug reactions and underlying literature. We compare the frequency of the composite endpoint among patients who encounter an actionable drug-gene interaction and adhered to the DPWG guidelines (group 2) to those who did not encounter an actionable drug-gene interactions associated adverse drug reactions(group 1), using binomial logistic regression in a non-inferiority analysis. We have set a non-inferiority at a margin of 1.2. Secondly, we compare the frequency of the composite endpoint among patients who encounter an actionable drug-gene interaction, but did not adhere to the DPWG guidelines (group 3), to those who did not encounter an actionable drug-gene interaction (group 1), using binomial logistic regression.

3. Results

3.1. IP3 Cohort and Follow-Up

Overall 200 patients were enrolled in the IP3 study between November 2014 and July 2016. Patient characteristics are presented in Table 1. The database containing the genotypes and predicted phenotypes is available at https://databases.lovd.nl/shared/individuals (patient IDs 184080-184279). 62 (31.0%) patients encountered an actionable drug-gene interaction for the drug of enrolment, as previously reported by Bank et al. [29]. Of these, health care providers chose to adhere to the DPWG guideline in 49 (79.0%) cases. Data collection was performed retrospectively between April 2018 and September 2018 in both pharmacy and GP EMRs; from pharmacy EMRs between May 4th 2018 and May 29th 2018; and from GP EMRs between April 3rd 2018 and September 28th 2018. Data could be retrospectively collected cross-sectionally from 200 (100%) and 177 (88.5%) pharmacy and GP EMRs, respectively (see Figure 2). The mean follow-up from pharmacy EMRs was 933 days (range 649–1279), approximately 2.5 years. The mean follow-up from GP EMRs was 917 days (range 622–1238).

Table 1. Summary of patient characteristics in Implementation of Pharmacogenetics into Primary care Project (IP3) cohort stratified by groups for analysis

			Groups for Analysis		
				Actionable Drug-Gene Interaction for the Drug of Enrolment ($n = 62, 31.0\%$)	
	Overall IP3 Study Cohort ($n = 200$)	1) No Drug-Gene Interaction for the Drug of Enrolment ($n = 138, 69.0\%$)	2) Health Care Provider Adhered to DPWG Guideline ($n = 49, 24.5\%$) *	3) Health Care Providers did not Adhere to DPWG Guideline ($n = 9, 4.5\%$) *
Gender					
Female, n (%)	103 (51.5)	74 (53.6)	25 (51.0)	3 (33.3)	
Male, n (%)	97 (48.5)	64 (46.4)	24 (49.0)	6 (66.8)	
Age in years, Mean (SD)	61.6 (11.2)	62.3 (11.0)	60.9 (11.5)	56.8 (13.3)	
BMI (kg/m^2), Mean (SD)	28.3 (14.9)	28.9 (17.7)	27.1 (4.5)	27.4 (2.4)	
Self-reported ethnicity father, n (%)					
Caucasian	187 (93.5)	128 (92.8)	47 (95.9)	9 (100.0)	
Other	13 (6.5)	10 (7.2)	2 (4.1)	0 (0.0)	
Self-reported ethnicity mother, n (%)					
Caucasian	188 (94.0)	129 (93.5)	47 (95.9)	9 (100.0)	
Other	12 (6.0)	9 (6.5)	2 (4.1)	0 (0.0)	
Drug of enrolment, n (%)					
Amitriptyline	15 (7.5)	9 (6.5)	5 (10.2)	0 (0.0)	
Atorvastatin	115 (57.5)	80 (58.0)	28 (57.1)	5 (55.6)	
Citalopram	7 (3.5)	5 (3.6)	1 (2.0)	0 (0.0)	
Escitalopram	3 (1.5)	2 (1.4)	1 (2.0)	0 (0.0)	
Nortriptyline	17 (8.5)	10 (7.2)	5 (10.2)	2 (22.2)	
Simvastatin	29 (14.5)	26 (18.8)	2 (4.1)	1 (11.1)	
Venlafaxine	14 (7.0)	6 (4.3)	7 (14.3)	1 (11.1)	
Number of comorbidities at baseline, Mean (SD) **	4.6 (2.5)	4.4 (2.4)	4.9 (2.6)	4.4 (2.3)	
Number of comedications at baseline, Mean (SD) **	4.0 (3.3)	3.93 (3.4)	4.0 (2.9)	4.4 (3.0)	

IP3: Implementation of Pharmacogenetics into Primary care Project; SD: standard deviation; BMI: body mass index; * Excluding others ($n = 4$): Recommendation given after drug was discontinued ($n = 1$); same dose ($n = 1$); dose increased and ECG unknown ($n = 1$); no drug-gene interaction and no action ($n = 1$). ** Based on $n = 177$ for whom data collection from GP records was completed.

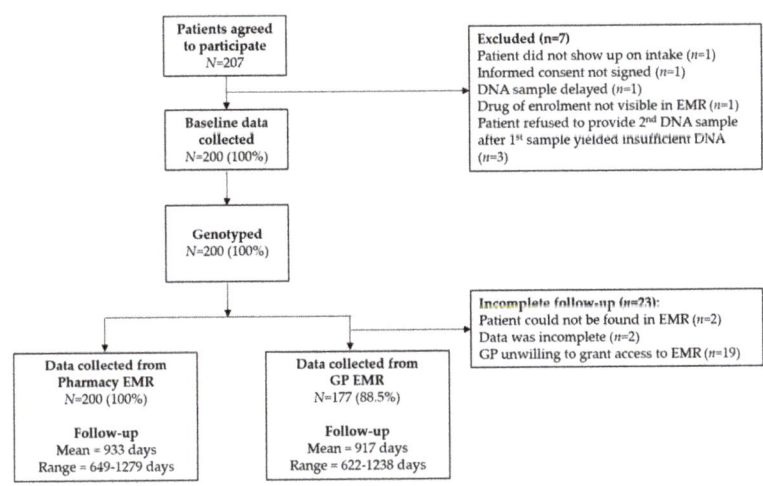

Figure 2. Flow chart or IP3 participant enrolment and follow-up.

3.2. Feasibility: Record of PGx Panel Results in the Pharmacy and GP EMRs

Record of PGx panel results by both pharmacists and GPs are shown in Figure 3. Pharmacists were able to record predicted phenotypes (including EMs) in 96.0% ($n = 192$) of pharmacy EMRs. In all cases they were recorded as contra-indications (100%, $n = 192$). Pharmacists failed to document the PGx results in 4.0% of cases ($n = 8$). The most common reason for failure of documentation (2.0%, $n = 4$) was merely due to PGx paper reports being lost in the pharmacy. The second most common reason was that the individual did not carry any aberrant variant, and was therefore predicted wildtype for all genes; this was the case for three patients (1.5%, $n = 3$). Pharmacists, therefore, felt it was not necessary to record EM phenotypes. Only one set of PGx results was failed to be documented in the EMR since the pharmacist did not know how to (0.5%). A discrepancy between the reported results and documented results was found in the records of two patients (1.0%). This was due to a manual error on account of the pharmacist.

General practitioners were able to record the PGx results in 67.8% ($n = 120$) of patient records. Of these, 34% ($n = 59$) were recorded as contra-indications and 35% ($n = 61$) in another format such as a PDF file.

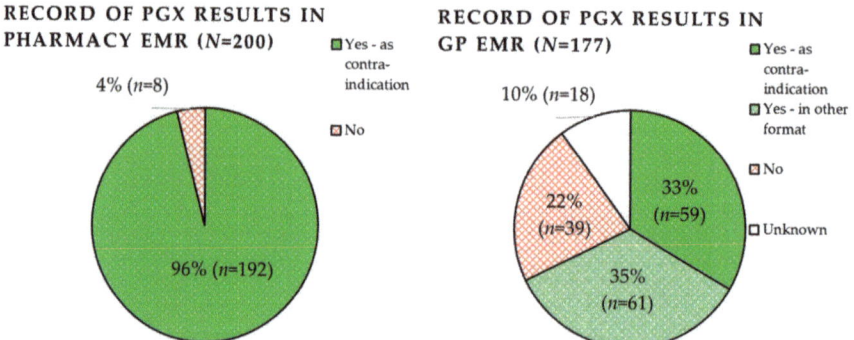

Figure 3. Record of pharmacogenetic panel results in the pharmacy and general practitioner (GP) electronic medical records (EMRs).

3.3. Real-World Impact: Frequency of Newly Prescribed Drugs for Which PGx Results Were Available in the EMR

Table 2 shows the frequency of newly initiated drugs for which there were potential drug-gene interactions and PGx results were available in the EMR. 97.0% ($n = 194$) of patients received at least one subsequent drug for which PGx results were in the EMR. Within the follow-up time, a mean of 2.71 drugs for which the PGx results were available were prescribed, of these 0.66 (24.2%) were actionable drug-gene interactions, requiring pharmacotherapy adjustment. The most commonly prescribed drugs for which PGx results were available were atorvastatin (14.4%), simvastatin (9.4%) and pantoprazole (9.4%). The most common drugs which were actionable drug-gene interactions, however, were atorvastatin (28.2%), metoprolol (13.0%) and amitriptyline (8.4%). To explore who may benefit most from PGx-panel testing, Table 3 presents baseline demographics stratified by an increasing number of newly initiated drugs for which there were potential drug-gene interaction. It seems that the number of newly initiated prescriptions increases with age, number of comorbidities and number of comedications, but this could not be statistically concluded.

Table 2. Frequency of newly initiated drugs for which there were potential drug-gene interactions in subsequent prescriptions after pharmacogenetics panel in 200 primary care patients with a mean follow-up of 933 days (=2.56 years).

	Number of Patients (%)	Three Most Commonly Prescribed with Potential Drug-Gene Interaction, N (%)	Actionable Drug-Gene Interaction (%)	Three Most Commonly Prescribed with Actionable Drug-Gene Interactions, N (%)
Subsequent drug 1	194 (97%)	1. atorvastatin, 69 (35.6%) 2. omeprazole, 26 (13.4%) 3. pantoprazole, 20 (10.3%)	47 (24.2%)	1. atorvastatin, 19 (40.4%) 2. amitriptyline, 11 (23.4%) 3. citalopram, 6 (12.8%)
Subsequent drug 2	166 (83%)	1. atorvastatin, 32 (19,3%) 2. metoprolol, 29 (17.5%) 3. simvastatin, 21 (12.7%)	46 (27.7%)	1. atorvastatin, 14 (30.4%) 2. metoprolol, 10 (21.7%) 3. codeine, 6 (13.0%)
Subsequent drug 3	115 (57.5%)	1. pantoprazole, 20 (17.4%) 2. omeprazole, 19 (16.5%) 3. simvastatin, 15 (13.0%)	23 (20.0%)	1. metoprolol, 7 (30.4%) 2. simvastatin, 4 (17.4%) 3. codeine/venlafaxine, 3 (13.0%)
Subsequent drug 4	66 (33%)	1. simvastatin, 15 (22.7%) 2. pantoprazole, 11 (16.7%) 3. atorvastatin, 9 (13.6%)	15 (22.7%)	1. atorvastatin, 4 (26.7%) 2. venlafaxine/simvastatin/clopidogrel, 2 (13.3%) 3. citalopram/omeprazole/codeine/flecainide/metoprolol, 1 (6.7%)
Overall	541	1. atorvastatin, 78 (14.4%) 2. simvastatin, 51 (9.4%) 3. pantoprazole, 51 (9.4%)	131 (24.2%)	1. atorvastatin, 37 (28.2%) 2. metoprolol, 17 (13.0%) 3. amitriptyline, 11 (8.4%)
Mean per patient (SD)	2.71 (1.1)	-	0.66 (0.8)	-

SD: standard deviation.

Table 3. IP3 cohort stratified by number of newly initiated drugs with a potential drug-gene interaction within follow-up.

	Overall IP3 Study Cohort (n = 200)	0 (n = 6, 3%)	1 (n = 27, 13.5%)	2 (n = 52, 26%)	3 (n = 50, 25%)	≥4 (n = 65, 32.5%)	p-Value *
Gender							0.775
Female, n (%)	103 (51.5)	4 (66.7)	12 (44.4)	24 (46.2)	27 (54.0)	36 (55.4)	
Male, n (%)	97 (48.5)	2 (33.3)	15 (55.6)	28 (53.8)	23 (46.0)	29 (44.6)	
Age in years, Mean (SD)	61.6 (11.2)	53.3 (16.3)	59.4 (10.6)	61.0 (11.5)	63.0 (10.5)	62.8 (11.1)	0.442
BMI (kg/m^2), Mean (SD)	28.3 (14.9)	25.6 (2.6)	29.1 (5.8)	27.4 (4.5)	27.6 (4.8)	29.6 (25.2)	0.854
Number of comorbidities at baseline, Mean (SD) **	4.6 (2.5)	3.4 (1.1)	4.0 (2.2)	4.0 (2.5)	4.6 (2.3)	5.4 (2.6)	0.232
Number of comedications at baseline, Mean (SD) **	4.0 (3.3)	3.0 (2.1)	3.4 (3.4)	3.3 (3.4)	3.8 (2.7)	5.1 (3.4)	0.279

SD: standard deviation; BMI: body mass index; * Univariate negative binomial regression; ** Based on n = 177 for whom data collection from GP records was completed.

3.4. Real-World Impact: Downstream Effects of Actionable Drug-Gene Interactions on Healthcare Utilization

Table 4 shows that patients who encountered an actionable drug-gene interaction and whose health care providers adhered to the DPWG guidelines had a similar healthcare utilization as a result of a drug-gene interactions associated adverse drug reaction (40.0%) to those who did not carry an actionable drug-gene interaction (30.0%). This in line with our initial hypothesis. The 95%-CIs of the incidence of composite endpoint drug-gene interactions associated adverse drug reaction of groups 1 and 2 overlap. We therefore observe that there is no difference between the two groups. However, we cannot demonstrate non-inferiority since the upper limit of the 95%-CI of the OR of group 1 is not lower than the non-inferiority margin of 1.2.

We observed a much lower healthcare utilization as a result of a drug-gene interactions associated adverse drug reactions among patients carrying an actionable drug-gene interaction but whose health care providers did not adhere to the DPWG guidelines (0.0%) to those who did not carry an actionable drug-gene interaction (30.0%). This is in contrast to our initial hypothesis.

Table 4. Healthcare utilization as a result of drug-gene interaction associated adverse drug reactions within 12 weeks of enrolment.

	Overall IP3 Study Cohort $n = 200$	1) No Drug-Gene Interaction for the Drug of Enrolment $n = 138$ (69.0%)	Actionable Drug-Gene Interaction for the Drug of Enrolment	
			2) Health Care Provider Adhered to DPWG Guideline $n = 49$ (24.5%)	3) Health Care Provider did not Adhere to DPWG Guideline $n = 9$ (4.5%)
GP EMR follow-up completed (%)	177 (88.5%)	120 (87.0%)	45 (91.8%)	8 (88.9%)
Number of patients experiencing drug-gene interactions associated adverse drug reactions	56 (31.6%)	37 (30.8%)	19 (43.2%)	0 (0.0%)
Composite endpoint drug-gene interactions associated adverse drug reactions				
Number of patients, n (%)	54 (30.5%)	36 (30.0%)	18 (40.0%)	0 (0.0%)
95% CI		66.0%–80.6%	47.1%–73.7%	
GP consults as a result of drug-gene interactions associated adverse drug reactions				
Number of patients, n (%)	52 (29.4%)	35 (29.2%)	17 (37.8%)	0 (0.0%)
Number of GP consults, Mean (SD)	53, 2.19 (2.11)	35, 2.06 (1.99)	18, 2.44 (2.36)	0, 0 (0)
ER visit as a result of drug-gene interactions associated adverse drug reactions				
Number of patients, n (%)	3 (1.7%)	1 (0.8%)	2 (4.4%)	0 (0%)
Number of ER visits, Mean (SD)	3, 1 (1)	1, 1 (1)	2, 1 (1)	0, 0 (0)
Hospitalization as a result of drug-gene interactions associated adverse drug reactions				
Number of patients, n (%)	1 (0.6%)	1 (0.6%)	0 (0.0%)	0 (0.0%)
Number of hosp., Mean (SD)	1, 1 (1)	1, 1 (1)	0, 0 (0)	0, 0 (0)
Binomial Logistic Regression (group 1 and 2) OR [95%CI] *		1.81 [0.89, 3.67]		

GP: general practitioner; OR: odd ratio; CI: confidence interval; * Including gender, age, and BMI as covariates.

4. Discussion

We report what is, to our knowledge, the first assessment of the real-world impact of pharmacist-initiated pre-emptive panel-based testing in primary care. This side-study demonstrates that recording of PGx panel results in the EMR is feasible and enables health care providers to (re)use these results to inform pharmacotherapy of newly initiated prescriptions. 96% of PGx panel results were successfully recorded in the pharmacy EMR, enabling 97% of patients to (re)use these results for at least one, and 33% of patients for up to four newly initiated prescriptions, within a relatively short 2.5-year follow-up. Of all newly initiated prescriptions with a potential drug-gene interaction ($n = 541$), 24.2% ($n = 131$) were actionable drug-gene interactions, requiring pharmacotherapy adjustment. We expect the potential impact of pre-emptive panel-based testing to further increase with time as the likelihood of additional subsequent prescriptions increases.

With their dedication to medication surveillance, pharmacists are leading candidates to manage requesting of PGx testing, recording of PGx results and application of the PGx guidelines. This is confirmed by other pilot studies performed in pharmacy settings [31–35]. However, we found that both pharmacists and GPs are very able to record PGx results in their EMRs as contra-indications (96% and 33% of pharmacists and GPs, respectively); enabling deployment of relevant guidelines by the clinical decision support system when a drug-gene interaction is encountered both at prescribing and dispensing. An advantage of applying this double-verification is the minimization of the risk of missing a drug-gene interaction. As a result, it is not disastrous that GPs also recorded them in other formats, thereby not enabling the clinical decision support system at prescribing, in 35% of cases. In contrast, a recent study showed that genotyping results were sparsely communicated and recorded correctly; only 3.1% and 5.9% of reported genotyping results were recorded by GPs and pharmacists, respectively, within a similar follow-up time [20]. The discrepancy between these could be due to the pilot study setting or differences in PGx reporting methods. IP3 study researchers have visited the participating IP3 pharmacies multiple times within the follow-up period; possibly unintentionally reminding or motivating pharmacists to record PGx results, which they may otherwise have not performed. However, it is important to note that GPs were outside the scope of the pilot study setting, as they were not the enrolling health care providers, and therefore provide a less biased perspective on recording frequency. Still, it is much higher than that reported by Simoons et al. [20]. Surprisingly, 1.5% of PGx results were not recorded by pharmacists because they did not include actionable genotypes. However, it is still of importance to document these results to avoid unnecessary re-testing of the patient. Finally, the fact that discrepancies between reported results and the recorded result were only observed in 1% of pharmacy EMR cases, indicates that the current manual system of recording is error prone. Regardless of the low error rate, PGx results are static and therefore life-long. It is therefore imperative that errors in the recording of PGx results are avoided. Future initiatives should focus on the development of automated sharing of PGx results across EMRs. In the Netherlands, such an initiative has been the launched but requires patient consent before it can be utilized. The National Exchange Point ("Landelijk Schakel Punt" (LSP)) is a nationwide secured EMR infrastructure to which nearly health care providers access [36]. Only when a patient has provided written consent for the LSP, can a professional summary of the local pharmacy or GP EMR, including PGx results, be downloaded by another treating health care provider in the same region; unless the patient chose to shield this information. Alternatively, providing the PGx results directly to patients may resolve the issue in terms of communicating and recording PGx results; for example, utilizing the Medication Safety-Code card [37,38].

In the face of a time in which health care providers are confronted with an increasing number of variables to optimize clinical decision making, it is of utmost importance that this information is presented in a structured fashion; this is achieved by a clinical decision support system [39,40]. PGx testing results differ from other laboratory testing results because they remain applicable over a patient's lifetime. We have demonstrated that, even within a relatively short follow-up, the real-world impact of a panel-based approach combined with a clinical decision support system is immense; almost all (97%) of patients used PGx results for at least one, and 33% of patients for up to four prescriptions within a relatively short 2.5-year follow-up. Of these, 24.2% ($n = 131$) were actionable drug-gene interactions. Similar proportions of actionable drug-gene interactions in primary care were found by Bank et al. (unpublished) [41]. Here, investigators overlaid the frequencies of phenotypes as observed within the IP3 cohort with nationwide prescription data spanning one year and found that 3.6 million incident prescriptions encountered a potential drug-gene interactions and of these, 856,002 (23.6%) encountered an actionable drug-gene interaction [41]. We observed drugs for which results were useful; these were primarily statins and proton pump inhibitors. This finding is in accordance with Samwald et al. [28]. The observed frequencies of potential drug-gene interactions, however, are much higher than reported by others previously [19,28]. Samwald et al. indicated half of the patients above 65 will use at least one of the drugs for which PGx guidelines are available during a four year period, and one fourth to one third will use two or more of these drugs [28]. Schildcrout et al. reported that 60% of the population would benefit from PGx guided prescribing within a 5-year period [19]. The higher frequency we observed could be a result of different target populations and drugs. Our sample consisted of patients selected by pharmacist and who initiated one of ten drugs, and therefore at higher risk for initiating subsequent drugs. Several promising studies indicate the effectiveness and effect of PGx panel-based testing on healthcare utilization in psychiatry and polypharmacy [22–27]. For example, Brixner et al. studied the effect of panel-based PGx testing with 6 genes on the healthcare utilization within polypharmacy patients. Results showed that the

PGx screened cohort had a lower rate of ER visits (RR = 0.29, 95% confidence interval (CI) = 0.15–0.55, $p = 0.0002$) and a lower rate of hospitalizations (relative risk (RR) of 0.61, 95% CI = 0.39–0.95, $p = 0.027$). With this decrease in ER visits and hospitalizations, the authors concluded that PGx panel-based testing could potentially lead to cost-savings [23]. These cost savings may be potentially higher than that observed in primary care since polypharmacy patients have a higher a priori risk of hospitalization, as it increases with the number of comedications [42]. In this study we aimed to assess the downstream effects of an actionable drug-gene interaction on healthcare utilization. Although we did not observe a statistically significant difference between groups 1 (40%) and 2 (30%), we were not able to conclude non-inferiority, since this is a side-study by design and therefore was underpowered for a non-inferiority analysis. In contrast to our initial hypothesis we observed a much lower healthcare utilization among group 3 (0%) patients when compared to group 2 (30%). However, this cannot be concluded, since the adherence rate of HCPs was high, thereby resulting in a relatively low number of patients carrying an actionable DGI but whose HCPs did not adhere to the DPWG guidelines. Another limitation to this analysis is the retrospectively collected data from GP EMRs, which is prone to reporting bias. Nonetheless, gold-standard evidence demonstrating (cost-)effectiveness of this approach is required to convince stakeholders of population-wide implementation. An RCT aiming to generate such evidence is underway [21].

However, questions regarding who should be tested, and when it is most cost effective to perform pre-emptive panel testing, remain unanswered. In this side-study, we have chosen to perform pre-emptive panel testing among those who received a first prescription for one of ten drugs. Here, there is an initial delay of PGx testing results for the first prescription, but PGx results can be used uninterrupted, if recorded in the EMR, when future drug-gene interactions are encountered. On the one hand, it may be more cost-effective to perform population-wide testing at birth, to ensure maximization of instances in which a PGx result is available when a drug-gene interaction is encountered. In contrast to our approach, not one prescription will be delayed as a result of PGx testing. On the other hand, some may never encounter drug-gene interactions, thereby unintentionally wasting resources on PGx testing. To shed light on this issue, some have predicted which patients may benefit from PGx testing in the near future algorithmically and using prescription data [43,44]. Others have modelled the cost-effectiveness of testing a 40-year old for life-long prevention of adverse drug reactions using a Markov model [45]. Overall, a consensus has not been reached regarding whom and when to test [16]. Within this side-study we observe the number of newly initiated prescriptions, and thus potential benefit of panel testing, increases with age, number of comorbidities and number of comedications, although this was not statistically significant. However, since 97% of this cohort made re-use of their panel results, we may conclude that the in- and exclusion criteria of this study may be successful criteria in selecting patients who will further benefit from panel testing. The most cost-effective target groups applicable for panel testing must be further investigated.

In addition to unanswered timing and application of testing, the variants selected to be included in a PGx panel also require additional curation. Recently, the DPWG has provided a suggested panel (van der Wouden et al., unpublished) [46]. Here, variants included in the panel reflect the entire set of existing DPWG guidelines and are continuously updated as the field of PGx expands. It will be of utmost importance to record the version number of the tested panel, so that it can be retrieved which variants were tested within a specific gene. Moreover, the most cost-effective technique used to determine the PGx profile is also undetermined. As the cost of next-generation sequencing decreases, we envision a future in which we may be able to extract relevant PGx variant alleles from sequencing data [47], possibly making genotype based testing redundant. If this is to come into fruition, the determining the cost-effectiveness of implementing PGx testing will become redundant, as the information on PGx variants become secondary findings, free of additional costs. In this case, only effectiveness will be of interest. Overall, the cost-effectiveness of a panel-approach is a dependant on many variables including the target population, timing, tested variants and testing technique.

5. Conclusions

Both pharmacists and GPs are very able to record PGx results into their respective EMRs, thereby maximizing the potential benefits of PGx results when deployed by the clinical decision support system in future prescriptions. Within this cohort, almost all patients were able to benefit from the availability of the PGx-panel results in their EMR, indicating that the real-world impact of a panel approach is immense. The downstream impact on healthcare utilization was unable to be concluded due to the small sample size. Ongoing research will quantify the effects of pre-emptive panel-based testing on patient outcomes [21]. Future research should focus on assessing the most cost-effective approach regarding timing, target population, variants and techniques for PGx testing. Regardless, we argue that in terms of logistics, delivery through a clinical decision support system is most feasible.

Supplementary Materials: The following are available online at http://www.mdpi.com/2073-4425/10/6/416/s1, Table S1: The tested PGx Panel in the IP3 pilot study. Table S2: Actionable drug-gene interactions relevant to the panel used. Table S3: Pre-defined drug-gene associated adverse drug reactions based on literature underlying the DPWG. Figure S1: Example report sent to physicians and pharmacists.

Author Contributions: Conceptualization, C.H.v.d.W., P.C.D.B., K.O., J.J.S. and H.J.G..; methodology, C.H.v.d.W., P.C.D.B., K.O., J.J.S. and H.J.G..; formal analysis, C.H.v.d.W., P.C.D.B., K.O., J.J.S. and H.J.G.; writing—original draft preparation, C.H.v.d.W.; writing—review and editing, C.H.v.d.W., P.C.D.B., K.O., J.J.S. and H.J.G.; visualization, C.H.v.d.W., P.C.D.B., K.O., J.J.S. and H.J.G.; supervision, J.J.S. and H.J.G.; project administration, C.H.v.d.W., P.C.D.B., K.O., J.J.S. and H.J.G.; funding acquisition, P.C.D.B., J.J.S., H.J.G.

Funding: The research leading to these results has received funding from the European Community's Horizon 2020 Programme under grant agreement No.668353 (U-PGx). This work was also supported by unrestricted grants from The Royal Dutch Pharmacist's Association, The Hague (KNMP), The Netherlands and Zorg en Zekerheid, Leiden, The Netherlands.

Acknowledgments: We would like to thank Stefan Böhringer for providing statistical advice. We would like to thank Rowena Schaap, Daniëlle Klootwijk, and Renée Baak-Pablo for their assistance in sample handling and analysis. We would also like to thank Noortje Stijntjes for her assistance in the collection of the follow-up data from pharmacy records. Finally, we would also like to thank Stephan Joosten for providing Figure 1.

Conflicts of Interest: The authors declare no conflict of interest.

References

1. Relling, M.V.; Evans, W.E. Pharmacogenomics in the clinic. *Nature* **2015**, *526*, 343–350. [CrossRef] [PubMed]
2. Weinshilboum, R.; Wang, L. Pharmacogenomics: Bench to bedside. *Nat. Rev. Drug Discov.* **2004**, *3*, 739–748. [CrossRef]
3. Wu, A.H. Pharmacogenomic testing and response to warfarin. *Lancet* **2015**, *385*. [CrossRef]
4. Pirmohamed, M. Personalized pharmacogenomics: Predicting efficacy and adverse drug reactions. *Annu. Rev. Genom. Hum. Genet.* **2014**, *15*, 349–370. [CrossRef]
5. Pirmohamed, M.; Burnside, G.; Eriksson, N.; Jorgensen, A.L.; Toh, C.H.; Nicholson, T.; Kesteven, P.; Christersson, C.; Wahlstrom, B.; Stafberg, C.; et al. A randomized trial of genotype-guided dosing of warfarin. *N. Engl. J. Med.* **2013**, *369*, 2294–2303. [CrossRef] [PubMed]
6. Verhoef, T.I.; Ragia, G.; de Boer, A.; Barallon, R.; Kolovou, G.; Kolovou, V.; Konstantinides, S.; Le Cessie, S.; Maltezos, E.; van der Meer, F.J.; et al. A randomized trial of genotype-guided dosing of acenocoumarol and phenprocoumon. *N. Engl. J. Med.* **2013**, *369*, 2304–2312. [CrossRef] [PubMed]
7. Coenen, M.J.; de Jong, D.J.; van Marrewijk, C.J.; Derijks, L.J.; Vermeulen, S.H.; Wong, D.R.; Klungel, O.H.; Verbeek, A.L.; Hooymans, P.M.; Peters, W.H.; et al. Identification of patients with variants in TPMT and dose reduction reduces hematologic events during thiopurine treatment of inflammatory bowel disease. *Gastroenterology* **2015**, *149*, 907–917. [CrossRef]
8. Mallal, S.; Phillips, E.; Carosi, G.; Molina, J.M.; Workman, C.; Tomazic, J.; Jagel-Guedes, E.; Rugina, S.; Kozyrev, O.; Cid, J.F.; et al. HLA-B*5701 screening for hypersensitivity to abacavir. *N. Engl. J. Med.* **2008**, *358*. [CrossRef]
9. Altman, R.B. Pharmacogenomics: "Noninferiority" is sufficient for initial implementation. *Clin. Pharmacol. Ther.* **2011**, *89*, 348–350. [CrossRef] [PubMed]

10. Pirmohamed, M.; Hughes, D.A. Pharmacogenetic tests: The need for a level playing field. *Nat. Rev. Drug Discov.* **2013**, *12*, 3–4. [CrossRef]
11. Swen, J.J.; Nijenhuis, M.; de Boer, A.; Grandia, L.; Maitland-van der Zee, A.H.; Mulder, H.; Rongen, G.A.; van Schaik, R.H.; Schalekamp, T.; Touw, D.J.; et al. Pharmacogenetics: From bench to byte—An update of guidelines. *Clin. Pharmacol. Ther.* **2011**, *89*, 662–673. [CrossRef]
12. Swen, J.J.; Wilting, I.; de Goede, A.L.; Grandia, L.; Mulder, H.; Touw, D.J.; de Boer, A.; Conemans, J.M.; Egberts, T.C.; Klungel, O.H.; et al. Pharmacogenetics: From bench to byte. *Clin. Pharmacol. Ther.* **2008**, *83*, 781–787. [CrossRef] [PubMed]
13. Relling, M.V.; Klein, T.E. CPIC: Clinical pharmacogenetics implementation consortium of the pharmacogenomics research network. *Clin. Pharmacol. Ther.* **2011**, *89*. [CrossRef] [PubMed]
14. Bank, P.; Caudle, K.E.; Swen, J.J.; Gammal, R.S.; Whirl-Carrillo, M.; Klein, T.E.; Relling, M.V.; Guchelaar, H.J. Comparison of the guidelines of the clinical pharmacogenetics implementation consortium and the dutch pharmacogenetics working group. *Clin. Pharmacol. Ther.* **2018**, *103*, 599–618. [CrossRef] [PubMed]
15. Weitzel, K.W.; Cavallari, L.H.; Lesko, L.J. Preemptive panel-based pharmacogenetic testing: The time is now. *Pharm. Res.* **2017**, *34*, 1551–1555. [CrossRef]
16. Roden, D.M.; Van Driest, S.L.; Mosley, J.D.; Wells, Q.S.; Robinson, J.R.; Denny, J.C.; Peterson, J.F. Benefit of preemptive pharmacogenetic information on clinical outcome. *Clin. Pharmacol. Ther.* **2018**, *103*, 787–794. [CrossRef]
17. Verbelen, M.; Weale, M.E.; Lewis, C.M. Cost-effectiveness of pharmacogenetic-guided treatment: Are we there yet? *Pharmacogenom. J.* **2017**. [CrossRef] [PubMed]
18. Swen, J.J.; Nijenhuis, M.; van Rhenen, M.; de Boer-Veger, N.J.; Buunk, A.-M.M.; Houwink, E.J.F.J.F.; Mulder, H.; Rongen, G.A.; van Schaik, R.H.N.H.N.; van der Weide, J.; et al. Pharmacogenetic information in clinical guidelines: The European perspective. *Clin. Pharmacol. Ther.* **2018**, *103*, 795–801. [CrossRef] [PubMed]
19. Schildcrout, J.S.; Denny, J.C.; Bowton, E.; Gregg, W.; Pulley, J.M.; Basford, M.A.; Cowan, J.D.; Xu, H.; Ramirez, A.H.; Crawford, D.C.; et al. Optimizing drug outcomes through pharmacogenetics: A case for preemptive genotyping. *Clin. Pharmacol. Ther.* **2012**, *92*, 235–242. [CrossRef] [PubMed]
20. Simoons, M.; Mulder, H.; Schoevers, R.A.; Ruhe, H.G.; van Roon, E.N. Availability of CYP2D6 genotyping results in general practitioner and community pharmacy medical records. *Pharmacogenomics* **2017**, *18*, 843–851. [CrossRef]
21. Van der Wouden, C.H.; Cambon-Thomsen, A.; Cecchin, E.; Cheung, K.C.; Dávila-Fajardo, C.L.; Deneer, V.H.; Dolžan, V.; Ingelman-Sundberg, M.; Jönsson, S.; Karlsson, M.O.; et al. Implementing pharmacogenomics in Europe: Design and implementation strategy of the ubiquitous pharmacogenomics consortium. *Clin. Pharmacol. Ther.* **2017**, *101*, 341–358. [CrossRef]
22. Elliott, L.S.; Henderson, J.C.; Neradilek, M.B.; Moyer, N.A.; Ashcraft, K.C.; Thirumaran, R.K. Clinical impact of pharmacogenetic profiling with a clinical decision support tool in polypharmacy home health patients: A prospective pilot randomized controlled trial. *PLoS ONE* **2017**, *12*, e0170905. [CrossRef] [PubMed]
23. Brixner, D.; Biltaji, E.; Bress, A.; Unni, S.; Ye, X.; Mamiya, T.; Ashcraft, K.; Biskupiak, J. The effect of pharmacogenetic profiling with a clinical decision support tool on healthcare resource utilization and estimated costs in the elderly exposed to polypharmacy. *J. Med. Econ.* **2015**, *19*, 213–228. [CrossRef]
24. Finkelstein, J.; Friedman, C.; Hripcsak, G.; Cabrera, M. Potential utility of precision medicine for older adults with polypharmacy: A case series study. *Pharmacogenom. Pers. Med.* **2016**, *9*, 31–45. [CrossRef]
25. Saldivar, J.-S.; Taylor, D.; Sugarman, E.; Cullors, A.; Garces, J.; Oades, K.; Centeno, J. Initial assessment of the benefits of implementing pharmacogenetics into the medical management of patients in a long-term care facility. *Pharmacogenom. Pers. Med.* **2016**, *9*, 1–6. [CrossRef]
26. Pérez, V.; Salavert, A.; Espadaler, J.; Tuson, M.; Saiz-Ruiz, J.; Sáez-Navarro, C.; Bobes, J.; Baca-García, E.; Vieta, E.; Olivares, J.M.M.; et al. Efficacy of prospective pharmacogenetic testing in the treatment of major depressive disorder: Results of a randomized, double-blind clinical trial. *BMC Psychiatry* **2017**, *17*, 250. [CrossRef] [PubMed]
27. Espadaler, J.; Tuson, M.; Lopez-Ibor, J.M.; Lopez-Ibor, F.; Lopez-Ibor, M.I. Pharmacogenetic testing for the guidance of psychiatric treatment: A multicenter retrospective analysis. *CNS Spectr.* **2017**, *22*, 315–324. [CrossRef] [PubMed]

28. Samwald, M.; Xu, H.; Blagec, K.; Empey, P.E.; Malone, D.C.; Ahmed, S.M.; Ryan, P.; Hofer, S.; Boyce, R.D. Incidence of exposure of patients in the United States to multiple drugs for which pharmacogenomic guidelines are available. *PLoS ONE* **2016**, *11*, e0164972. [CrossRef]
29. Bank, P.C.; Swen, J.J.; Schaap, R.D.; Klootwijk, D.B.; Baak-Pablo, R.F.; Guchelaar, H.J. A pilot study of the implementation of pharmacogenomic pharmacist initiated pre-emptive testing in primary care. *Eur. J. Hum. Genet.* **2019**. Accepted.
30. Link, E.; Parish, S.; Armitage, J.; Bowman, L.; Heath, S.; Matsuda, F.; Gut, I.; Lathrop, M.; Collins, R. SLCO1B1 variants and statin-induced myopathy—A genomewide study. *N. Engl. J. Med.* **2008**, *359*, 789–799. [CrossRef] [PubMed]
31. Dawes, M.; Aloise, M.N.; Ang, S.J.; Cullis, P.; Dawes, D.; Fraser, R.; Liknaitzky, G.; Paterson, A.; Stanley, P.; Suarez-Gonzalez, A.; et al. Introducing pharmacogenetic testing with clinical decision support into primary care: A feasibility study. *CMAJ Open* **2016**, *4*. [CrossRef] [PubMed]
32. Swen, J.J.; van der Straaten, T.; Wessels, J.A.; Bouvy, M.L.; Vlassak, E.E.; Assendelft, W.J.J.; Guchelaar, H.J.J. Feasibility of pharmacy-initiated pharmacogenetic screening for CYP2D6 and CYP2C19. *Eur. J. Clin. Pharmacol.* **2012**, *68*, 363–370. [CrossRef] [PubMed]
33. Ferreri, S.P.; Greco, A.J.; Michaels, N.M.; O'Connor, S.K.; Chater, R.W.; Viera, A.J.; Faruki, H.; McLeod, H.L.; Roederer, M.W. Implementation of a pharmacogenomics service in a community pharmacy. *J. Am. Pharm. Assoc.* **2014**, *54*, 172–180. [CrossRef] [PubMed]
34. Haga, S.B.; LaPointe, N.M.; Cho, A.; Reed, S.D.; Mills, R.; Moaddeb, J.; Ginsburg, G.S. Pilot study of pharmacist-assisted delivery of pharmacogenetic testing in a primary care setting. *Pharmacogenomics* **2014**, *15*, 1677–1686. [CrossRef]
35. Murray, M.E.; Barner, J.C.; Pope, N.D.; Comfort, M.D. Impact and feasibility of implementing a systematic approach for medication therapy management in the community pharmacy setting: A pilot study. *J. Pharm. Pract.* **2018**. [CrossRef]
36. Track your own healthcare with 'Volgjezorg'. Available online: https://www.volgjezorg.nl/en (accessed on 18 January 2019).
37. Samwald, M.; Minarro-Giménez, J.A.A.; Blagec, K.; Adlassnig, K.-P.P. Towards a global IT system for personalized medicine: The Medicine Safety Code initiative. *Stud. Health Technol. Inform.* **2014**, *205*, 261–265.
38. Blagec, K.; Koopmann, R.; Crommentuijn-van Rhenen, M.; Holsappel, I.; van der Wouden, C.H.; Konta, L.; Xu, H.; Steinberger, D.; Just, E.; Swen, J.J.; et al. Implementing pharmacogenomics decision support across seven European countries: The Ubiquitous Pharmacogenomics (U-PGx) project. *J. Am. Med. Inform. Assoc.* **2018**. [CrossRef]
39. Overby, C.L.; Erwin, A.L.; Abul-Husn, N.S.; Ellis, S.B.; Scott, S.A.; Obeng, A.O.; Kannry, J.L.; Hripcsak, G.; Bottinger, E.P.; Gottesman, O. Physician attitudes toward adopting genome-guided prescribing through clinical decision support. *J. Pers. Med.* **2014**, *4*. [CrossRef]
40. Bell, G.C.; Crews, K.R.; Wilkinson, M.R.; Haidar, C.E.; Hicks, J.K.; Baker, D.K.; Kornegay, N.M.; Yang, W.; Cross, S.J.; Howard, S.C.; et al. Development and use of active clinical decision support for preemptive pharmacogenomics. *J. Am. Med. Inform. Assoc.* **2014**. [CrossRef]
41. Bank, P.; Swen, J.; Guchelaar, H J. Nation-wide impact of implementing a pre-emptive pharmacogenetics panel approach to guide drug prescribing in primary care in The Netherlands (in submission). **2019**.
42. Leendertse, A.J.; Van Den Bemt, P.M.; Poolman, J.B.; Stoker, L.J.; Egberts, A.C.; Postma, M.J. Preventable hospital admissions related to medication (HARM): Cost analysis of the HARM study. *Value Health* **2011**, *14*, 34–40. [CrossRef]
43. Pulley, J.M.; Denny, J.C.; Peterson, J.F.; Bernard, G.R.; Jones, C.L.; Ramirez, A.H.; Delaney, J.T.; Bowton, E.; Brothers, K.; Johnson, K. Operational implementation of prospective genotyping for personalized medicine: The design of the Vanderbilt PREDICT project. *Clin. Pharmacol. Ther.* **2012**, *92*, 87–95. [CrossRef]
44. Grice, G.R.; Seaton, T.L.; Woodland, A.M.; McLeod, H.L. Defining the opportunity for pharmacogenetic intervention in primary care. *Pharmacogenomics* **2006**, *7*, 61–65. [CrossRef]
45. Alagoz, O.; Durham, D.; Kasirajan, K. Cost-effectiveness of one-time genetic testing to minimize lifetime adverse drug reactions. *Pharmacogenom. J.* **2015**, *16*, 129–136. [CrossRef]

46. Van der Wouden, C.H.; Van Rhenen, M.H.; Jama, W.; Ingelman-Sundberg, M.; Lauschke, V.M.; Konta, L.; Schwab, M.; Swen, J.; Guchelaar, H.J. Development of the PGx-passport: A panel of actionable germline genetic variants for pre-emptive pharmacogenetic testing (manuscript in preparation). 2019.
47. Yang, W.; Wu, G.; Broeckel, U.; Smith, C.A.; Turner, V.; Haidar, C.E.; Wang, S.; Carter, R.; Karol, S.E.; Neale, G.; et al. Comparison of genome sequencing and clinical genotyping for pharmacogenes. *Clin. Pharmacol. Ther.* **2016**, *100*. [CrossRef]

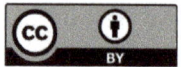

© 2019 by the authors. Licensee MDPI, Basel, Switzerland. This article is an open access article distributed under the terms and conditions of the Creative Commons Attribution (CC BY) license (http://creativecommons.org/licenses/by/4.0/).

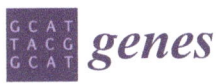

Review

Pharmacogenetics in the Treatment of Cardiovascular Diseases and Its Current Progress Regarding Implementation in the Clinical Routine

Cristina Lucía Dávila-Fajardo [1,*], Xando Díaz-Villamarín [1], Alba Antúnez-Rodríguez [2], Ana Estefanía Fernández-Gómez [1], Paloma García-Navas [1], Luis Javier Martínez-González [2], José Augusto Dávila-Fajardo [3] and José Cabeza Barrera [1]

[1] Department of Clinical Pharmacy, San Cecilio University Hospital, Institute for Biomedical Research, ibs.GRANADA, 18016 Granada, Spain; xandodv@gmail.com (X.D.-V.); estefania_fergo@hotmail.com (A.E.F.-G.); palomichi_96@hotmail.com (P.G.-N.); jose.cabeza.sspa@juntadeandalucia.es (J.C.B.)
[2] Genomics Unit, Centro Pfizer-Universidad de Granada-Junta de Andalucía de Genómica e Investigación Oncológica (Genyo), 18016 Granada, Spain; albantunez@gmail.com (A.A.-R.); luisjavier.martinez@genyo.es (L.J.M.-G.)
[3] English Department, Official Language School Leganes, 28915 Leganés, Madrid, Spain; josehood11@hotmail.com
* Correspondence: cristinal.davila.sspa@juntadeandalucia.es

Received: 8 February 2019; Accepted: 26 March 2019; Published: 1 April 2019

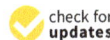

Abstract: There is a special interest in the implementation of pharmacogenetics in clinical practice, although there are some barriers that are preventing this integration. A large part of these pharmacogenetic tests are focused on drugs used in oncology and psychiatry fields and for antiviral drugs. However, the scientific evidence is also high for other drugs used in other medical areas, for example, in cardiology. In this article, we discuss the evidence and guidelines currently available on pharmacogenetics for clopidogrel, warfarin, acenocoumarol, and simvastatin and its implementation in daily clinical practice.

Keywords: pharmacogenetics; clopidogrel; warfarin; acenocoumarol

---

1. Introduction

In recent years, there have been important advances to understand how genetic variations are associated with the efficacy and/or toxicity of medicines. Some of these studies have been randomized clinical trials (RCT) for a variety of drug–gene combinations that have shown that the performance of pharmacogenetic tests before prescribing a medication can improve patient health outcomes [1–5]. For this reason, nowadays, there is an important need to generalize the clinical implementation of genomic medicine and pharmacogenetics (PGx).

There are some barriers that are preventing the integration of PGx in daily clinical practice [6]. Among them, we can highlight the lack of correlation between the different PGx guidelines and those published by other professional organizations (oncology, cardiology, etc.) [7], the lack of a clinically relevant PGx test panel, the need for training of health personnel and patients, and the lack of information on cost-effectiveness studies [8,9]. All of those reasons prevent physicians from demanding a proactive approach to PGx.

The most important PGx-based drug dosing guidelines are published by the Clinical Pharmacogenetics Implementation Consortium (CPIC), the Royal Dutch Association for the Advancement of Pharmacy—Pharmacogenetics Working Group (DPWG), and the Canadian

Pharmacogenomics Network for Drug Safety (CPNDS). In general, there is enough agreement between the guidelines in terms of pharmacotherapeutic recommendations, but there are some aspects in which there are discrepancies due to the methodology used to support the dose recommendations that should be taken into account [10]. A large part of these PGx tests are focused on drugs used in oncology, antiviral drugs [11], and psychiatry fields. However, the scientific evidence is also high for other drugs used in other medical areas, for example, in cardiology. In our opinion, clinical pharmacists are ideal candidates to translate the PGx to clinical practice since they are qualified to lead efforts to guide optimal drug selection and drug dosing based on those results. However, most of them are not fully aware of the advance in the knowledge of PGx and some advanced pharmacist functions in applying clinical pharmacogenetic may require specialized education, training, or experience.

In this article we discuss the most relevant evidence currently available on PGx of cardiovascular drugs, focusing on those drugs with available PGx information and genetic tests, and its implementation into daily clinical practice. In order to provide a thorough analysis, we chose well-defined criteria. We decided to use the Pharmacogenomics Knowledgebase (PharmGKB) [12], where strength of evidence is rated in levels ranging from 1–4, with level 1 meeting the highest criteria. Thus, for this review, we focused on clopidogrel, warfarin, acenocoumarol, and simvastatin, as all of them are considered as level 1 for at least one variant (Table 1).

Table 1. Drug-genes interactions reported in this article and the corresponding PGx guidelines and the level of evidence. CPIC: Clinical Pharmacogenetics Implementation Consortium, DPWG: Dutch Pharmacogenetics Working Group, CPNDS: Canadian Pharmacogenomics Network for Drug Safety.

Drugs	Genes	PGx Guidelines	Level of Evidence
Clopidogrel	CYP2C19	CPIC, DPWG	1A
Warfarin	CYP2C9, VKORC1	CPIC, CPNDS	1A
Acenocoumarol	CYP2C9, VKORC1, CYP4F2	DPWG	1B
Simvastatin	SLCO1B1	CPIC	1A

2. The Most Relevant Evidence in Pharmacogenetics of Drugs Used in Cardiology

2.1. Clopidogrel

Clopidogrel is a prodrug used as an antiplatelet in combination with acetylsalicylic acid in the treatment of acute coronary syndrome (ACS), including patients undergoing stent implantation after percutaneous coronary intervention (PCI) [13,14]. However, there is significant interpatient variability in the response of clopidogrel as a significant number of patients show high incidence of secondary cardiovascular events [15]. Several mechanisms were proposed for explaining the variable response to the drug, particularly when patients undergo PCI [16]. Subsequently, different genetic variants were associated with variability in response to the drug. The higher level of evidence is focused on the *CYP2C19* polymorphisms [17–21].

After absorption, 85% of the prodrug is inactivated by plasma esterases, and the remaining prodrug is activated in the liver by hepatic cytochrome isoenzymes. The conversion to its active metabolite depends partially on the CYP2C19 enzyme. Loss of function (LOF) *CYP2C19* alleles (*2 (rs424485), *3 (rs4986893), *4 (rs28399504), *5 (rs56337013), *6 (rs72552267), *7 (rs72558186), *8 (rs41291556), *9 (rs17884712), *10 (rs6413438), *22 (rs140278421), *24 (rs118203757), and *35 (rs12769205), mainly the *CYP2C19*2* variant due to the higher frequency, were associated with lower levels of active clopidogrel metabolite, reduced platelet inhibition, and higher rates of cardiovascular events [22]. The variant *CYP2C19*17* (rs12248560) is associated with a higher enzymatic activity, which means a lower on-treatment platelet reactivity [23–26] in response to clopidogrel when compared with homozygous wild-type carriers. However, *CYP2C19*2/*17* carriers exhibited an increased platelet reactivity in response to clopidogrel, as compared with CYP2C19*1/*1 carriers [27], although data need to be consistently replicated.

For this reason, in 2010, The US Food and Drug Administration (FDA)-approved drug label for clopidogrel warned that tests are available to identify patients who were CYP2C19 poor metabolizers and suggested an alternative treatment in these patients, as they may have reduced effectiveness of the drug, therefore increasing the chance of secondary cardiovascular event rates in ACS and PCI patients, compared with patients with normal CYP2C19 function [28]. The European Medicines Agency (EMA) was positioned in a very similar way.

Nowadays, there have been some published clinical trials, meta-analyses, intervention studies, and many observational studies supporting the evidence of genotyping patients for clopidogrel use in ACS and PCI (Tables 2 and 3).

Table 2. Main characteristics from the large scale clopidogrel studies included in this review. MACE: major adverse cardiovascular events, CV: cardiovascular, LOF: loss of function alleles, ST: stent thrombosis, PCI: percutaneous coronary intervention.

Ref	Year	Ethnic	Population Studied	n	PCI-Stent (%)	Follow up	Endpoint	Polymorphisms	Outcomes (LOF vs. no LOF)
High-risk patients (PCI-stent)									
Collet [29]	2009	Europeans	ACS	259	86	>4 years	MACE (CV death, ACS, urgent PCI)	CYP2C19*2	HR 5.38 (2.32-12.47) $p \leq 0.0001$
Mega [22]	2009	84% Europeans	ACS stent (TRITON)	1477	100	15 months	ST definite	CYP2C19*2	HR 6.04 (1.75-20.80) $p = 0.004$
							MACE (CV death, ACS, stroke)	CYP2C19*2	HR 1.53 (1.07-2.19) $p = 0.01$
							ST definite	CYP2C19*2	HR 3.09 (1.19-8.0) $p = 0.02$
Mega [17]	2010	84% Europeans	ACS stent (TRITON)	2905	100	15 months	MACE (CV death, ACS, stroke)	CYP2C19*2 and ABCB1	ABCB1 TT vs. CT/CC: HR 1.72 (1.22-2.44) $p = 0.002$ CYP2C19*2 + ABCB1 HR 1.97 (1.38-2.82) $p = 0.0002$
Simon [30]	2009	Europeans	ACS	2208	68.7	12 months	MACE (death any cause, ACS, stroke)	CYP2C19 and ABCB1	CYP2C19: HR 1.98 (1.10-3.58) ABCB1: HR 1.72 (1.20-2.47)
Sorich [31]	2010	84% Europeans	ACS stent (TRITON)	13608	100	15 months	MACE (CV death, ACS, stroke)	CYP2C19 LOF	OR 1.63 (1.45-1.81) $p < 0.0001$
Shuldiner [32]	2009	Europeans	PCI	227	100	12 months	MACE (CV death, ACS, stroke, PCI)	CYP2C19*2	HR 2.42 (1.18-4.99) $p = 0.02$
Wallentin [33]	2010	Europeans	ACS	10285	60	12 months	MACE (CV death, ACS, stroke)	CYP2C19	HR at 30 days: $p = 0.028$
								CYP2C19 and ABCB1	HR 1.2 (1.0-1.4) $p = 0.047$**
Low-risk patients									
Pare [34]	2010	Europeans-latin american	ACS stable	5059	14.5	12 months	MACE (CV death, ACS, stroke)	CYP2C19*2	$p = 0.32$

Data are showed as: OR: odds ratio, HR: hazard ratio, (95%CI), p-value, ** Data obtained from the frequencies of the groups.

Table 3. Main characteristics from the non RCT and RCT about clopidogrel included in this review. MACE: major adverse cardiovascular events, CV: cardiovascular, LOF: loss of function alleles, ST: stent thrombosis, MI: myocardial infarction.

Ref	Year	Ethnic	Population Studied	n	PCI-Stent (%)	Follow up	Endpoint	Polymorphisms	Outcomes (Intervention Group vs. Control Group)
Non RCT									
Sánchez-Ramos [35]	2016	Europeans	ACS-PCI-stent	719	100	1 year	MACE (CV death, ACS, stroke)	CYP2C19*2, *3 and ABCB1	HR 0.63 (0.41-0.97) p = 0.037 HR 0.61 (0.39-0.94) p = 0.02**
							ST definite	CYP2C19*2, *3 and ABCB1	HR 1.27 (0.08-20.2) p = 0.87
							Urgent revascularization*	CYP2C19*2, *3 and ABCB1	HR 0.63 (0.31-1.28) p = 0.20
RCT									
Shen [36]	2016	Asians	CAD-PCI	628	100	1 month 6 months 12 months	MACE (composite of death from any cause, myocardial infarction, or target vessel revascularization)	CYP2C19*2	1.3% vs. 5.6%, p = 0.003 3.2% vs. 7.8%, p = 0.012 4.2% vs. 9.4%, p = 0.010
Roberts (Rapid Gene) [37]	2012	Europeans	ACS or stable angina/stent	187	100	7 days	high on-treatment platelet reactivity	CYP2C19*2	0% vs. 30% p = 0.0092
Roberts (RAPID STEMI study) [38]	2015	Europeans	STEMI-stent	102	100	1 month	high on-treatment platelet reactivity	CYP2C19*2, *17 and ABCB1 TT	OR −0.15 p = 0.03
Xie [39]	2013	Asians	CAD-PCI	600	100	180 days	MACE (death from any cause, MI, stroke, ischemia)	CYP2C19*2, *3	1.0% and 6.2%, p < 0.01
Notarangelo Pharmclo [40]	2015	Europeans	ACS	888	No data	12 months	MACE (CV death, nonfatal IM, nonfatal stroke)	CYP2C19*2, *17 and ABCB1	HR 0.58 (0.43-0.78) p < 0.001
Bergmeijer (Popular genetics) [41]	ongoing	Europeans	STEMI-stent	2500	100	15 months	MACE (CV death, ACS, stroke)	CYP2C19*2, *3	
Tailor-PCI (NCT01742117)	ongoing	Europeans	ACS or CAD/stent	5000	100	12 months	MACE (non-fatal MI, non-fatal stroke, severe recurrent ischemia, CV death, and ST)	CYP2C19*2, *17	

Data are showed as: OR: odds ratio, HR: hazard ratio, (95%CI), p-value, * Urgent revascularization non related with ST, ** adjusted in multivariate analysis.

2.1.1. Large-Scale Studies in High-Risk Patients

Several large-scale studies in high-risk patients (PCI–stent) have evaluated the clinical implications of genetic variations in patients with coronary artery disease (CAD). In an article published at the beginning of 2009, Collet et al. [29] examined 259 patients <45 years with a first ACS with clopidogrel for at least one month, with 73% undergoing PCI. CYP2C19*2 carriers had a higher risk of death, ACS, and urgent revascularization ($p = 0.0005$, HR = 3.69) compared with non-carriers.

During this period, 2208 patients were enrolled in the French Registry of Acute ST-elevation and non-ST-elevation Myocardial Infarction (FAST-MI) [30], with 68.7% undergoing PCI. They evaluated whether some genes previously associated with altered pharmacokinetics of clopidogrel were also associated with cardiovascular events during the first year after ACS. Patients with two allelic variations *ABCB1* (TT) had a higher risk of cardiovascular events than those without allelic variation (CC) (Hazard ratio, HR = 1.72, 95%CI: 1.20–2.47). The risk of death, ACS, or stroke in patients with PCI was 3.58 times higher in patients who carry two copies *CYP2C19* LOF alleles compared to subjects without this allele.

In a Genome Wide Association Study (GWAS) performed in a large Amish population [32], it was seen that patients with increased age, greater BMI, higher triglycerides levels, and lower high-density lipoprotein cholesterol were associated with a poorer clopidogrel response; these variables explained less than 10% of the variation. In contrast, the heritability of ADP-stimulated platelet aggregation in response to clopidogrel was 73%, suggesting a substantial genetic component. They showed that in 277 ACS–PCI patients, the *CYP2C19*2* polymorphism was associated with poorer cardiovascular outcomes (HR = 2.42, 95%CI: 1.18–4.99, $p = 0.02$).

Genetic Post-Hoc Substudies of the TRITON 38 Trial

The efficacies of clopidogrel and prasugrel were compared in the TRITON 38 trial [42] where 13,608 ACS–PCI–stent patients were included. Prasugrel reduced the percentage of cardiovascular death, ACS, or stroke at 15 months post-ACS, although it increased cases of bleeding.

Two genetic post-hoc studies of the TRITON-TIMI trial have been published by Mega et al. [17,22]. In a first approach [22], they evaluated the association between genetic polymorphisms in *CYP450* and secondary cardiovascular events in the clopidogrel subgroup. Patients who carried LOF alleles showed higher risk of cardiovascular death, ACS, or stroke compared with non-carriers (HR 1.53, 95%IC: 1.07–2.19, $p = 0.01$) and a higher risk of stent thrombosis (HR = 3.09, 95%CI: 1.19–8.00, $p = 0.02$). Months later, in a second article [17], they assessed the effect of the *ABCB1* polymorphism by itself and alongside variants in *CYP2C19* on cardiovascular outcomes. Both variants (*CYP2C19*2* and *ABCB1*) were significant independent predictors of cardiovascular death, ACS, or stroke (*ABCB1* 3435 TT vs. CT/CC, HR 2.01, 95% CI: 1.30–3.11, $p = 0.0017$; *CYP2C19* LOF alleles carriers vs. non-carriers, HR 1.77, IC95%: 1.11–2.80, $p = 0.0155$). When the participants were divided into four groups on the basis of *ABCB1* 3435 C > T and *CYP2C19* status, those who did not carry at-risk genotypes in either gene had a significantly lower rate of cardiovascular death, ACS, or stroke at 15 months compared to those who were either carriers of *CYP2C19* LOF alleles, *ABCB1* 3435 TT homozygotes, or both ($p = 0.0002$).

During this period, another post-hoc study was published by Sorich et al. [31]. Individuals with a *CYP2C19* LOF genotype had a higher risk of cardiovascular death, ACS, or stroke than non-carriers in the clopidogrel group (RR 1.62, 95%CI: 1.27–2.06).

Genetics Post-Hoc Substudy of PLATO

In the PLATO trial [43], ticagrelor and clopidogrel were compared in patients with ACS, of whom only 64% had undergone PCI. In the genetic substudy including 10285 [33], PLATO demonstrated an increased rate of cardiovascular events in *CYP2C19* LOF carriers in the first 30 days of treatment with clopidogrel than in those with normal alleles, but they didn't find significant difference in outcomes over the full follow-up period. Although *ABCB1* polymorphism was also genotyped, the combination of both variants (*CYP2C19* and *ABCB1*) comparing LOF carriers versus non-carriers in the clopidogrel group was not compared.

2.1.2. Meta-Analyses of Large-Scale Studies

These studies and others were combined in several meta-analyses. In 2015, a systematic review of them was published by Osnabrugge et al. [44]. Most of the studies included in the meta-analysis showed statistical significance between polymorphisms and clinical endpoints, e.g., major adverse cardiovascular events (MACE) and stent thrombosis. However, the meta-analysis concluded that the association between *CYP2C19* LOF alleles and clinical efficacy of clopidogrel differed widely with regard to assessment, interpretation of high heterogeneity, and publication bias. Also, personalizing antiplatelet management based on genotyping is not supported by the currently available evidence [44].

2.1.3. Non-Randomized Clinical Trials

Others prospective, non-RCTs of *CYP2C19* genotype-guided clopidogrel therapy with clinical outcomes have been performed. In 2016, our group published a study with the aim of analyzing if the *CYP2C19/ABCB1* genotype-guided approach, in which the choice of antiplatelet therapy is based on the genetic test, could reduce the rates of cardiovascular events and bleeding compared to a non-tailored approach in 719 patients (more than 86% with ACS) who had undergone PCI with stent [35,45]. The primary endpoint (composite of cardiovascular death, ACS, or stroke during 12 months after intervention) occurred in 10.1% in the genotyping group and in 14.1% in the control group (HR 0.63, 95% CI (0.41–0.97), $p = 0.037$). The results showed that there was no difference in major and minor bleeding between the two groups (4.1% vs. 4.7%, HR = 0.80, 95%CI (0.39–1.63), $p = 0.55$) [35].

2.1.4. Clinical Trials

In 2016, Shen et al. published a study where 628 CAD patients undergoing PCI were divided into a control group (n = 319) and an intervention group ($n = 309$), which were tested for *CYP2C19* [36]. In the intervention group, extensive metabolizer patients received 75 mg daily of clopidogrel, intermediate metabolizer patients received 150 mg daily of clopidogrel, and poor metabolizer patients received ticagrelor 90 mg twice daily. The control group received clopidogrel 75 mg daily. The rates of MACE in the intervention group were lower than those in the control group at 1, 6, and 12 months ($P = 0.010$). There were no differences in the rates of bleeding between both groups ($P > 0.05$).

In 2012, a clinical trial testing this strategy was published (RAPID GENE Study, NCT01184300) using a novel point-of-care genetic test to identify carriers of the *CYP2C19*2* allele, which aimed to assess a pharmacogenetic approach to dual antiplatelet treatment after PCI [37]. The *CYP2C19*2*-pharmacogenetic strategy after PCI was effective in reducing high on-treatment platelet reactivity at day 7 in *CYP2C19*2* carriers. Recently, the same group confirmed that the identification of these genetic variants in patients with STEMI receiving PCI is feasible at the bedside and demonstrated that treatment of *CYP2C19*2*, *17, and *ABCB1* TT carriers with prasugrel resulted in a significant reduction in high platelet reactivity after 1 month compared to an augmented dosing of clopidogrel [38].

In 2013, 600 patients with CAD undergoing PCI randomly received a personalized antiplatelet therapy or conventional antiplatelet treatment and followed for the 180-day period after randomization. In the intervention group, the antiplatelet therapy was chosen according to CYP2C19 phenotype. In the control group, the patients received conventional antiplatelet treatment. The incidence of the primary end point (MACE) was 9.03% for patients assigned to conventional treatment and 2.66% for patients assigned to personalized therapy ($p < 0.01$), without differences in bleeding events between the 2 groups [39].

The PHARMCLO RCT is another clopidogrel pharmacogenetic study published in 2018 [40]. It is a prospective, multicenter RCT achieved in Italy between 2013 and 2015. 888 patients hospitalized for ACS were randomly assigned to standard of care or the PGx intervention arm, which included the genotyping of *ABCB1*, *CYP2C19*2*, and *CYP2C19*17* using an ST Q3 system that provides data within 70 min at each patient's bedside. The patients were followed up for 12 months for the primary composite endpoint of cardiovascular death and the first occurrence of nonfatal myocardial infarction, nonfatal stroke, and major bleeding was defined according to Bleeding Academic Research Consortium type 3 to 5 criteria. The study was prematurely stopped at only 25% of prespecified enrollment, because of the lack of in vitro diagnosis certification of the genotyping instrument. However, despite only enrolling a fraction of the anticipated sample size, the primary endpoint occurred in 15.9% in the intervention arm and in 25.9% in the standard-of-care arm (HR: 0.58; 95% CI: 0.43 to 0.78; $p < 0.001$).

In the Netherlands, a multicenter trial named Cost-effectiveness of Genotype Guided Treatment With Antiplatelet Drugs in STEMI Patients: Optimization of Treatment (POPular Genetics, NCT01761786) started in 2011 to assess the efficacy, safety, and cost-effectiveness of the *CYP2C19* genotype-guided antiplatelet treatment strategy, using clopidogrel in non-carriers of the *CYP2C19**2 or *3 allele and ticagrelor or prasugrel in carriers of the *CYP2C19**2 or *3 allele in 2500 STEMI patients. [41]. Similarly, the Tailored Antiplatelet Therapy Following PCI (TAILOR-PCI) is a multi-site, open label, prospective, randomized trial, where 5000 patients with ACS or stable CAD who underwent PCI with stent will be recruited and randomized to receive a conventional therapy or a *CYP2C19* genotype-based anti-platelet therapy approach (NCT01742117).

2.1.5. Meta-Analyses

In 2018, a meta-analysis performed by Kheiri et al. [46] was published, including six RCTs with a total of 2371 patients. Of those studies, only three trials included ACS patients [39,40,47], Tuteja et al. [48] was not published and included CAD patients, Tomaniak et al. [49] included stable CAD patients, and Robert et al. [37] mainly included CAD (only 37% ACS). The results showed that the rate of MACEs was not significantly different between intervention groups and control groups (8.9% vs. 12.8%, RR0.67 IC 0.35–1.27, $p = 0.22$, $I^2 = 74\%$). The high heterogeneity was due to inconsistency in definitions of MACE among the trials, different follow-up times, different genotype testing systems with varied tested alleles, and a variety of dosing algorithms. Sensitivity analysis by excluding the unpublished trial [48] resulted in a significant reduction of MACE in favor to the genotype-guided group with almost no heterogeneity (RR 0.55, 95%CI 0.41–0.74, $p < 0.01$, I2 = 2%). Similarly, a sensitive analysis by including only the three trials that assessed genotype testing exclusively in ACS patients suggested a significant reduction of MACE.

2.1.6. Guidelines

Taking into account all the commented information, clopidogrel should be considered as an ideal target for pharmacogenetic intervention, at least in high-risk patients, due to the high level of evidence associated with the reduction of cardiovascular events rates and because there are other alternatives of antiplatelet drugs which are not affected by *CYP2C19* polymorphisms. This is supported by CIPC and DPGW guidelines, which have labelled the clopidogrel–CYP2C19 interaction as 1A. The CPIC and the DPWG recommend the use of genetic information to guide clopidogrel therapy, especially in ACS patients who have undergone PCI [50–53]. Both guidelines recommend considering an alternative drug for CYP2C19 poor or intermediate metabolizers due to increased risk for reduced response to clopidogrel.

In low-risk patients (no PCI–stent), no relationship was found between *CYP2C19**2 status and adverse outcomes [34,54]. Despite the evidence and the PGx guidelines, the current guidelines for the treatment of ACS by the American Heart Association/American College of Cardiology (AHA/ACC) and the guideline recommendations by European Society of Cardiology do not make references to the possibility of carrying out the pharmacogenetic test even in high-risk patients (ACS–PCI–stent) and, in consequence, they contradict the CPIC and DPGW guidelines and the FDA and EMA recommendations. A recent and very good review of the lack of updating of the American and European cardiology guidelines of ACS with respect to the clopidogrel test has been published by Luzum and Cheung [7]. The AHA/ACC recommends against routine pharmacogenetic testing for clopidogrel because no RCTs have demonstrated the testing improves patient's outcomes [55]. According to the authors of this article [7], the level of evidence supporting by *CYP2C19* genotype-guided clopidogrel therapy in patients that received PCI is at least as strong as the other genetic tests recommended by the AHA/ACC. Fortunately, several institutions have implemented pharmacogenetic testing for clopidogrel despite the negative recommendation by AHA/ACC [35,45,56,57] and they found improvement in the clinical results of patients [58,59].

2.1.7. Cost-Effectiveness Studies

There are different cost-effectiveness studies supporting that preventive genotyping test of *CYP2C19* is cost-effective and could be applicable in clinical practice [60–63]. In collaboration with The Golden Helix Foundation, in 2018 we performed a cost-effectiveness analysis of pharmacogenomic-guided antiplatelet treatment using the data published [60] by our team regarding Spanish ACS patients who underwent PCI [35]. This study is one of the very few that aims to compare the cost-effectiveness of antiplatelet treatment modalities retrospectively versus prospectively genotyped patients for the *CYP2C19*2*, *CYP2C19*3*, and *CYP2C19*17* alleles. Our analysis suggests that the prospective treatment strategy costs slightly less and has a marginally higher effectiveness compared to the retrospective group.

In 2015, Johnson et al. [64] estimated the financial impact of *CYP2C19* genotyping in a theoretical cohort of 1000 patients with ACS who received PCI–stent implantation and were treated with clopidogrel, prasugrel, or ticagrelor in a managed care setting. The budget-impact analysis used published event rates from primary literature to estimate costs of events analysis for three different scenarios: Scenario A, no *CYP2C19* genotyping; Scenario B, 50% of patients received *CYP2C19* genotyping with appropriate treatment based on genotype; and Scenario C, 100% of patients received *CYP2C19* genotyping with appropriate treatment based on genotype. They concluded that important financial benefits may be realized through use of genotype-guided antiplatelet therapy to reserve prasugrel or ticagrelor use for patients with reduced CYP2C19 activity to avoid costs associated with adverse cardiac events.

A systematic review of economic evaluation of pharmacogenetic testing for prevention of adverse drug reactions was published in 2016 [65]. There was evidence supporting the cost effectiveness of testing for different drugs, including clopidogrel.

2.2. Warfarin

Warfarin is an anticoagulant widely used for the prevention of thromboembolic and hemorrhagic episodes [66,67]. The drug decreases the activation of vitamin K-dependent coagulation factors by inhibiting the enzyme epoxide reductase [68]. Due to the great variability in the individual response and a narrow therapeutic window, there is a significant risk of thromboembolism if the doses are less than adequate, or of hemorrhage in case of overdose [69] for patients with the same International Normalized Ratio (INR) target [67].

Different algorithms based on clinical parameters such as age, weight, and height were published, but these are inaccurate and explain only 12–22% of the dose variation [70]. In recent years, different algorithms also including genetic polymorphisms that affect enzymes that mediate the metabolism of the drug were published. The most popular variants are the genes that encode CYP2C9 and the epoxide reductase of vitamin K in the *VKORC1* gene, which affect the properties pharmacokinetics and pharmacodynamics of warfarin [71].

The *CYP2C9* gene has many allelic variants. Individuals homozygous for the wild-type allele (*CYP2C9*1*) have a "normal metabolism" of S-warfarin, the most potent form of this drug. The *2 (rs1799853) and *3 (rs1057910) alleles have a reduced enzymatic activity for the excretion of the drug, which entails a decrease of around 30% and 80%, respectively [67].

On the other hand, the enzyme encoded by *VKORC1* catalyzes the reduction of vitamin K, a necessary step to activate the coagulation factors. Its polymorphism, -1639G > A (rs9923231), is associated with an increased sensitivity to warfarin and the decrease in the amount required [67].

2.2.1. Genotype-Guided Algorithms

Gage et al. [72] published the first warfarin genotype-guided algorithm, including 369 patients who had a stable dose of warfarin. As genetic variants they only included *CYP2C9*2* and *3 and as demographic and clinical variants they included age, body surface area, gender race, target INR, and comedication (amiodarone and simvastatin). The algorithm presented a coefficient of determination (R^2) of 39%. In 2008, the same group published a new algorithm [70] which improved the $R^2 = 54\%$. They increased the number of patients to 1015 and included another genetic variant, *VKORC1* 1639G>A, smoking status, and the indication of the drug [70].

For these reasons, in 2007, the FDA approved the inclusion in the drug's data sheet of a dosage table that recommends taking into account polymorphisms -1639G>A in the *VKORC1* gene and *2 and *3 in the *CYP2C9* gene, to set the initial dose [73]. The decision was made because many studies showed that these polymorphisms were associated with great variability in the response to warfarin.

Other pharmacogenetic algorithms have been proposed that take into account both the genetic polymorphisms and the clinical variables of the patients to estimate the maintenance dose of warfarin [70,74–76], which seem to have greater accuracy than the tables in the technical data sheet [77]. However, they do not evaluate whether the pharmacogenetic algorithm can lead to the improvement of clinical results, such as % INR out of range, time to reach the INR, and frequency of appearance of thrombotic or hemorrhagic events. These algorithms explain about 50% of the dose variation [70,77], with greater benefit at the end of the dosage [74].

2.2.2. Clinical Trials

Different clinical trials have been published in recent years, measuring in these cases clinical outcomes such as thrombotic and hemorrhagic adverse events, time to reach the INR, and time in therapeutic range (Table 4). Among all of them we would like to highlight two pharmacogenetic trials of warfarin therapy, European Pharmacogenetics of Anticoagulant Therapy (EU-PACT), and Clarification of Optimal Anticoagulation through Genetics (COAG), reported by Pirmohamed et al. [3] and Kimmel et al. [78], respectively, that were published at the same time with contradictory messages. Pirmohamed et al. [3] recruited 455 patients with atrial fibrillation (AF) or venous thromboembolism. For patients assigned to the genotype-guided group, warfarin doses were prescribed according to a PGx algorithm for the first five days. Patients in the control group received a 3-day loading-dose regime (fixed-dose strategy). After the initiation period, the treatment of all patients was managed according to routine clinical practice. The primary outcome was the percentage of time in the therapeutic range (TTR) of 2.0 to 3.0 for the INR during the first 12 weeks after warfarin initiation. The mean percentage of time in the therapeutic range was 67.4% in the genotype group as compared with 60.3% in the control group ($p < 0.001$). The mean time to reach a therapeutic INR was 21 days in the genotype group as compared with 29 days in the control group ($p < 0.001$).

Kimmel et al. [78] recruited 1015 patients, 80% with AF or deep-vein thrombosis or pulmonary embolism. The dose of warfarin during the first five days of therapy was determined according to a dosing algorithm that included both clinical variables and genotype data, or to one that included clinical variables only. The primary outcome was the percentage of TTR from day 4 or 5 through day 28 of therapy. At 4 weeks, the mean percentage of TTR was 45.2% in the genotype group and 45% in the control group ($p = 0.91$). In North Africans patients, the mean percentage of time in the therapeutic range was less in the genotype group than in the control group.

One possible explanation could be the difference observed in the genotyping results [79], as the prevalence of homozygotes, who required the most significant dosing changes, was 17% in EU-PACT versus 11% in the COAG trial for the *VKORC1* variant and 3.4% in EU-PACT versus 1% in the COAG trial for the *CYP2C9*2* and *CYP2C9*3* variants. According to Shaw et al. [80] some key differences between the two studies were length of follow-up time (12 weeks for EU-PACT and 4 weeks for COAG), determination of dose in the non-genotype group (fixed dose in EUPACT and clinical dosing algorithm in COAG), patient ancestry (2% non-European in EU-PACT and 33% non-European in COAG), and the availability of genetic test results (EU-PACT genotype results were available in approximately 2 h, COAG genotype results were not available before the first dose for 55% of patients). Another possible explanation could be the different diseases affecting the patients which could also affect the warfarin dosing.

After these trials, others have been published in which it was demonstrated that the pharmacogenetic algorithm could reduce the time to reach the maintenance dose [81] or that a lower number of thrombotic or hemorrhagic events was achieved [82]. In 2017, the GIFT randomized clinical trial was published [82] to determine if genotype-guided dosing improves the safety of warfarin initiation among undergoing hip or knee arthroplasty. The results showed that genotype-guided warfarin dosing, compared with clinically guide dosing, reduced the combined risk of major bleeding, INR of 4 or greater, venous thromboembolism, and death. Further research is necessary to determine the cost-effectiveness of personalized warfarin dose.

Table 4. Main characteristics from the RCT about warfarin included in this review.

Ref	Year	Ethnic	Population Studied	n	Follow up	Endpoint	Polymorphisms	Homozygotes Action Required	Outcomes (Intervention Group vs. Control Group)	Availability Test	Dose in Non-Genotype Group
Pirmohamed (EU-PACT) [3]	2015	2% non-European	AF (72.1%) VT (27.9%)	455	12 weeks	%TTR	CYP2C9*2,*3 VKORC1	VKORC1: 17% CYP2C9*2 and *3: 3.4%	67.4% vs. 60.3%, p < 0.001	2h	Fixed-dose strategy
Kimel (COAG) [79]	2015	33% non-European	AF (23%) DVT or PE (56%)	1015	4 weeks	%TTR	CYP2C9*2, *3 VKORC1	VKORC1: 11% CYP2C9*2 and *3: 1%	45.2% vs. 45% p = 0.91	Not before the 1st dose for 55% of patients	Clinical dosing algorithm
Gage (GIFT) [82]	2017	91% European	Hip or knee arthroplasty	1650	30 and 60 days	Composite (major bleeding, INR ≥ 4, VT, death)	CYP2C9*2, *3 CYP4F2	NA	RR 0.73 (0.56-0.95) p = 0.02	NA	NA

AF: atrial fibrillation, DVT: Deep-vein thrombosis, PE: pulmonary embolism. %TTR: percentage time in therapeutic range. NA: Not applicable.

2.2.3. Meta-Analyses

The efficacy of the different algorithms published has been analyzed in different meta-analyses. In 2014, Goulding et al. [83] performed a meta-analysis including nine RCTs which evaluated genotype-guided warfarin dosing. Analysis of the percentage of TTR showed a statistically significant benefit in favor of genotype-guided warfarin dosing (mean difference = 6.67; 95% CI 1.34, 12.0, I^2 = 80%). Similarly, they found a statistically significant reduction in minor bleeding, major bleeding, and thromboembolism associated with genotype-guided warfarin dosing, RR 0.57 (95% CI 0.33, 0.99; I^2 = 60%). As conclusion, they considered that the genotype-guided warfarin dosing algorithm could improve the clinical effectiveness.

In 2015, Liao et al. [84] performed a meta-analysis including seven trials. In total, 1910 patients were included, 960 patients who received genotype plus clinical algorithm of warfarin dosing and 950 patients who received clinical algorithm only. The results showed that the percentage of TTR in the genotype-guided group improved compared with the standard group in the RCTs when the initial standard dose was fixed (95% CI 0.09–0.40; I^2 = 47.8%), but not when the studies were using no fixed initial doses. They did not find any difference in the incidences of adverse events (RR 0.94, 95% CI 0.84–1.04; I^2 = 0%, p = 0.647) and death rates (RR 1.36, 95% CI 0.46–4.05; I2 = 10.4%, p = 0.328) between the two groups.

In 2014, Tang et al. [85] performed a systematic review and meta-analysis including ten studies with a total of 5299 patients. The control groups were treated with fixed dose or clinical algorithms. The results showed that patients in the genotype-guided group had higher percentage of TTR than the control group (I^2 = 84%) and reduced risk for hemorrhagic complications (I^2 = 0%).

In 2015, Belley-Cote et al. [86] performed a systematic review and a meta-analysis including 12 studies (3217 patients) (11 studies with warfarin and 1 study with acenocoumarol and phenprocoumon). The control group was treated with fixed dose or clinical algorithms. They concluded that the genotype-guide approach compared to the non-genotype guide was not found to decrease a composite of death, thromboembolism, and major bleeding (I^2 = 10%), but the results improved the TTR (I^2 = 79%) in comparison with fixed vitamin K-antagonist dosing, but not with the clinical algorithms.

In 2015, Li et al. [87] conducted a meta-analysis of the published RCTs comparing PGx algorithm-based warfarin dosing with clinical variants or standard protocols (control group). A total of ten RCTs were retrieved for the meta-analysis, including 2601 participants. No heterogeneity was found for the primary or subgroup analyses of major bleeding and thromboembolic events ($I^2 \leq 25\%$). The results showed that major bleeding and thromboembolic events were significantly lower in the PGx group than in the control group. Similarly, there was a trend towards increased percentage of TTR (p = 0.05) in the PGx group, but no difference was observed for over-anticoagulation (INR > 4).

In 2015, Dahal et al. [88] performed a meta-analysis including ten RCTs, which included 2505 patients, and compared PGx algorithm-based warfarin dosing with clinical variants or standard protocols (control group). After one month, improved percentage of TTR and major bleeding incidence (I^2 = 26%) was observed, making this a cost-effective strategy in patients requiring longer anticoagulation therapy.

In 2015, Shi et al. [89] included 11 trials involving 2678 patients in a meta-analysis. The results showed that the PGx approach did not improve the TTR compared to control group (I^2 = 82%), although it significantly shortened the time to maintenance dose and the time to first therapeutic INR. Moreover, the PGx approach significantly reduced the risk of adverse events and major bleeding (I^2 = 15%).

2.2.4. Guidelines

In 2017 an update of the CPIC guidelines for pharmacogenetics-guided warfarin dosing was published [90]. Evidence from the literature has permitted including another variant (*CYP4F2* rs12777823), related to the limitation of the excessive accumulation of vitamin K that improves the accuracy of dose prediction [91]. Similarly, the CPNDS clinical recommendation group has published guidelines for the use of pharmacogenetic testing for variants in *VKORC1* and *CYP2C9* in adult and pediatric patients with an indication for warfarin [80]. They recommend testing for the *VKORC1* SNP (Single nucleotide polymorphism) -1639G>A (rs9923231) and the *CYP2C9* alleles *2 and *3 in order to better guide warfarin dosage.

2.2.5. Cost-Effectiveness Studies

Similar to clopidogrel, there are different cost-effectiveness studies supporting that preventive genotype testing for warfarin is cost-effective. Most of the studies have demonstrated that the genotype-guided dosing approach can lead to reduced bleeding and improve quality-adjusted life-years (QALYs) gained. In 2009, Eckman et al. [92] examined the cost-effectiveness of genotype-guided dosing (*CYP2C9*2, CYP2C9*3*, and/or *VKORC1*) versus standard induction of warfarin therapy for patients with nonvalvular AF using the Markov decision model. Effectiveness was measured in QALYs. They concluded that warfarin-related genotyping is unlikely to be cost-effective for typical patients with nonvalvular AF, but may be cost-effective in patients at high risk for hemorrhage who are starting warfarin therapy.

In 2009, Leey et al. [93] evaluated the potential clinical and economic outcomes of genotype-guided warfarin therapy in elderly patients newly diagnosed with AF. A decision tree was designed to represent the medical decision (pharmacogenetic testing or not) and the main clinical outcomes (embolic stroke, bleeding). They found that any reduction in major bleeding as a result of pharmacogenetic testing would lead to improved utility.

In 2013, Pink et al. [94] compared the cost-effectiveness of a variety of clinical dosing algorithms, pharmacogenetic dosing algorithms, and new anticoagulant-based therapies. Warfarin pharmacogenetic algorithms were more cost-effective than clinical-based dosing algorithms. Neither dabigatran nor rivaroxaban were cost-effective options, but apixaban appeared to be the most cost-effective treatment when warfarin therapy was poorly controlled.

2.3. Acenocumarol

Acenocoumarol is a vitamin K epoxide reductase inhibitor. The drug inhibits recycling of the inactive oxidized to the active reduced form of vitamin K. It is used for the prevention of thromboembolic and hemorrhagic episodes [95]. As with warfarin, different polymorphisms in *CYP2C9* and *VKORC1* genes have been associated with the efficacy of the drug.

2.3.1. Pharmacogenetics Algorithms

In the last years, several pharmacogenetics algorithms have also been published for acenocoumarol in diverse populations. Verde et al. constructed an "acenocoumarol-dose genotype score" based on the number of alleles associated with a higher acenocoumarol dosage carried by each participant for each polymorphism [96]. They concluded that this approach could discriminate patients requiring high acenocoumarol doses to achieve the target. Rathore et al. [97] and Krishna et al. [98] published two algorithms for Indian populations, including demographic, clinical, and genetic variants, and the coefficients of determinations obtained were 41% and 61.5%, respectively [97,98]. Four algorithms were developed for European populations. In 2011, the European Pharmacogenetics of Anticoagulant Therapy (EU-PACT) study group published an algorithm including *CYP2C9* and *VKORC1* variants and clinical variables (age, sex, weight, height, and amiodarone use). The PGx algorithm explained 52.6% of the dosage variance, whereas the non-genotype algorithm explained 23.7% [99]. Borobia et al. [100] developed an algorithm for a cohort of 147 patients with thromboembolic venous disease who were on stable doses including clinical variables (age, body mass index (BMI), amiodarone use, and enzyme-inducer use) and genetic variations of *CYP2C9*, *VKORC1*, *CYP4F2*, and *APOE*. The clinical factors explained 22% of the dose variability, which increased to 60.6% when pharmacogenetic information was included ($p < 0.001$) [100]. Cerezo-Manchado et al. [101] published an algorithm including 973 patients undergoing anticoagulation therapy. The algorithm was composite of clinical factors (age and BMI) and genetic variants (*VKORC1*, *CYP2C9*, and *CYP4F2* variants). The algorithm explained 50% of the variance in the acenocoumarol dosage, whereas the clinical algorithm explained 16% [101].

In 2016, a new algorithm including clinical (age, weight, amiodarone use, enzyme inducer status, international normalized ratio target range) and genetic variables (*CYP2C9*2* (rs1799853), *CYP2C9*3* (rs1057910), *VKORC1* (rs9923231), and *CYP4F2* (rs2108622)) to predict the most appropriate acenocoumarol dosage for stable anticoagulation in a cohort of 685 Spanish patients was published by our team in collaboration with Hospital de la Paz [102]. The R^2 explained by the algorithm was 52.8% in the generation cohort and 64% in the validation cohort. When the patients were classified into three dosage groups according to the stable dosage (<11 mg/week, 11–21 mg/week, >21 mg/week), the percentage of correctly classified patients was higher in the intermediate group, whereas differences between pharmacogenetic and clinical algorithms increased in the extreme dosage groups.

The utility of PGx-guided acenocoumarol and phenprocoumon prescribing during therapy initiation was investigated in a prospective trial: EU-PACT [2]. The genotype-guided dosing algorithm included clinical variables and genotyping for *CYP2C9* and *VKORC1* and the control-dosing algorithm included only clinical variables for the initiation of acenocoumarol or phenprocoumon treatment in patients with AF or venous thromboembolism. The primary outcome was the percentage of TTR in the 12-week period after the initiation of therapy. The intervention arm showed no statistically significant difference in the mean percentage of time in the therapeutic INR range compared with the control group. ($p = 0.52$). Some years later, to explore the potential reasons for these findings, the same team performed subanalyses stratifying the data by the *VKORC1* and *CYP2C9* genotypes [103]. They realized that the EU-PACT genetic-guided dose initiation algorithms for acenocoumarol and phenprocumon could have predicted the dose overcautiously in the *VKORC1* AA-*CYP2C9*1/*1* subgroup.

2.3.2. Meta-Analyses

Recently, a meta-analysis has been published [104] including 15,754 patients. The *CYP4F2*3* polymorphism was consistently associated with an increase in mean coumarin dose (+9% (95% CI 7–10%), with a larger effect in females, in patients taking acenocoumarol, and in Europeans. The inclusion of the *CYP4F2*3* in dosing algorithms slightly improved the prediction of stable coumarin dose. New pharmacogenetic equations potentially useful for clinical practice were derived [104].

2.3.3. Guidelines

The DPWG recommends checking INR more frequently after initiating or discontinuing NSAIDs in individuals taking acenocoumarol with at least one *CYP2C9*2* or **3* allele. While *VKORC1* genotype has been found to contribute to acenocoumarol dose variability, there are no dosing recommendations at this time because of strict INR monitoring by the Dutch Thrombosis Service. They recommend checking INR more frequently in patients with the AA genotype [52,53].

2.4. Simvastatin

Simvastatin is a lipid-modifying agent used in the treatment of different kinds of hypercholesterolemia, one of the most significant risk factors in cardiovascular disease. Furthermore, it has shown a decrease of morbimortality in atherosclerotic cardiovascular disease patients, even those with normal cholesterol levels.

Simvastatin has been significantly associated with skeletal muscle toxicity (myalgia, myopathy, and rhabdomyolysis) [105], especially a high risk of myopathy with a dose of 80 mg daily [106].

Simvastatin inhibits the cholesterol production by competitive inhibition of HMG-CoA reductase, increasing the number of LDL receptors on liver cells. Its metabolism is mediated by many CYP isoenzymes (CYP3A4, CYP3A5, CYP2C9, CYP2C19, etc.) and its movement depends on SLCO1B1 and ABCB isoforms [12]. The FDA approved a drug label for simvastatin indicating that simvastatin is a substrate for the transport protein SLCO1B1. Genetic variants contained in genes encoding these transporters and metabolic enzymes expression may affect a patient's simvastatin response.

2.4.1. Observational Studies

The SLCO1B1 enzyme, encoded by the *SLCO1B1* gene, is involved in the simvastatin carriage from intestinal to liver cells [12]. In this gene, there may be a variant, the *c.521T>C* (rs4149056), considered in *SLCO1B1*5*, **15*, and **17* haplotypes, which is the only one which has reached the highest level of evidence about its association with interindividual differences in simvastatin patients' responses [107].

Among healthy individuals, the *SLCO1B1* 521 CC genotype has been associated with higher plasma concentration of simvastatin [108,109]. This genotype has been also significantly related to an increased likelihood of muscular disease in patients treated with simvastatin after ACS (OR = 16.9; 95%CI = 4.7–61.1; p = 6.0E-4) and with a higher risk of muscular disease in occlusive vascular disease or diabetes patients (RR = 2.6; 95%CI = 1.3–5; p = 0.004) [110] when compared with *CT* or *TT* genotypes. Furthermore, *CC* compared to *CT* genotype confirmed these results, with *SLCO1B1*5 CC* individuals showing a higher risk of muscular disease.

2.4.2. Clinical Trials

The STRENGTH study was a pharmacogenetics study of statin efficacy and safety. 509 patients were randomized to atorvastatin, simvastatin, or pravastatin. The composite adverse event (discontinuation for any side effect, myalgia, or CK > 3× baseline during follow-up) occurred in 99 subjects. *SLCO1B1*5* genotype and female sex were associated with mild statin-induced side effects. In patients with hypercholesterolemia, the *C* allele was associated with increased risk of adverse drug events when treated with atorvastatin, pravastatin, or simvastatin (OR = 1.7; 95%CI = 1.04–2.08; p = 0.03) [111]. Furthermore, regarding patients with hyperlipidemia treated with simvastatin only, carrying the *SLCO1B1*5* (*CC/CT* vs. *TT*) allele was associated with higher risk of muscular diseases [112].

2.4.3. Guidelines

The FDA recommends against 80 mg daily simvastatin dosage. In patients with the C allele at *SLCO1B1* rs4149056, there are modest increases in myopathy risk even at lower simvastatin doses (40 mg daily); if optimal efficacy is not achieved with a lower dose, alternate agents should be considered. This annotation is based on the CPIC guideline for simvastatin and *SLCO1B1* [107].

3. Discussion

There are many barriers that hinder the implementation of PGx in daily clinical practice. In our opinion, once the regulatory agencies recommend doing the pharmacogenetic test, their implementation should not be delayed. However, as we have shown in this review, it is not performing at the expected rate as there is a disconnection between drug labels and the standard of care in daily clinical practice.

Regulators are often confronted with challenges involved in translating data from pharmacogenomic studies into clinically relevant and meaningful product information, starting with the level of scientific evidence required to justify the inclusion of PGx data in the product information [11]. In case of the new drugs, there are two guidelines on pharmacogenomics during drug development and the post-authorization phase, respectively [113].

With them, the EMA intends further to enable the potential of PGx during drug development and surveillance and to gain insight into the associated scientific challenges and discuss potential solutions. The guidelines are expected to improve genomic data-informed drug development and clinical experience, thereby promoting understanding of interindividual drug response variations and, consequently, providing guidance towards more personalized treatments in the interest of patients and the public.

However, older drugs, such as warfarin, acenocoumarol, simvastatin, and clopidogrel, have been subject to pharmacogenomic scrutiny by the EMA after their authorization [11]. So, the implementation of the PGx test should be easy.

Knowing the evidence commented above for clopidogrel, it would appear therefore that genotype-directed therapy with clopidogrel would more likely benefit a population with the greatest risk (PCI–stent). Administration of stronger antiplatelet drugs in low-risk patients would probably not reduce the thrombotic risk, but would increase the risk of bleedings [114]. However, prescribing stronger antiplatelet drugs only to the high-risk patients resistant to clopidogrel could add to a new era of personalized medicine. The old "one size fits all" regime should come to an end; tailored antiplatelet therapy is taking over, based on the patient's individual risk factors for atherothrombotic events such as HPR (High platelet reactivity), diabetes, ACS, and genetic polymorphisms.

The AHA/ACC guidelines recommend against routine pharmacogenetic testing because there are no clinical trials published yet [14,55], but, before the no recommendation to do the PGx test of clopidogrel by the AHA/ACC due to the lack of RCT, there was already one published by Xie et al. [39], in which it was shown that the incidence of secondary cardiovascular events was lower in the intervention group with respect to the control group, as we have commented in this review. It is probably necessary to wait for the clinical results of the rest of RCTs discussed in this review and wait for the next update of the AHA/ACC.

In our opinion, the level of evidence supporting *CYP2C19* genotype-guided clopidogrel therapy in patients undergoing PCI is high enough and endorsed by the regulatory agencies for the AHA/ACC guide to include it, given that the AHA/ACC recommends other PGx tests in absence of prospective clinical trials. The evidence showed by large-scale observational studies in high-risk patients suggests that the *CYP2C19* LOF alleles are associated with MACE. The meta-analysis published by Osnabrugge et al. [44] showed that there is high heterogeneity between studies and publication bias and since the validity of the overall conclusion of a meta-analysis depends, to a large extent, on the homogeneity of the studies included, in our opinion this should be considered as an important limitation of the meta-analysis [115]. Regarding clinical trials, one non-RCT [35] and five RCTs [36,37,39–41] (and TAILOR-PCI) show that PGx tests can improve results in the health of patients. Similarly, the meta-analysis including these RCTs [46] showed high heterogeneity due to inconsistency in definitions of MACE, different follow-up time, different genotype systems, etc. Despite this, when an unpublished article [48] was excluded from the meta-analysis, there was almost no heterogeneity and the results showed that the intervention group reduced MACE and was statistically significant. Moreover, several studies have shown that the application of PGx to clopidogrel is cost-effective.

Regarding warfarin, several PGx algorithms, including clinical variables, have been published and considered efficient methods for determining individual stable warfarin dose. Although there is enough information to show the association between genetic variants and warfarin dose, the results published in RCTs are controversial, mainly because of the complexity, the important differences in the design, the differences observed in the prevalence of the genotyping results [79], and the different diseases included, all of which could affect warfarin dosing. In spite of this, most of the meta-analyses of RCTs show at least an improvement of percentage of TTR when using the pharmacogenetic algorithm compared with the standard protocol.

Sample size in genotyping trials (e.g., Tailored Antiplatelet Initiation to Lessen Outcomes Due to Decreased Clopidogrel Response after Percutaneous Coronary Intervention [TAILOR-PCI trial, ClinicalTrials.gov number, NCT01742117) should probably be calculated on the basis of the prevalence of reduced-function or loss-of-function alleles that affect the phenotype, since we do not anticipate a difference in outcomes in patients without such mutations [116].

In our opinion, the greatest benefit of the implementation of the PGx test for warfarin would be in those patients who initiate the treatment; then we could anticipate if the drug is going to work or if it is better to prescribe a new oral anticoagulant drug and in those patients who, after a reasonable period, do not manage to maintain the INR in order to justify that it is due to poor metabolism of the drug.

Observational evidence suggests that the use of a genotype-guided dosing algorithm may increase the effectiveness and safety of acenocoumarol therapy. Although it's important to note that the published algorithms differ in the kind of patients and diseases, the clinical and genetic included variables, and the methods used to develop the predictive models.

However, the only clinical trial achieved reported initially that genotype-guided dosing of acenocoumarol (and phenprocoumon) did not improve the percentage of time in the therapeutic INR range during the 12 weeks after the initiation of therapy. After performing subanalyses stratifying the data by the *VKORC1* and *CYP2C9* genotypes [103], they realized that the EU-PACT genetic-guided dose initiation algorithms for acenocoumarol (and phenprocumon) could have predicted the dose overcautiously in the *VKORC1* AA-*CYP2C9**1/*1 subgroup.

This trial had limitations that could have influenced the final result; on the one hand, it is important to know that the CYP2C9 enzyme has much less influence on the pharmacokinetics of phenprocoumon than on the pharmacokinetics of warfarin [117], but on the other hand, the number of patients included was lower than the number required according to the power calculation.

In our opinion, those patients who fail to reach or maintain the INR after a period of treatment could benefit from the PGx test. More studies are necessary to implement the PGx test before the prescription for guiding the dose of acenocoumarol.

Regarding simvastatin, an RCT showed that *SLCO1B1**5 genotype and female sex were associated mild statin-induced side effects. As the FDA and CPIC guidelines recommend the PGx test, this should at least be used when symptomatology of myopathy starts.

In conclusion, PGx tests for clopidogrel in high-risk patients and warfarin in patients including all indications could begin to be implemented in daily clinical practice, similar to simvastatin tests. Acenocoumarol should be limited to patients who do not reach the INR after a certain time of treatment. The algorithm could improve acenocoumarol dosage selection for patients who will begin treatment with this drug, especially in extreme-dosage patients. Further studies are necessary to confirm that the PGx test for acenocoumarol is ready for use.

Funding: This research received no external funding.

Conflicts of Interest: The authors declare no conflict of interest.

References

1. Mallal, S.; Phillips, E.; Carosi, G.; Molina, J.M.; Workman, C.; Tomazic, J.; Jagel-Guedes, E.; Rugina, S.; Kozyrev, O.; Cid, J.F.; et al. Hla-b*5701 screening for hypersensitivity to abacavir. *N. Engl. J. Med.* **2008**, *358*, 568–579. [CrossRef]
2. Verhoef, T.I.; Ragia, G.; de Boer, A.; Barallon, R.; Kolovou, G.; Kolovou, V.; Konstantinides, S.; Le Cessie, S.; Maltezos, E.; van der Meer, F.J.; et al. A randomized trial of genotype-guided dosing of acenocoumarol and phenprocoumon. *N. Engl. J. Med.* **2013**, *369*, 2304–2312. [CrossRef] [PubMed]
3. Pirmohamed, M.; Burnside, G.; Eriksson, N.; Jorgensen, A.L.; Toh, C.H.; Nicholson, T.; Kesteven, P.; Christersson, C.; Wahlstrom, B.; Stafberg, C.; et al. A randomized trial of genotype-guided dosing of warfarin. *N. Engl. J. Med.* **2013**, *369*, 2294–2303. [CrossRef] [PubMed]
4. Wu, A.H. Pharmacogenomic testing and response to warfarin. *Lancet* **2015**, *385*, 2231–2232. [CrossRef]
5. Coenen, M.J.; de Jong, D.J.; van Marrewijk, C.J.; Derijks, L.J.; Vermeulen, S.H.; Wong, D.R.; Klungel, O.H.; Verbeek, A.L.; Hooymans, P.M.; Peters, W.H.; et al. Identification of patients with variants in tpmt and dose reduction reduces hematologic events during thiopurine treatment of inflammatory bowel disease. *Gastroenterology* **2015**, *149*, 907–917. [CrossRef] [PubMed]
6. Bank, P.C.D.; Swen, J.J.; Guchelaar, H.J. Implementation of pharmacogenomics in everyday clinical settings. *Adv. Pharmacol.* **2018**, *83*, 219–246.
7. Luzum, J.A.; Cheung, J.C. Does cardiology hold pharmacogenetics to an inconsistent standard? A comparison of evidence among recommendations. *Pharmacogenomics* **2018**, *19*, 1203–1216. [CrossRef]
8. Van der Wouden, C.H.; Cambon-Thomsen, A.; Cecchin, E.; Cheung, K.C.; Davila-Fajardo, C.L.; Deneer, V.H.; Dolzan, V.; Ingelman-Sundberg, M.; Jonsson, S.; Karlsson, M.O.; et al. Implementing pharmacogenomics in europe: Design and implementation strategy of the ubiquitous pharmacogenomics consortium. *Clin. Pharmacol. Ther.* **2017**, *101*, 341–358. [CrossRef]

9. Van der Wouden, C.H.; Cambon-Thomsen, A.; Cecchin, E.; Cheung, K.C.; Davila-Fajardo, C.L.; Deneer, V.H.; Dolzan, V.; Ingelman-Sundberg, M.; Jonsson, S.; Karlsson, M.O.; et al. Corrigendum: Implementing pharmacogenomics in europe: Design and implementation strategy of the ubiquitous pharmacogenomics consortium. *Clin. Pharmacol. Ther.* **2017**, *102*, 152. [CrossRef] [PubMed]
10. Bank, P.C.D.; Caudle, K.E.; Swen, J.J.; Gammal, R.S.; Whirl-Carrillo, M.; Klein, T.E.; Relling, M.V.; Guchelaar, H.J. Comparison of the guidelines of the clinical pharmacogenetics implementation consortium and the dutch pharmacogenetics working group. *Clin. Pharmacol. Ther.* **2018**, *103*, 599–618. [CrossRef] [PubMed]
11. Ehmann, F.; Caneva, L.; Papaluca, M. European medicines agency initiatives and perspectives on pharmacogenomics. *Br. J. Clin. Pharmacol.* **2014**, *77*, 612–617. [CrossRef]
12. Whirl-Carrillo, M.; McDonagh, E.M.; Hebert, J.M.; Gong, L.; Sangkuhl, K.; Thorn, C.F.; Altman, R.B.; Klein, T.E. Pharmacogenomics knowledge for personalized medicine. *Clin. Pharmacol. Ther.* **2012**, *92*, 414–417. [CrossRef]
13. King, S.B., 3rd; Smith, S.C., Jr.; Hirshfeld, J.W., Jr.; Jacobs, A.K.; Morrison, D.A.; Williams, D.O.; Feldman, T.E.; Kern, M.J.; O'Neill, W.W.; Schaff, H.V.; et al. 2007 focused update of the acc/aha/scai 2005 guideline update for percutaneous coronary intervention: A report of the american college of cardiology/american heart association task force on practice guidelines. *J. Am. Coll. Cardiol.* **2008**, *51*, 172–209. [CrossRef]
14. Kushner, F.G.; Hand, M.; Smith, S.C., Jr.; King, S.B., 3rd; Anderson, J.L.; Antman, E.M.; Bailey, S.R.; Bates, E.R.; Blankenship, J.C.; Casey, D.E., Jr.; et al. 2009 focused updates: ACC/AHA guidelines for the management of patients with ST-elevation myocardial infarction (updating the 2004 guideline and 2007 focused update) and ACC/AHA/SCAI guidelines on percutaneous coronary intervention (updating the 2005 guideline and 2007 focused update): A report of the American College of Cardiology Foundation/American Heart Association Task Force on Practice Guidelines. *J. Am. Coll. Cardiol.* **2009**, 2205–2241.
15. Snoep, J.D.; Hovens, M.M.; Eikenboom, J.C.; van der Bom, J.G.; Jukema, J.W.; Huisman, M.V. Clopidogrel nonresponsiveness in patients undergoing percutaneous coronary intervention with stenting: A systematic review and meta-analysis. *Am. Heart J.* **2007**, *154*, 221–231. [CrossRef]
16. Giusti, B.; Gori, A.M.; Marcucci, R.; Saracini, C.; Vestrini, A.; Abbate, R. Determinants to optimize response to clopidogrel in acute coronary syndrome. *Pharmgenomics Pers. Med.* **2010**, *3*, 33–50. [CrossRef]
17. Mega, J.L.; Close, S.L.; Wiviott, S.D.; Shen, L.; Walker, J.R.; Simon, T.; Antman, E.M.; Braunwald, E.; Sabatine, M.S. Genetic variants in abcb1 and CYP2C19 and cardiovascular outcomes after treatment with clopidogrel and prasugrel in the triton-timi 38 trial: A pharmacogenetic analysis. *Lancet* **2010**, *376*, 1312–1319. [CrossRef]
18. Fuster, V.; Sweeny, J.M. Clopidogrel and the reduced-function CYP2C19 genetic variant: A limited piece of the overall therapeutic puzzle. *JAMA* **2010**, *304*, 1839–1840. [CrossRef]
19. Giusti, B.; Gori, A.M.; Marcucci, R.; Abbate, R. Current status of clopidogrel pharmacogenomics. *Pharmacogenomics* **2012**, *13*, 1671–1674. [CrossRef]
20. Wang, X.Q.; Shen, C.L.; Wang, B.N.; Huang, X.H.; Hu, Z. Genetic polymorphisms of CYP2C19*2 and abcb1 c3435t affect the pharmacokinetic and pharmacodynamic responses to clopidogrel in 401 patients with acute coronary syndrome. *Gene* **2015**, *558*, 200–207. [CrossRef]
21. Su, J.; Xu, J.; Li, X.; Zhang, H.; Hu, J.; Fang, R.; Chen, X. Abcb1 c3435t polymorphism and response to clopidogrel treatment in coronary artery disease (cad) patients: A meta-analysis. *PLoS ONE* **2012**, *7*, e46366. [CrossRef]
22. Mega, J.L.; Close, S.L.; Wiviott, S.D.; Shen, L.; Hockett, R.D.; Brandt, J.T.; Walker, J.R.; Antman, E.M.; Macias, W.; Braunwald, E.; et al. Cytochrome p-450 polymorphisms and response to clopidogrel. *N. Engl. J. Med.* **2009**, *360*, 354–362. [CrossRef]
23. Sibbing, D.; Koch, W.; Gebhard, D.; Schuster, T.; Braun, S.; Stegherr, J.; Morath, T.; Schomig, A.; von Beckerath, N.; Kastrati, A. Cytochrome 2c19*17 allelic variant, platelet aggregation, bleeding events, and stent thrombosis in clopidogrel-treated patients with coronary stent placement. *Circulation* **2010**, *121*, 512–518. [CrossRef]
24. Sibbing, D.; Gebhard, D.; Koch, W.; Braun, S.; Stegherr, J.; Morath, T.; Von Beckerath, N.; Mehilli, J.; Schomig, A.; Schuster, T.; et al. Isolated and interactive impact of common CYP2C19 genetic variants on the antiplatelet effect of chronic clopidogrel therapy. *J. Thromb. Haemost.* **2010**, *8*, 1685–1693. [CrossRef]

25. Frere, C.; Cuisset, T.; Gaborit, B.; Alessi, M.C.; Hulot, J.S. The CYP2C19*17 allele is associated with better platelet response to clopidogrel in patients admitted for non-st acute coronary syndrome. *J. Thromb. Haemost.* **2009**, *7*, 1409–1411. [CrossRef]
26. Tiroch, K.A.; Sibbing, D.; Koch, W.; Roosen-Runge, T.; Mehilli, J.; Schomig, A.; Kastrati, A. Protective effect of the CYP2C19 *17 polymorphism with increased activation of clopidogrel on cardiovascular events. *Am. Heart J.* **2010**, *160*, 506–512. [CrossRef]
27. Harmsze, A.M.; van Werkum, J.W.; Hackeng, C.M.; Ruven, H.J.; Kelder, J.C.; Bouman, H.J.; Breet, N.J.; Ten Berg, J.M.; Klungel, O.H.; de Boer, A.; et al. The influence of CYP2C19*2 and *17 on on-treatment platelet reactivity and bleeding events in patients undergoing elective coronary stenting. *Pharmacogenet. Genomics* **2012**, *22*, 169–175. [CrossRef]
28. US Department of Health and Human Services. *FDA Drug Safety Communication: Reduced Effectiveness of Plavix (Clopidogrel) in Patients Who Are Poor Metabolizers of the Drug*; US Food and Drug Administration: Silver Spring, MD, USA, 2010.
29. Collet, J.P.; Hulot, J.S.; Pena, A.; Villard, E.; Esteve, J.B.; Silvain, J.; Payot, L.; Brugier, D.; Cayla, G.; Beygui, F.; et al. Cytochrome p450 2c19 polymorphism in young patients treated with clopidogrel after myocardial infarction: A cohort study. *Lancet* **2009**, *373*, 309–317. [CrossRef]
30. Simon, T.; Verstuyft, C.; Mary-Krause, M.; Quteineh, L.; Drouet, E.; Meneveau, N.; Steg, P.G.; Ferrieres, J.; Danchin, N.; Becquemont, L.; et al. Genetic determinants of response to clopidogrel and cardiovascular events. *N. Engl. J. Med.* **2009**, *360*, 363–375. [CrossRef]
31. Sorich, M.J.; Vitry, A.; Ward, M.B.; Horowitz, J.D.; McKinnon, R.A. Prasugrel vs. Clopidogrel for cytochrome p450 2c19-genotyped subgroups: Integration of the triton-timi 38 trial data. *J. Thromb. Haemost.* **2010**, *8*, 1678–1684. [CrossRef]
32. Shuldiner, A.R.; O'Connell, J.R.; Bliden, K.P.; Gandhi, A.; Ryan, K.; Horenstein, R.B.; Damcott, C.M.; Pakyz, R.; Tantry, U.S.; Gibson, Q.; et al. Association of cytochrome p450 2c19 genotype with the antiplatelet effect and clinical efficacy of clopidogrel therapy. *JAMA* **2009**, *302*, 849–857. [CrossRef]
33. Wallentin, L.; James, S.; Storey, R.F.; Armstrong, M.; Barratt, B.J.; Horrow, J.; Husted, S.; Katus, H.; Steg, P.G.; Shah, S.H.; et al. Effect of CYP2C19 and abcb1 single nucleotide polymorphisms on outcomes of treatment with ticagrelor versus clopidogrel for acute coronary syndromes: A genetic substudy of the plato trial. *Lancet* **2010**, *376*, 1320–1328. [CrossRef]
34. Pare, G.; Mehta, S.R.; Yusuf, S.; Anand, S.S.; Connolly, S.J.; Hirsh, J.; Simonsen, K.; Bhatt, D.L.; Fox, K.A.; Eikelboom, J.W. Effects of CYP2C19 genotype on outcomes of clopidogrel treatment. *N. Engl. J. Med.* **2010**, *363*, 1704–1714. [CrossRef]
35. Sanchez-Ramos, J.; Davila-Fajardo, C.L.; Toledo Frias, P.; Diaz Villamarin, X.; Martinez-Gonzalez, L.J.; Martinez Huertas, S.; Burillo Gomez, F.; Caballero Borrego, J.; Bautista Paves, A.; Marin Guzman, M.C.; et al. Results of genotype-guided antiplatelet therapy in patients who undergone percutaneous coronary intervention with stent. *Int. J. Cardiol.* **2016**, *225*, 289–295. [CrossRef]
36. Shen, D.L.; Wang, B.; Bai, J.; Han, Q.; Liu, C.; Huang, X.H.; Zhang, J.Y. Clinical value of CYP2C19 genetic testing for guiding the antiplatelet therapy in a chinese population. *J. Cardiovasc. Pharmacol.* **2016**, *67*, 232–236. [CrossRef]
37. Roberts, J.D.; Wells, G.A.; Le May, M.R.; Labinaz, M.; Glover, C.; Froeschl, M.; Dick, A.; Marquis, J.F.; O'Brien, E.; Goncalves, S.; et al. Point-of-care genetic testing for personalisation of antiplatelet treatment (rapid gene): A prospective, randomised, proof-of-concept trial. *Lancet* **2012**, *379*, 1705–1711. [CrossRef]
38. So, D.Y.; Wells, G.A.; McPherson, R.; Labinaz, M.; Le May, M.R.; Glover, C.; Dick, A.J.; Froeschl, M.; Marquis, J.F.; Gollob, M.H.; et al. A prospective randomized evaluation of a pharmacogenomic approach to antiplatelet therapy among patients with st-elevation myocardial infarction: The rapid stemi study. *Pharmacogenomics J.* **2016**, *16*, 71–78. [CrossRef]
39. Xie, X.; Ma, Y.T.; Yang, Y.N.; Li, X.M.; Zheng, Y.Y.; Ma, X.; Fu, Z.Y.; Ba, B.; Li, Y.; Yu, Z.X.; et al. Personalized antiplatelet therapy according to CYP2C19 genotype after percutaneous coronary intervention: A randomized control trial. *Int. J. Cardiol.* **2013**, *168*, 3736–3740. [CrossRef]
40. Notarangelo, F.M.; Maglietta, G.; Bevilacqua, P.; Cereda, M.; Merlini, P.A.; Villani, G.Q.; Moruzzi, P.; Patrizi, G.; Malagoli Tagliazucchi, G.; Crocamo, A.; et al. Pharmacogenomic approach to selecting antiplatelet therapy in patients with acute coronary syndromes: The pharmclo trial. *J. Am. Coll. Cardiol.* **2018**, *71*, 1869–1877. [CrossRef]

41. Bergmeijer, T.O.; Janssen, P.W.; Schipper, J.C.; Qaderdan, K.; Ishak, M.; Ruitenbeek, R.S.; Asselbergs, F.W.; van't Hof, A.W.; Dewilde, W.J.; Spano, F.; et al. CYP2C19 genotype-guided antiplatelet therapy in st-segment elevation myocardial infarction patients-rationale and design of the patient outcome after primary pci (popular) genetics study. *Am. Heart J.* **2014**, *168*, 16-22.e1. [CrossRef]
42. Wiviott, S.D.; Braunwald, E.; McCabe, C.H.; Montalescot, G.; Ruzyllo, W.; Gottlieb, S.; Neumann, F.J.; Ardissino, D.; De Servi, S.; Murphy, S.A.; et al. Prasugrel versus clopidogrel in patients with acute coronary syndromes. *N. Engl. J. Med.* **2007**, *357*, 2001–2015. [CrossRef]
43. Wallentin, L.; Becker, R.C.; Budaj, A.; Cannon, C.P.; Emanuelsson, H.; Held, C.; Horrow, J.; Husted, S.; James, S.; Katus, H.; et al. Ticagrelor versus clopidogrel in patients with acute coronary syndromes. *N. Engl. J. Med.* **2009**, *361*, 1045–1057. [CrossRef]
44. Osnabrugge, R.L.; Head, S.J.; Zijlstra, F.; ten Berg, J.M.; Hunink, M.G.; Kappetein, A.P.; Janssens, A.C. A systematic review and critical assessment of 11 discordant meta-analyses on reduced-function CYP2C19 genotype and risk of adverse clinical outcomes in clopidogrel users. *Genet. Med.* **2015**, *17*, 3–11. [CrossRef]
45. Davila-Fajardo, C.L.; Sanchez-Ramos, J.; Villamarin, X.D.; Martinez-Gonzalez, L.J.; Frias, P.T.; Huertas, S.M.; Gomez, F.B.; Borrego, J.C.; Paves, A.B.; Guzman, M.C.; et al. The study protocol for a non-randomized controlled clinical trial using a genotype-guided strategy in a dataset of patients who undergone percutaneous coronary intervention with stent. *Data Brief.* **2017**, *10*, 518–524. [CrossRef] [PubMed]
46. Kheiri, B.; Osman, M.; Abdalla, A.; Haykal, T.; Pandrangi, P.V.; Chahine, A.; Ahmed, S.; Osman, K.; Bachuwa, G.; Hassan, M.; et al. CYP2C19 pharmacogenetics versus standard of care dosing for selecting antiplatelet therapy in patients with coronary artery disease: A meta-analysis of randomized clinical trials. *Catheter. Cardiovasc. Interv.* **2018**. [CrossRef] [PubMed]
47. Tam, C.C.; Kwok, J.; Wong, A.; Yung, A.; Shea, C.; Kong, S.L.; Tang, W.H.; Siu, D.; Chan, R.; Lee, S. Genotyping-guided approach versus the conventional approach in selection of oral p2y12 receptor blockers in chinese patients suffering from acute coronary syndrome. *J. Int. Med. Res.* **2017**, *45*, 134–146. [CrossRef] [PubMed]
48. American College of Cardiology Annual Scientific Session. *Assessment of Prospective CYP2C19 Genotype Guided Dosing of Anti-Platelet Therapy in Percutaneous Coronary Intervention (Adapt)*; American College of Cardiology Annual Scientific Session (ACC 2018): Orlando, FL, USA, 2018.
49. Tomaniak, M.; Koltowski, L.; Kochman, J.; Huczek, Z.; Rdzanek, A.; Pietrasik, A.; Gasecka, A.; Gajda, S.; Opolski, G.; Filipiak, K.J. Can prasugrel decrease the extent of periprocedural myocardial injury during elective percutaneous coronary intervention? *Pol. Arch. Intern. Med.* **2017**, *127*, 730–740.
50. Scott, S.A.; Sangkuhl, K.; Gardner, E.E.; Stein, C.M.; Hulot, J.S.; Johnson, J.A.; Roden, D.M.; Klein, T.E.; Shuldiner, A.R.; Clinical Pharmacogenetics Implementation Consortium. Clinical pharmacogenetics implementation consortium guidelines for cytochrome p450-2c19 (CYP2C19) genotype and clopidogrel therapy. *Clin. Pharmacol. Ther.* **2011**, *90*, 328–332. [CrossRef]
51. Scott, S.A.; Sangkuhl, K.; Stein, C.M.; Hulot, J.S.; Mega, J.L.; Roden, D.M.; Klein, T.E.; Sabatine, M.S.; Johnson, J.A.; Shuldiner, A.R.; et al. Clinical pharmacogenetics implementation consortium guidelines for CYP2C19 genotype and clopidogrel therapy: 2013 update. *Clin. Pharmacol. Ther.* **2013**, *94*, 317–323. [CrossRef]
52. Swen, J.J.; Wilting, I.; de Goede, A.L.; Grandia, L.; Mulder, H.; Touw, D.J.; de Boer, A.; Conemans, J.M.; Egberts, T.C.; Klungel, O.H.; et al. Pharmacogenetics: From bench to byte. *Clin. Pharmacol. Ther.* **2008**, *83*, 781–787. [CrossRef]
53. Swen, J.J.; Nijenhuis, M.; de Boer, A.; Grandia, L.; Maitland-van der Zee, A.H.; Mulder, H.; Rongen, G.A.; van Schaik, R.H.; Schalekamp, T.; Touw, D.J.; et al. Pharmacogenetics: From bench to byte—An update of guidelines. *Clin. Pharmacol. Ther.* **2011**, *89*, 662–673. [CrossRef] [PubMed]
54. Bhatt, D.L.; Pare, G.; Eikelboom, J.W.; Simonsen, K.L.; Emison, E.S.; Fox, K.A.; Steg, P.G.; Montalescot, G.; Bhakta, N.; Hacke, W.; et al. The relationship between CYP2C19 polymorphisms and ischaemic and bleeding outcomes in stable outpatients: The charisma genetics study. *Eur. Heart J.* **2012**, *33*, 2143–2150. [CrossRef] [PubMed]

55. Levine, G.N.; Bates, E.R.; Bittl, J.A.; Brindis, R.G.; Fihn, S.D.; Fleisher, L.A.; Granger, C.B.; Lange, R.A.; Mack, M.J.; Mauri, L.; et al. 2016 ACC/AHA guideline focused update on duration of dual antiplatelet therapy in patients with coronary artery disease: A report of the american college of cardiology/american heart association task force on clinical practice guidelines. *J. Am. Coll. Cardiol.* **2016**, *68*, 1082–1115. [CrossRef]
56. Weitzel, K.W.; Elsey, A.R.; Langaee, T.Y.; Burkley, B.; Nessl, D.R.; Obeng, A.O.; Staley, B.J.; Dong, H.J.; Allan, R.W.; Liu, J.F.; et al. Clinical pharmacogenetics implementation: Approaches, successes, and challenges. *Am. J. Med. Genet. C Semin. Med. Genet.* **2014**, *166C*, 56–67. [CrossRef] [PubMed]
57. Pulley, J.M.; Denny, J.C.; Peterson, J.F.; Bernard, G.R.; Vnencak-Jones, C.L.; Ramirez, A.H.; Delaney, J.T.; Bowton, E.; Brothers, K.; Johnson, K.; et al. Operational implementation of prospective genotyping for personalized medicine: The design of the vanderbilt predict project. *Clin. Pharmacol. Ther.* **2012**, *92*, 87–95. [CrossRef]
58. Cavallari, L.H.; Franchi, F.; Rollini, F.; Been, L.; Rivas, A.; Agarwal, M.; Smith, D.M.; Newsom, K.; Gong, Y.; Elsey, A.R.; et al. Clinical implementation of rapid CYP2C19 genotyping to guide antiplatelet therapy after percutaneous coronary intervention. *J. Transl. Med.* **2018**, *16*, 92. [CrossRef]
59. Lee, C.R.; Sriramoju, V.B.; Cervantes, A.; Howell, L.A.; Varunok, N.; Madan, S.; Hamrick, K.; Polasek, M.J.; Lee, J.A.; Clarke, M.; et al. Clinical outcomes and sustainability of using CYP2C19 genotype-guided antiplatelet therapy after percutaneous coronary intervention. *Circ. Genom. Precis. Med.* **2018**, *11*, e002069. [CrossRef]
60. Fragoulakis, V.; Bartsakoulia, M.; Diaz-Villamarin, X.; Chalikiopoulou, K.; Kehagia, K.; Ramos, J.G.S.; Martinez-Gonzalez, L.J.; Gkotsi, M.; Katrali, E.; Skoufas, E.; et al. Cost-effectiveness analysis of pharmacogenomics-guided clopidogrel treatment in spanish patients undergoing percutaneous coronary intervention. *Pharmacogenomics J.* **2019**. [CrossRef]
61. Reese, E.S.; Daniel Mullins, C.; Beitelshees, A.L.; Onukwugha, E. Cost-effectiveness of cytochrome p450 2c19 genotype screening for selection of antiplatelet therapy with clopidogrel or prasugrel. *Pharmacotherapy* **2012**, *32*, 323–332. [CrossRef]
62. Kazi, D.S.; Garber, A.M.; Shah, R.U.; Dudley, R.A.; Mell, M.W.; Rhee, C.; Moshkevich, S.; Boothroyd, D.B.; Owens, D.K.; Hlatky, M.A. Cost-effectiveness of genotype-guided and dual antiplatelet therapies in acute coronary syndrome. *Ann. Intern. Med.* **2014**, *160*, 221–232. [CrossRef]
63. Jiang, M.; You, J.H. Cost-effectiveness analysis of personalized antiplatelet therapy in patients with acute coronary syndrome. *Pharmacogenomics* **2016**, *17*, 701–713. [CrossRef]
64. Johnson, S.G.; Gruntowicz, D.; Chua, T.; Morlock, R.J. Financial analysis of CYP2C19 genotyping in patients receiving dual antiplatelet therapy following acute coronary syndrome and percutaneous coronary intervention. *J. Manag. Care Spec. Pharm.* **2015**, *21*, 552–557. [CrossRef]
65. Plumpton, C.O.; Roberts, D.; Pirmohamed, M.; Hughes, D.A. A systematic review of economic evaluations of pharmacogenetic testing for prevention of adverse drug reactions. *Pharmacoeconomics* **2016**, *34*, 771–793. [CrossRef]
66. Carlquist, J.F.; Horne, B.D.; Muhlestein, J.B.; Lappe, D.L.; Whiting, B.M.; Kolek, M.J.; Clarke, J.L.; James, B.C.; Anderson, J.L. Genotypes of the cytochrome p450 isoform, cyp2c9, and the vitamin k epoxide reductase complex subunit 1 conjointly determine stable warfarin dose: A prospective study. *J. Thromb. Thrombolysis* **2006**, *22*, 191–197. [CrossRef]
67. Johnson, J.A.; Gong, L.; Whirl-Carrillo, M.; Gage, B.F.; Scott, S.A.; Stein, C.M.; Anderson, J.L.; Kimmel, S.E.; Lee, M.T.; Pirmohamed, M.; et al. Clinical pharmacogenetics implementation consortium guidelines for cyp2c9 and vkorc1 genotypes and warfarin dosing. *Clin. Pharmacol. Ther.* **2011**, *90*, 625–629. [CrossRef]
68. Stehle, S.; Kirchheiner, J.; Lazar, A.; Fuhr, U. Pharmacogenetics of oral anticoagulants: A basis for dose individualization. *Clin. Pharmacokinet.* **2008**, *47*, 565–594. [CrossRef]
69. Kamali, F.; Wynne, H. Pharmacogenetics of warfarin. *Annu. Rev. Med.* **2010**, *61*, 63–75. [CrossRef]
70. Gage, B.F.; Eby, C.; Johnson, J.A.; Deych, E.; Rieder, M.J.; Ridker, P.M.; Milligan, P.E.; Grice, G.; Lenzini, P.; Rettie, A.E.; et al. Use of pharmacogenetic and clinical factors to predict the therapeutic dose of warfarin. *Clin. Pharmacol. Ther.* **2008**, *84*, 326–331. [CrossRef]
71. Wadelius, M.; Pirmohamed, M. Pharmacogenetics of warfarin: Current status and future challenges. *Pharm. J.* **2007**, *7*, 99–111. [CrossRef]

72. Gage, B.F.; Eby, C.; Milligan, P.E.; Banet, G.A.; Duncan, J.R.; McLeod, H.L. Use of pharmacogenetics and clinical factors to predict the maintenance dose of warfarin. *Thromb. Haemost.* **2004**, *91*, 87–94.
73. *Coumadin- (Warfarin Sodium) Tablet [Package Insert]*; Bristol-Myers Squibb Pharma Company: Princeton, NJ, USA, 2015.
74. International Warfarin Pharmacogenetics Consortium; Klein, T.E.; Altman, R.B.; Eriksson, N.; Gage, B.F.; Kimmel, S.E.; Lee, M.T.; Limdi, N.A.; Page, D.; Roden, D.M.; et al. Estimation of the warfarin dose with clinical and pharmacogenetic data. *N. Engl. J. Med.* **2009**, *360*, 753–764.
75. Santos, P.C.; Marcatto, L.R.; Duarte, N.E.; Gadi Soares, R.A.; Cassaro Strunz, C.M.; Scanavacca, M.; Krieger, J.E.; Pereira, A.C. Development of a pharmacogenetic-based warfarin dosing algorithm and its performance in brazilian patients: Highlighting the importance of population-specific calibration. *Pharmacogenomics* **2015**, *16*, 865–876. [CrossRef]
76. Wei, M.; Ye, F.; Xie, D.; Zhu, Y.; Zhu, J.; Tao, Y.; Yu, F. A new algorithm to predict warfarin dose from polymorphisms of cyp4f2, cyp2c9 and vkorc1 and clinical variables: Derivation in han chinese patients with non valvular atrial fibrillation. *Thromb. Haemost.* **2012**, *107*, 1083–1091. [CrossRef]
77. Finkelman, B.S.; Gage, B.F.; Johnson, J.A.; Brensinger, C.M.; Kimmel, S.E. Genetic warfarin dosing: Tables versus algorithms. *J. Am. Coll. Cardiol.* **2011**, *57*, 612–618. [CrossRef]
78. Kimmel, S.E.; French, B.; Kasner, S.E.; Johnson, J.A.; Anderson, J.L.; Gage, B.F.; Rosenberg, Y.D.; Eby, C.S.; Madigan, R.A.; McBane, R.B.; et al. A pharmacogenetic versus a clinical algorithm for warfarin dosing. *N. Engl. J. Med.* **2013**, *369*, 2283–2293. [CrossRef] [PubMed]
79. Kimmel, S.E.; French, B.; Geller, N.L.; Investigators, C. Genotype-guided dosing of vitamin k antagonists. *N. Engl. J. Med.* **2014**, *370*, 1763–1764.
80. Shaw, K.; Amstutz, U.; Kim, R.B.; Lesko, L.J.; Turgeon, J.; Michaud, V.; Hwang, S.; Ito, S.; Ross, C.; Carleton, B.C.; et al. Clinical practice recommendations on genetic testing of cyp2c9 and vkorc1 variants in warfarin therapy. *Ther. Drug Monit.* **2015**, *37*, 428–436. [CrossRef] [PubMed]
81. Jiang, N.X.; Ge, J.W.; Xian, Y.Q.; Huang, S.Y.; Li, Y.S. Clinical application of a new warfarin-dosing regimen based on the cyp2c9 and vkorc1 genotypes in atrial fibrillation patients. *Biomed. Rep.* **2016**, *4*, 453–458. [CrossRef]
82. Gage, B.F.; Bass, A.R.; Lin, H.; Woller, S.C.; Stevens, S.M.; Al-Hammadi, N.; Li, J.; Rodriguez, T., Jr.; Miller, J.P.; McMillin, G.A.; et al. Effect of genotype-guided warfarin dosing on clinical events and anticoagulation control among patients undergoing hip or knee arthroplasty: The gift randomized clinical trial. *JAMA* **2017**, *318*, 1115–1124. [CrossRef] [PubMed]
83. Goulding, R.; Dawes, D.; Price, M.; Wilkie, S.; Dawes, M. Genotype-guided drug prescribing: A systematic review and meta-analysis of randomized control trials. *Br. J. Clin. Pharmacol.* **2015**, *80*, 868–877. [CrossRef] [PubMed]
84. Liao, Z.; Feng, S.; Ling, P.; Zhang, G. Meta-analysis of randomized controlled trials reveals an improved clinical outcome of using genotype plus clinical algorithm for warfarin dosing. *J. Thromb. Thrombolysis* **2015**, *39*, 228–234. [CrossRef]
85. Tang, Q.; Zou, H.; Guo, C.; Liu, Z. Outcomes of pharmacogenetics-guided dosing of warfarin: A systematic review and meta-analysis. *Int. J. Cardiol.* **2014**, *175*, 587–591. [CrossRef]
86. Belley-Cote, E.P.; Hanif, H.; D'Aragon, F.; Eikelboom, J.W.; Anderson, J.L.; Borgman, M.; Jonas, D.E.; Kimmel, S.E.; Manolopoulos, V.G.; Baranova, E.; et al. Genotype-guided versus standard vitamin k antagonist dosing algorithms in patients initiating anticoagulation. A systematic review and meta-analysis. *Thromb. Haemost.* **2015**, *114*, 768–777. [CrossRef] [PubMed]
87. Li, X.; Yang, J.; Wang, X.; Xu, Q.; Zhang, Y.; Yin, T. Clinical benefits of pharmacogenetic algorithm-based warfarin dosing: Meta-analysis of randomized controlled trials. *Thromb. Res.* **2015**, *135*, 621–629. [CrossRef] [PubMed]
88. Dahal, K.; Sharma, S.P.; Fung, E.; Lee, J.; Moore, J.H.; Unterborn, J.N.; Williams, S.M. Meta-analysis of randomized controlled trials of genotype-guided vs standard dosing of warfarin. *Chest* **2015**, *148*, 701–710. [CrossRef]
89. Shi, C.; Yan, W.; Wang, G.; Wang, F.; Li, Q.; Lin, N. Pharmacogenetics-based versus conventional dosing of warfarin: A meta-analysis of randomized controlled trials. *PLoS ONE* **2015**, *10*, e0144511. [CrossRef] [PubMed]

90. Johnson, J.A.; Caudle, K.E.; Gong, L.; Whirl-Carrillo, M.; Stein, C.M.; Scott, S.A.; Lee, M.T.; Gage, B.F.; Kimmel, S.E.; Perera, M.A.; et al. Clinical pharmacogenetics implementation consortium (cpic) guideline for pharmacogenetics-guided warfarin dosing: 2017 update. *Clin. Pharmacol. Ther.* **2017**, *102*, 397–404. [CrossRef] [PubMed]
91. Borgiani, P.; Ciccacci, C.; Forte, V.; Sirianni, E.; Novelli, L.; Bramanti, P.; Novelli, G. Cyp4f2 genetic variant (rs2108622) significantly contributes to warfarin dosing variability in the italian population. *Pharmacogenomics* **2009**, *10*, 261–266. [CrossRef]
92. Eckman, M.H.; Rosand, J.; Greenberg, S.M.; Gage, B.F. Cost-effectiveness of using pharmacogenetic information in warfarin dosing for patients with nonvalvular atrial fibrillation. *Ann. Intern. Med.* **2009**, *150*, 73–83. [CrossRef]
93. Leey, J.A.; McCabe, S.; Koch, J.A.; Miles, T.P. Cost-effectiveness of genotype-guided warfarin therapy for anticoagulation in elderly patients with atrial fibrillation. *Am. J. Geriatr. Pharmacother.* **2009**, *7*, 197–203. [CrossRef]
94. Pink, J.; Pirmohamed, M.; Lane, S.; Hughes, D.A. Cost-effectiveness of pharmacogenetics-guided warfarin therapy vs. Alternative anticoagulation in atrial fibrillation. *Clin. Pharmacol. Ther.* **2014**, *95*, 199–207. [CrossRef]
95. Trailokya, A.; Hiremath, J.S.; Sawhney, J.; Mishra, Y.K.; Kanhere, V.; Srinivasa, R.; Tiwaskar, M. Acenocoumarol: A review of anticoagulant efficacy and safety. *J. Assoc. Physicians India* **2016**, *64*, 88–93.
96. Verde, Z.; Ruiz, J.R.; Santiago, C.; Valle, B.; Bandres, F.; Calvo, E.; Lucia, A.; Gomez Gallego, F. A novel, single algorithm approach to predict acenocoumarol dose based on cyp2c9 and vkorc1 allele variants. *PLoS ONE* **2010**, *5*, e11210. [CrossRef]
97. Rathore, S.S.; Agarwal, S.K.; Pande, S.; Singh, S.K.; Mittal, T.; Mittal, B. Therapeutic dosing of acenocoumarol: Proposal of a population specific pharmacogenetic dosing algorithm and its validation in north indians. *PLoS ONE* **2012**, *7*, e37844. [CrossRef]
98. Krishna Kumar, D.; Shewade, D.G.; Loriot, M.A.; Beaune, P.; Sai Chandran, B.V.; Balachander, J.; Adithan, C. An acenocoumarol dosing algorithm exploiting clinical and genetic factors in south indian (dravidian) population. *Eur. J. Clin. Pharmacol.* **2015**, *71*, 173–181. [CrossRef]
99. Van Schie, R.M.; Wessels, J.A.; le Cessie, S.; de Boer, A.; Schalekamp, T.; van der Meer, F.J.; Verhoef, T.I.; van Meegen, E.; Rosendaal, F.R.; Maitland-van der Zee, A.H.; et al. Loading and maintenance dose algorithms for phenprocoumon and acenocoumarol using patient characteristics and pharmacogenetic data. *Eur. Heart J.* **2011**, *32*, 1909–1917. [CrossRef]
100. Borobia, A.M.; Lubomirov, R.; Ramirez, E.; Lorenzo, A.; Campos, A.; Munoz-Romo, R.; Fernandez-Capitan, C.; Frias, J.; Carcas, A.J. An acenocoumarol dosing algorithm using clinical and pharmacogenetic data in spanish patients with thromboembolic disease. *PLoS ONE* **2012**, *7*, e41360. [CrossRef]
101. Cerezo-Manchado, J.J.; Rosafalco, M.; Anton, A.I.; Perez-Andreu, V.; Garcia-Barbera, N.; Martinez, A.B.; Corral, J.; Vicente, V.; Gonzalez-Conejero, R.; Roldan, V. Creating a genotype-based dosing algorithm for acenocoumarol steady dose. *Thromb. Haemost.* **2013**, *109*, 146–153. [CrossRef]
102. Tong, H.Y.; Davila-Fajardo, C.L.; Borobia, A.M.; Martinez-Gonzalez, L.J.; Lubomirov, R.; Perea Leon, L.M.; Blanco Banares, M.J.; Diaz-Villamarin, X.; Fernandez-Capitan, C.; Cabeza Barrera, J.; et al. A new pharmacogenetic algorithm to predict the most appropriate dosage of acenocoumarol for stable anticoagulation in a mixed spanish population. *PLoS ONE* **2016**, *11*, e0150456. [CrossRef]
103. Baranova, E.V.; Verhoef, T.I.; Ragia, G.; le Cessie, S.; Asselbergs, F.W.; de Boer, A.; Manolopoulos, V.G.; Maitland-van der Zee, A.H.; EU-PACT group. Dosing algorithms for vitamin k antagonists across vkorc1 and cyp2c9 genotypes. *J. Thromb. Haemost.* **2017**, *15*, 465–472. [CrossRef]
104. Danese, E.; Raimondi, S.; Montagnana, M.; Tagetti, A.; Langaee, T.; Borgiani, P.; Ciccacci, C.; Carcas, A.J.; Borobia, A.M.; Tong, H.Y.; et al. The effect of CYP4F2, VKORC1 and CYP2C9 in influencing coumarin dose. A single patient data meta-analysis in more than 15,000 individuals. *Clin. Pharmacol. Ther.* **2018**. [CrossRef]
105. Wilke, R.A.; Lin, D.W.; Roden, D.M.; Watkins, P.B.; Flockhart, D.; Zineh, I.; Giacomini, K.M.; Krauss, R.M. Identifying genetic risk factors for serious adverse drug reactions: Current progress and challenges. *Nat. Rev. Drug Discov.* **2007**, *6*, 904–916. [CrossRef]

106. Group, S.S.C.; Bowman, L.; Armitage, J.; Bulbulia, R.; Parish, S.; Collins, R. Study of the effectiveness of additional reductions in cholesterol and homocysteine (search): Characteristics of a randomized trial among 12064 myocardial infarction survivors. *Am. Heart J.* **2007**, *154*, 815–823, 823.e1–823.e6.
107. Ramsey, L.B.; Johnson, S.G.; Caudle, K.E.; Haidar, C.E.; Voora, D.; Wilke, R.A.; Maxwell, W.D.; McLeod, H.L.; Krauss, R.M.; Roden, D.M.; et al. The clinical pharmacogenetics implementation consortium guideline for slco1b1 and simvastatin-induced myopathy: 2014 update. *Clin. Pharmacol. Ther.* **2014**, *96*, 423–428. [CrossRef]
108. Tsamandouras, N.; Dickinson, G.; Guo, Y.; Hall, S.; Rostami-Hodjegan, A.; Galetin, A.; Aarons, L. Development and application of a mechanistic pharmacokinetic model for simvastatin and its active metabolite simvastatin acid using an integrated population pbpk approach. *Pharm. Res.* **2015**, *32*, 1864–1883. [CrossRef]
109. Pasanen, M.K.; Neuvonen, M.; Neuvonen, P.J.; Niemi, M. Slco1b1 polymorphism markedly affects the pharmacokinetics of simvastatin acid. *Pharmacogenet. Genomics* **2006**, *16*, 873–879. [CrossRef]
110. Group, S.C.; Link, E.; Parish, S.; Armitage, J.; Bowman, L.; Heath, S.; Matsuda, F.; Gut, I.; Lathrop, M.; Collins, R. Slco1b1 variants and statin-induced myopathy—A genomewide study. *N. Engl. J. Med.* **2008**, *359*, 789–799.
111. Voora, D.; Shah, S.H.; Spasojevic, I.; Ali, S.; Reed, C.R.; Salisbury, B.A.; Ginsburg, G.S. The slco1b1*5 genetic variant is associated with statin-induced side effects. *J. Am. Coll. Cardiol.* **2009**, *54*, 1609–1616. [CrossRef]
112. Brunham, L.R.; Lansberg, P.J.; Zhang, L.; Miao, F.; Carter, C.; Hovingh, G.K.; Visscher, H.; Jukema, J.W.; Stalenhoef, A.F.; Ross, C.J.; et al. Differential effect of the rs4149056 variant in slco1b1 on myopathy associated with simvastatin and atorvastatin. *Pharmacogenomics J.* **2012**, *12*, 233–237. [CrossRef]
113. EMA: Guideline on the Use of Pharmacogenetic Methodologies in the Pharmacokinetic Evaluation of Medical Products. Available online: https://www.ema.europa.eu/en/use-pharmacogenetic-methodologies-pharmacokinetic-evaluation-medicinal-products (accessed on 2 February 2012).
114. Bergmeijer, T.O.; ten Berg, J.M. Value of CYP2C19 *2 and *17 genotyping in clinical practice. Promising but not ready yet. *Rev. Esp. Cardiol. (Engl. Ed.)* **2012**, *65*, 205–207. [CrossRef]
115. Higgins, J.P.; Thompson, S.G.; Deeks, J.J.; Altman, D.G. Measuring inconsistency in meta-analyses. *BMJ* **2003**, *327*, 557–560. [CrossRef]
116. Koller, E.A.; Roche, J.C.; Rollins, J.A. Genotype-guided dosing of vitamin k antagonists. *N. Engl. J. Med.* **2014**, *370*, 1761.
117. Kirchheiner, J.; Ufer, M.; Walter, E.C.; Kammerer, B.; Kahlich, R.; Meisel, C.; Schwab, M.; Gleiter, C.H.; Rane, A.; Roots, I.; et al. Effects of CYP2C9 polymorphisms on the pharmacokinetics of r- and s-phenprocoumon in healthy volunteers. *Pharmacogenetics* **2004**, *14*, 19–26. [CrossRef]

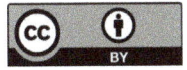

© 2019 by the authors. Licensee MDPI, Basel, Switzerland. This article is an open access article distributed under the terms and conditions of the Creative Commons Attribution (CC BY) license (http://creativecommons.org/licenses/by/4.0/).

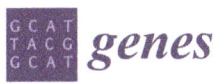

Review

Pharmacogenomic and Pharmacotranscriptomic Profiling of Childhood Acute Lymphoblastic Leukemia: Paving the Way to Personalized Treatment

Sonja Pavlovic [1,*], Nikola Kotur [1], Biljana Stankovic [1], Branka Zukic [1], Vladimir Gasic [1] and Lidija Dokmanovic [2,3]

1. Laboratory for Molecular Biomedicine, Institute of Molecular Genetics and Genetic Engineering, University of Belgrade, 11000 Belgrade, Serbia; nikola0104@gmail.com (N.K.); bi.stankovic@gmail.com (B.S.); branka.petrucev@gmail.com (B.Z.); vlada.gasic42@gmail.com (V.G.)
2. University Children's Hospital, 11000 Belgrade, Serbia; lidija.dokmanovic@udk.bg.ac.rs
3. Faculty of Medicine, University of Belgrade, 11000 Belgrade, Serbia
* Correspondence: sonya@sezampro.rs

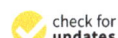

Received: 4 February 2019; Accepted: 25 February 2019; Published: 1 March 2019

Abstract: Personalized medicine is focused on research disciplines which contribute to the individualization of therapy, like pharmacogenomics and pharmacotranscriptomics. Acute lymphoblastic leukemia (ALL) is the most common malignancy of childhood. It is one of the pediatric malignancies with the highest cure rate, but still a lethal outcome due to therapy accounts for 1–3% of deaths. Further improvement of treatment protocols is needed through the implementation of pharmacogenomics and pharmacotranscriptomics. Emerging high-throughput technologies, including microarrays and next-generation sequencing, have provided an enormous amount of molecular data with the potential to be implemented in childhood ALL treatment protocols. In the current review, we summarized the contribution of these novel technologies to the pharmacogenomics and pharmacotranscriptomics of childhood ALL. We have presented data on molecular markers responsible for the efficacy, side effects, and toxicity of the drugs commonly used for childhood ALL treatment, i.e., glucocorticoids, vincristine, asparaginase, anthracyclines, thiopurines, and methotrexate. Big data was generated using high-throughput technologies, but their implementation in clinical practice is poor. Research efforts should be focused on data analysis and designing prediction models using machine learning algorithms. Bioinformatics tools and the implementation of artificial intelligence are expected to open the door wide for personalized medicine in the clinical practice of childhood ALL.

Keywords: pharmacogenomics; pharmacotranscriptomics; high-throughput analysis; childhood acute lymphoblastic leukemia

1. Introduction

Emerging high-throughput technologies, which enable the analysis of individual genomes, epigenomes, transcriptomes, proteomes, metabolomes, and microbiomes, so called "omics", have brought great advancements in the field of biomedical sciences [1]. Moreover, multiple genomic, epigenomic, transcriptomic, and proteomic markers have already been included in routine diagnostic, prognostic, and therapeutic protocols for a great number of diseases [2,3]. This is important for designing new therapies, like molecular and gene therapy, which is the basis of personalized medicine.

Pharmacogenetics and pharmacogenomics are staples of personalized medicine. The goal of pharmacogenomics is to create an effective therapy strategy based on the genomic profile of a patient. Pharmacotranscriptomics is a field of study which investigates associations between variations in the transcriptome with the pharmacokinetics and the pharmacodynamics of drugs to detect interindividual differences between patients, so that a more efficient dose regimen of a drug can be established.

There are two main approaches in pharmacogenomics and pharmacotranscriptomics: One based on candidate pharmacogenes/pharmacotranscripts, the other based on testing the entire genome/transcriptome (genome-wide association studies/transcriptome-wide association studies (GWAS/TWAS)) for pharmacogenomic/pharmacotranscriptomic markers. Candidate genes/transcripts studies have high statistical power, but their weakness is the fact that they lack the capacity to discover new genes or transcripts. On the contrary, the strength of GWAS/TWAS lies in the ability to identify relevant pharmacogenomic or pharmacotranscriptomic markers regardless of whether their function was previously known, but they have low statistical power due to the number of independent tests performed [4].

Acute lymphoblastic leukemia (ALL) is the most common malignancy of childhood, accounting for around 30% of all childhood cancers and around 80% of all childhood leukemia. It is one of the pediatric malignancies with the highest cure rate [5]. However, more than 10% of patients experience an unfavorable outcome.

Considering that more efficient treatment of pediatric ALL has not been achieved by the introduction of novel drugs into the treatment protocols, but instead by trying to diminish the adverse effects of the drugs that are already included in the protocols, it is understandable that pharmacogenomics and pharmacotranscriptomics have become very important in this field.

In the current review, we present the results of pharmacogenomics and pharmacotranscriptomics studies conducted in pediatric ALL using high-throughput technologies. We aim to summarize the contributions of these novel technologies in this field to find out what additional opportunities they offer and to suggest future directions.

2. Childhood Acute Lymphoblastic Leukemia

Acute lymphoblastic leukemia (ALL) is a rare disease, representing about one fourth of all cancers in children. The incidence rate of ALL among children aged up to 14 years is about 41:1,000,000, with a peak in children aged 2–7 years. Biologically, the disease originates from T- and B-lymphoid precursors of the bone marrow [6].

In childhood ALL, almost all patients achieve remission, and about 85% of the patients are expected to be cured with modern treatment protocols [7]. The treatment of the patients with ALL is usually tailored according to risk group stratification defined by clinical and laboratory features [8]. Standard treatment options for childhood ALL encompass historically validated cytotoxic agents grouped into so called therapeutic phases or elements. These include remission induction chemotherapy agents—vincristine, a corticosteroid drug, anthracyclines, and asparaginase [9]. Post-induction (or consolidation) treatment options for childhood ALL include cyclophosphamide, cytarabine, 6-mercaptopurine, and high-dose methotrexate. Most protocols also include an intensification phase, utilizing the same drugs, namely vincristine, corticosteroids, anthracyclines, and cytarabine, combined with another thiopurine, such as 6-thioguanine [10]. After completing intensive treatment phases, the patient is due for maintenance therapy, whose backbone is based on daily oral 6-mercaptopurine and weekly oral methotrexate.

Hematopoietic stem cell transplantation also has a role in the treatment of ALL patients, such as those with unfavorable clinical and laboratory features as well as patients with relapsed disease.

Efficient therapy causes side effects in 75% of childhood ALL patients [11]. Aside from this, chemotherapy leads to delayed side effects and even permanent sequelae [12,13]. It is estimated that 1–3% of pediatric ALL patients have a lethal outcome due to the consequences of treatment side effects and not due to the consequence of the disease [8,14].

It is necessary to emphasize that a patient with a malignancy has two genomes: The constitutional genome, characteristic for all cells except the tumor clone; the other is the tumor genome that contains acquired genetic variants and which changes during the evolution of tumor clones. Variants in the constitutional genome and germinative variants influence the transport and the metabolism of drugs, making them responsible for the efficacy of the drugs and the side effects, while somatic mutations are responsible for the resistance of the tumor to drugs [15].

The side effects of therapy in pediatric ALL are a consequence of the insufficient specificity of drugs, the small therapeutic index of drugs, and the high exposure and long-term application of drugs. The most frequent complications are hypersensitive reactions, neuro-, cardio-, and hepatotoxicity, the toxicity of the digestive tract and kidneys, as well as myelosuppression and osteonecrosis [11]. General toxicity can be diminished by patient stratification, while individual patient toxicity caused by genetic variants of the genes responsible for drug metabolism can be prevented with specific genetic tests and individually tailored chemotherapy [16,17].

3. Glucocorticoid Drugs

Synthetics glucocorticoids (GCs) are some of the most frequently used drugs in the treatment of immune or inflammatory diseases, like inflammatory bowel disease, asthma, allergic rhinitis, etc. The capability of GCs to induce apoptosis in thymocytes, monocytes, and peripheral T cells makes them a central component in chemotherapeutic protocols in the treatment of leukemia, lymphomas, and myelomas. GCs drugs, prednisone and dexamethasone, represent the basis of chemotherapy in childhood ALL. The cytotoxic effect of GCs is connected with their antiproliferative effect, which is realized in specific cell types using the glucocorticoid receptor (GR) [18]. A proposed mechanism of action of GCs in lymphoblasts is that they activate the Bim protein, which induces apoptosis and deactivates NF-κB and AP1, thus leading to a negative modulation in cell survival [19]. The most important side effects of GCs drugs are osteonecrosis, sepsis, diabetes, myopathy, hypertension, and behavioral disorders.

The mechanisms of the GCs response in childhood ALL are not well-known yet. Despite confusing results of candidate genes studies, some variants in pharmacogenes could be considered as possible pharmacogenomic markers of the GCs response in ALL.

One of the most important pharmacogenes is the *NR3C1* gene that encodes the GR. Most frequently studied variants in this pharmacogene, like rs6189/rs6190 (ER22/23EK) and rs56149945 (N363S), have not shown a significant association with the therapeutic response to GCs in ALL [20,21]. Another extensively studied variant, rs41423247 (*BclI* variant), has shown an association with the therapeutic response [22].

It has been shown that the presence of the minor allele of variant rs6198 in the 3'UTR region of the *NR3C1* gene is associated with a poor response to GCs in pediatric ALL [23]. The variants, rs33389 and rs33388, have shown to affect the GCs response only when they act as a haplotype [23,24]. On the other hand, the rs33389 C allele and rs33388 T allele as a part of *NR3C1* ACT haplotype (rs41423247-rs33389-rs33388) are strongly associated with GCs sensitivity.

ABCB1 is another pharmacogene relevant to the GCs response that has deserved special attention in candidate gene studies. It encodes for a membrane transporter, P-glycoprotein, an efflux transporter that ejects xenobiotics. The haplotype, *ABCB1* CGT (rs1128503-rs2032582-rs1045641), was found to be associated with a poor GCs response and increased the risk of relapse in the induction remission phase of childhood ALL therapy [25,26]. Until now, only the *ABCB1* C3435T variant was associated with adverse effects, i.e., bone marrow toxicity [25] and grade 1 and grade 2 infections [27].

Glutathione S-transferases (*GSTs*) are genes of the same gene family that encode detoxification enzymes, which initiate the process of elimination of xenobiotics. Three enzymes of this enzyme family have been studied extensively in the context of the GCs response in childhood ALL: GSTM1, GSTT1, and GSTP1. When it came to *GSTT1*, conflicting results were reported [23,28–30]. Variants in *GSTM1* were shown to be associated with the severity of infections [27] and an increased risk of relapse [30]. In one study, it was shown that the *GSTP1* GCs (rs1695-rs1138272) haplotype was associated with a good response to GCs in the remission induction phase of childhood ALL therapy [23].

A variant, rs1876829, in the *CRHR1* gene was shown to be associated with GCs-induced hypertension in childhood ALL [31]. While there are other candidate genes (*ST13*, *STIP1*, *FKBP5*) whose products participate in the GCs pathway, they have not been studied in the context of the GCs response in childhood ALL. Generally, there are not many pharmacogenomics studies related to the GCs response in childhood ALL using the candidate gene approach.

As for candidate transcripts studies, they are even fewer. A higher expression of *ABCB1*, related to the *ABCB1* CGT (rs1128503-rs2032582-rs1045641) haplotype, was found to be associated with GCs resistance [23].

Unlike the candidate gene approach, using high throughput methods in association studies of the GCs response could point to relevant variants or clusters of variants that could be quite important in determining the differences in the GCs response between childhood ALL patients. Novel pharmacogene variants in pediatric ALL could be essential as prognostic and/or predictive biomarkers for selecting the best dose and the right time for GCs treatment of this malignancy [32].

In one GWAS study [33], 440,044 single nucleotide polymorphisms (SNPs) which contributed to the risk of relapse were studied in 2535 childhood ALL patients, after adjusting the studied cohort of patients for genetic ancestry and therapeutic regimens. Of the 134 newly found SNPs associated with the risk of relapse, four SNPs (rs6007758, rs41488548, rs10264856, rs4728709) were found to be associated with a higher clearance of dexamethasone, two of which (rs10264856, rs4728709) were located in the *ABCB1* gene, which was also considered as a pharmacogene for GCs therapy using the candidate gene approach.

In another GWAS [34], it was found that the single region of chromosome 14, which contains *SERPINA6*/*SERPINA1* genes, accounts for around 1% of the variance of plasma cortisol levels. Using an Illumina Exome chip and the meta-analysis of GWAS, one SNP, rs12589136, was found to influence the binding activity of the reactive center loop of the corticosteroid-binding globulin. This led to higher plasma cortisol levels and higher cortisol binding activity. Thus, variant rs12589136 was shown to influence plasma cortisol levels, which could be a future potential target of investigation when it comes to GCs therapy outcomes in childhood ALL patients.

The toxicity of GCs treatment is a generally acknowledged problem in the remission induction therapy of childhood ALL. Osteonecrosis due to the administration of dexamethasone for treating high-risk ALL patients is one of the most dangerous toxicity events of GCs treatment in childhood ALL. One GWAS study [35] found that the SNP, rs10989692, near the glutamate receptor gene, *GRIN3A*, was associated with osteonecrosis. This association was supported by two replication studies of independent cohorts of patients treated with GCs for various medical conditions. The SNP, rs10989692, could be a germline genetic variant that predisposes to glucocorticoid-induced osteonecrosis. In another GWAS study, SNPs in the *ACP1* gene (acid phosphatase 1) were associated with an increased risk of osteonecrosis during dexamethasone treatment of pediatric ALL [36]. The gene, *ACP1*, is important for regulating cholesterol and triglyceride levels [37], meaning that lipid levels are possibly relevant in the pathology of osteonecrosis in pediatric ALL.

Research in the field of pharmacotranscriptomic markers of the GCs response in childhood ALL is still new and insufficient. However, some results have been reported. The long noncoding RNA GAS5 was shown to be associated with a poor GCs response in childhood ALL during remission induction therapy [38]. GAS5 imitates the glucocorticoid response element (GRE) sequence, which is a DNA sequence to which the GC-GR complex needs to bind to in order to realize its effect, thus GAS5 can bind the GC-GR complex and stop it from binding to the GRE sequence [39]. Additionally, the association between two microRNAs, hsa-miR-142-3p and hsa-miR-17-5p, and GCs resistance in pediatric ALL was found using a semantics-oriented computational approach [40].

Microarray gene expression analyses have shown that the modified expression of genes coding for several proteins or transcription factors can be associated with GCs resistance in pediatric ALL. Epithelial membrane protein 1 (EMP1) expression was shown to be higher in prednisone poor responders, unlike in prednisone good responders [41]. EMP1 is a protein that promotes phosphorylation of Src and FAK [42]. The Src kinase family is essential in lymphocyte receptor signaling [43,44]. In another microarray study, the expression of caspase 1 (CASP1) and its activator, NLRP3, was shown to be increased as a result of poor methylation of their promoters. The elevated level of CASP1 results in intensive cleavage of the GR and increased GCs resistance [45].

Genes involved in chromatin remodeling represent another group that shows potential in contributing to the outcome of the GCs response in childhood ALL. One study using microarrays has shown that a decreased expression of three subunits of the SWI/SNF complex (SMARCA4, ARID1A, and SMARCB1) is associated with GR resistance [46]. Furthermore, when CREBBP, a gene which encodes the transcription coactivator and histone-acetyltransferase CREB-binding protein, was investigated using sequencing analysis, later confirmed with gene expression arrays, it was found that damaging mutations in the CREBBP gene contributed to GCs resistance [12].

4. Vincristine

The vinca alkaloid vincristine (VCR) is widely used as an anticancer drug in both solid tumors and other malignancies. VCR's cytotoxic effects are achieved by the disruption of the mitotic spindle microtubules as VCR binds to tubulin dimers. In this way, mitotic arrest is induced and leukemic cells die during metaphase [47]. The toxicity of VCR consists of a peripheral neuropathy described by neuropathic pain and sensory and motor dysfunction, causing the necessary decrease of the VCR dose, the discontinuation of the ALL treatment, and morbidity.

A number of candidate genes involved in different aspects of VCR metabolism have been assessed for an association with both sensory and motor peripheral neuropathies related to VCR treatment in pediatric ALL patients. However, this kind of study has produced inconsistent data on genetic variants associated with an increased risk of VCR-related neuropathy and also on their significance [13,48–55]. Nevertheless, evidence from multiple studies demonstrated that the CYP3A family of enzymes is responsible for the metabolism of the VCR. The most important among them is the CYP3A5 enzyme, and variations in the CYP3A5 gene could be essential for VCR-related side effects in pediatric patients with ALL [49,56]. Namely, the most VCR-toxicity related CYP3A5 allelic variant in Caucasians includes CYP3A5*3, with a single nucleotide change in intron 3 leading to a premature termination codon. Patients that are carriers of the CYP3A5*3/*3 genotype with essentially no CYP3A5 expression have severe VCR-related neurotoxicity side effects [57].

An agnostic approach was applied in GWAS, and the results showed that an inherited variant in the promoter region of the CEP72 gene (rs924607, risk genotype TT) was associated with a higher prevalence and severity of VCR-related peripheral neuropathy in children with ALL, during the two years of continuation therapy [58]. Homozygous carriers of the CEP72 rs924607 risk TT genotype had a cumulative risk of neuropathy that was significantly higher and the mean severity of neuropathy was significantly greater compared with all other patients. CEP72 encodes a centrosomal protein indispensable for microtubule formation. This genomic variant generates a binding site for a NKX-6.3 transcriptional repressor in the CEP72 gene promoter and consequently affects the decrease of CEP72 mRNA expression, endangering microtubule stability. The same study employed shRNA impairment of the CEP72 mRNA expression in in vitro model systems and confirmed findings that reduced CEP72 expression in induced pluripotent stem neuronal cells as well as in leukemia cells increases their sensitivity to VCR. The same findings were confirmed using primary ALL cells from ALL patients who were homozygous carriers of the CEP72 rs924607 TT risk genotype.

The retrospective replication study showed no association between VCR-related neurotoxicity during the induction phase of the ALL treatment and the CEP72 rs924607 risk TT genotype [59]. The distinctive genetic background of the two analyzed populations and/or possible mechanisms causing peripheral neurotoxicity in the early or late phases of ALL treatment could be the reason. Also, the precise number of VCR doses and the overall length of VCR treatment should be considered when assessing VCR-related neurotoxicity [60]. It is possible that other genetic markers in CEP72 or other genes (like CYP3A5) [61] were not taken into account when the replication study was done. It is important to notice that the end points' or "phenotypes'" precise definitions are equally vital to understand when assessing the pharmacogenetics potential of a given marker, as well as the sole genetic variations associated with the phenotype [62].

A study using targeted sequencing and RNA-sequencing revealed that genetic variants in the VCR transporter gene, *ABCC2* (rs3740066 GG and rs12826 GG risk genotypes), were associated with VCR-related neurotoxicity during the induction phase in pediatric ALL patients [63]. Furthermore, a statistically significant protective haplotype, formed by rs3740066–rs3740065–rs12826–rs12762549–rs11190298 (ATAGG) in the *ABCC2* gene, was identified.

Recently, a whole-exome sequencing analysis combined with an exome-wide association study was performed to find out genetic risk factors for VCR-related neurotoxicity [64]. The study identified two variants significantly associated with an increased risk of high-grade VCR-related neurotoxicity, rs2781377 in the *SYNE2* gene and rs10513762 in the *MRPL47* gene. Additionally, variant rs3803357 in the *BAHD1* gene played a protective role regarding neurotoxicity. The *SYNE2* gene or *Nesprin*-2 codes for a protein with an important role in various cellular and nuclear functions [65]. The *MRPL47* gene codes for the mitochondrial ribosomal proteins involved in the oxidative phosphorylation system and, through reduced adenosine triphosphate (ATP) production, the variants in this gene could affect neuropathies, myopathies, and developmental disorders [66]. The *BAHD1* gene, an important regulator of gene silencing, already associated with tumor suppression and inflammation [67], could be connected to sensory and autonomic neuropathy via an epigenetic mechanism [68].

A recent GWAS identified genetic variants, rs1045644 in the coagulation factor C homology (*COCH*) gene and rs7963521 associated with the regulation of chemerin plasma levels, as being significantly associated with VCR-related neuropathy in ALL children [69]. Variant rs1045644 in the *COCH* gene has already been associated with progressive hearing loss and vestibular imbalance [70]. Variant rs7963521, acting through chemerin protein, influences the chemokine like receptor 1, G protein-coupled receptor 1, and the C-C chemokine-like receptor 2, thus affecting various processes, including angiogenesis, adipogenesis, osteoblastogenesis, diabetes, and inflammatory reactions [71]. The involvement of the *CEP72* gene previously reported in VCR-related toxicity [58] was not confirmed in this study [69].

An initial microRNA expression study pointed out involvement of miR-125b, miR-99a, and miR-100 in resistance to VCR and daunorubicine treatment in different major subtypes of pediatric acute leukemia [72]. MiR-125b was expressed significantly higher in patients resistant to VCR or daunorubicine, specifically in *ETV6-RUNX1*-positive ALL patients. Both miR-99a and miR-100 showed an increased expression in ALL children with VCR and daunorubicine resistance, similar to miR-125b. MiR-125b, miR-99a, and miR-100 are co-expressed in acute pediatric ALL [72]. Interestingly, the individual overexpression of these miRNAs did not induce VCR resistance, but miR-125b in combination with miR-99a or miR-100 induced a significant resistance to VCR, resulting in the concept of the synergistic drug resistance modifying effect of combined miRNAs expression [73]. Eleven genes, including four genes encoding ribosomal proteins, were significantly downregulated in *ETV6-RUNX1*-positive cells expressing high levels of miR-125b together with miR-100 and/or miR-99a [73].

A microarray analysis was used in the study, which revealed the association of the rs12894467 risk allele T with the premature mir-300 and toxicity in the induction phase of ALL treatment [74]. In fact, the rs12894467 risk allele T leads to an upregulation of miR-300, whose target among others are the transporters, ABCB1 and ABCC1, involved in VCR detoxification. An association between rs639174 in *DROSHA* and vomiting was also found.

A recent high-throughput study [75] identified the A allele of rs12402181 in the seed region of miR-3117-3p that could increase the efflux of the VCR through the *ABCC1* and *RALBP1* gene, and C allele of rs7896283 in a pre-mature sequence of miR-4481, which could be involved in the regulation of the axon guidance pathway genes and peripheral nerve regeneration, processes that are significantly associated with VCR-related neurotoxicity. The *ABCC1* gene codes for the multidrug resistance protein

1, which mediates the efflux of a broad range of antineoplastic drugs, including VCR and variants that alter the transporter functions and have already been associated with VCR-related neurotoxicity [76].

5. Asparaginase

Asparaginase is an enzyme that catalyzes the hydrolysis of the amino acid, asparagine (Asn), into aspartic acid (Asp) and ammonia. In general, leukemic cells do not synthesize Asn like normal cells, and are therefore dependent on its exogenous input [77]. The introduction of asparaginase leads to a circulating Asn deficit, depriving the leukemic cell of exogenous Asn, and resulting in leukemic cell death.

An asparaginase enzyme comes from various bacterial sources. However, only *Escherichia coli* and *Erwinia chrysanthemi* asparaginase are used in medicine. *Erwinia* asparaginase has been found to have less toxicity, but also less efficacy than native *E. coli* asparaginase [78]. Polyethylene glycol (PEG) asparaginase, native *E. coli* asparaginase covalently linked to PEG, decreases proteolysis, increases the drug's half-life, and decreases the immunogenicity of the native *E. coli* asparaginase with a corresponding efficacy [79].

Toxicities, like hypersensitivity, pancreatitis, coagulation abnormalities, encephalopathy, and liver dysfunction, were reported to be related to asparaginase treatment. In cases of serious adverse drug reactions, asparaginase therapy may be altered or withdrawn in some patients.

Early candidate gene approach studies identified certain genetic variants associated with adverse drug reactions in children with ALL that received asparaginase during standard treatment ALL protocol. An analysis of the genes coding for proteins in the asparaginase pathway (asparagine synthetase—ASNS, the basic region leucine zipper activating transcription factor 5—ATF5, and arginosuccinate synthase 1—ASS1) identified the genetic variation in the *ATF5* gene, T1562C, that affects the activation of endogenous asparaginase transcription after nutrition deprivation, influencing ATF function and responses to treatment in ALL children [80]. Further study of asparaginase action pathway genes revealed that the 3R3R *ASNS* genotype was correlated with pancreatitis and allergies in ALL patients [81].

A "hypothesis-free" exome-wide association study (EWAS) was performed on whole exome sequencing (WES) data [82], indicating that the rs3809849 in the *MYBBP1A* gene was associated with an allergy, pancreatitis, and thrombosis related to asparaginase use. The same genetic variant was also associated with a reduction in event free survival and overall survival. The *MYBBP1A* gene encodes the MYB binding protein 1a, involved in many essential cellular processes, including cell cycle control, mitosis, the nuclear stress response, and tumor suppression [83]. This protein is also a co-repressor of NF-kB nuclear factor [84]. Furthermore, rs11556218 in the *IL16* and rs34708521 in the *SPEF2* genes were both associated with thrombosis and pancreatitis related to asparaginase use. The *IL16* gene codes for interleukin-16, a cytokine with known roles in cancer development and inflammatory and autoimmune responses [85]. The *SPEF2* (Sperm Flagellar 2) gene codes for a protein that is required for correct axoneme development, influencing protein dimerization activity [86]. A concept that synergistic interactions between the genetic variants identified in this study is related to asparagine-related toxicities (rs3809849 *MYBBP1A*, rs11556218 *IL16*, and rs34708521 *SPEF2* genes) was proposed [82].

An unbiased transcriptome-wide RNA targeted sequencing discovered that ALL patient leukemic cells with relatively high levels of opioid receptor μ1 (OPRM1) are more sensitive to asparaginase treatment compared to OPRM1-depleted leukemic cells [87]. Stimulation of the opioid receptor leads to the activation of inhibitory Gi-proteins that influence cAMP levels and subsequently induces apoptosis by caspase activation in leukemia cells [88]. It is proposed that OPRM1 can be targeted for effective treatment of asparaginase-resistant ALL patients.

Using a GWAS approach, a single-genetic variant rs738409 in *PNPLA3*, which was strongly associated with hepatotoxicity after induction therapy in pediatric ALL patients, was identified [89]. Patatin-like Phospholipase Domain Containing Protein 3 (PNPLA3 or adiponutrin) is an enzyme involved in triacylglycerol metabolism and signaling [90] and the genetic variant identified in this study leads to the increase of hepatic triglycerides and the induction of fatty liver, thus conferring an increased risk of hepatotoxicity. This finding was confirmed in a mice model in the same study. The validation study confirmed the association of rs738409 in *PNPLA3* with hepatotoxicity during the induction phase of pediatric ALL therapy [75].

In another GWA study, a germline genetic variant, rs4958351, in the *GRIA1* gene, associated with an asparaginase allergy in pediatric ALL patients, was identified [91]. This genetic locus was previously associated with asthma and atopy [92] and the findings strongly support the hypothesis that an asparaginase allergy and asthma share a range of genes that might cause adverse reactions. *GRIA1* encodes a subunit of the AMPA (α-amino-3-hydroxyl-5-methyl-4-isoxazole-propionate) receptor, an ion channel that transmits glutamatergic signals in the brain. The same variant was found to influence some neurologic disorders [93].

The correlation between the *GRIA1* variant, rs4958351, and *E. coli* asparaginase hypersensitivity was confirmed in different childhood ALL subsets [94]. Namely, carriers of at least one A allele at rs4958351 and the T-ALL subtype were at a deceased risk for asparaginase-related hypersensitivity in comparison to the GG genotype. Patients with B-ALL subtypes and the same alleles were at a higher hypersensitivity risk. Interestingly, a lower frequency of asparaginase hypersensitivity was detected among ALL patients with Down syndrome. Moreover, the association between the *GRIA1* variant, rs4958351, and *E. coli* asparaginase hypersensitivity was confirmed in 146 Slovenian pediatric ALL patients [95]. The same association of rs4958351 in the *GRIA1* gene with an asparaginase allergy in pediatric ALL patients was confirmed in another GWAS study, with the additional observation that the risk of allergy was higher in patients treated with native *E. coli* asparaginase than in patients treated with PEGylated *E. coli* asparaginase [77].

A microarray study identified an association of the *HLA-DRB1*07:01* allele with asparaginase hypersensitivity and with anti-asparaginase antibodies [96]. Furthermore, *HLA-DRB1*07:01* was predicted to have high-affinity binding for asparaginase epitopes. A mechanism was proposed of how an allergy could develop, suggesting that inherited *HLA-DRB1* variant alleles produce amino acid variations of the protein whose interaction with asparaginase epitopes is aberrant, leading to a higher frequency of asparaginase hypersensitivity [96].

Also, the *HLA-DRB1*07:01* variant allele was confirmed to be associated with asparaginase hypersensitivity using an exome array approach [96]. Moreover, the association of *HLA-DRB1*07:01* and asparaginase hypersensitivity, identified in European ALL pediatric patients [96], was confirmed in non-European ALL patients [77].

In the study using next-generation sequencing, it was found that *HLA-DRB1*07:01* and *HLA-DQB1*02:02* alleles were associated with an increased risk of the development of asparaginase hypersensitivity [97]. Furthermore, the *HLA-DRB1*07:01-DQA1*02:01-DQB1*02:02* haplotype carriers were positively and significantly associated with an increased risk to asparaginase hypersensitivity. The findings from the previous study were confirmed [96], but after haplotype reconstruction, only the *HLA-DRB1*07:01-DQB1*02:02* haplotype was associated with asparaginase hypersensitivity [97].

In the study using a genome wide approach, an association of the intronic rs6021191 variant in the *NFATC2* gene with a higher risk of asparaginase hypersensitivity in pediatric ALL patients was found [77]. The presence of the same variant was correlated with higher *NFATC2* mRNA expression [77]. The *NFATC2* gene codes for a cytoplasmic component of the nuclear factor of the activated T cells (NFAT) transcription factor family [98], but its role in asparaginase hypersensitivity is still unclear. It is known that NFATC2 could affect the development and function of regulatory T cells, thus influencing the immune response [99]. Furthermore, a strong association was identified for rs62228256 *NFATC2* and asparaginase-associated pancreatitis [100].

A very recent large GWAS study found and validated variants in the *PRSS1-PRSS2* locus (rs4726576; rs10273639) to be associated with the risk of asparaginase-associated pancreatitis in children with ALL [100]. The pathogenesis of aparaginase-associated pancreatitis in ALL children is the same as in non-asparaginase associated pancreatitis, developed because of alcohol or hyperlipidemia exposure. It is a consequence of the activation of trypsin within pancreatic acinar cells [100].

The non-coding *CNOT3* variant, rs73062673, was confirmed to be strongly associated with a PEG-asparaginase allergy in ALL children in the GWAS [101]. This is the first study taking into account asparaginase enzyme activity measurements to identify asparaginase hypersensitivity. It has been shown that *CNOT3* influences the transcription of MHC class II genes [102]. Moreover, the study pointed out two more genetic variants related to *HLA-DQA1* rs9272131, previously indicted to be involved in allergies, together with variants in the *TAP2* gene, located in close proximity to the *HLA-DQA1* variant, also with previously reported connections with asthma and allergy [103]. The association between the *HLA* region and asparaginase hypersensitivity has been described previously [77,96,97], but the potential contribution of an *HLA*-regulating gene is novel.

6. Anthracyclines

Anthracyclines (doxorubicin, daunorubicin, epirubicin, and idarubicin) are used to treat a wide range of cancers, including childhood ALL. Daunorubicin and doxorubicin (DOX) are isolated from a natural soil-dwelling bacterium, *Streptomyces peucetius* var. caesius, and from a mutated strain of the same bacterium, respectively [104]. Anthracyclines exert their action through a number of different mechanisms. They inhibit topoisomerase 2-α (TOP2A), which cause double stranded DNA breaks and relax DNA supercoiling during processes of DNA replication and transcription. Anthracyclines interfere with TOP2A dissociation from DNA after making a DNA brake and stop re-ligation [105]. Anthracyclines also intercalate with DNA directly, thus inhibiting biosynthesis of macromolecules, inducing the formation of free radicals and DNA damages and lipid peroxidation, and affecting DNA-binding and alkylation and DNA cross-linking. These combined effects eventually lead to programmed cell death [106].

The benefit of anthracyclines' use in complex treatment protocols is compromised by cumulative dose-dependent cardiotoxicity [107]. Acute anthracycline-induced cardiotoxicity happens often immediately after the first dose, but delayed chronic anthracycline-induced cardiotoxicity could be presented within one year, a few years, or even decades after the first anthracycline dose.

A number of candidate gene studies brought encouraging results about genes and genetic variants involved in anthracycline-related cardiotoxicity, such as *ABCC1*, *ABCC2*, *ABCC5*, *ABCB1*, *ABCB4*, *CBR3*, *RAC2*, *NCF4*, *CYBA*, *GSTP1*, *CAT*, *SULT2B1*, *POR*, *HAS3*, *SLC22A7*, *SLC22A17*, *HFE*, and *NOS3* [108]. However, large scale studies have pointed out few genetic markers that need to be validated in different cohorts of patients and also in various populations.

A microarray study showed that a synonymous coding variant (L461L) in the *SLC28A3* gene (or human concentrative nucleoside transporter (*hCNT3*)) was highly associated with anthracycline-induced cardiotoxicity [109]. Previous investigations on this nucleoside transporter provided evidence that supports a functional role of this genetic variant in anthracycline-induced cardiotoxicity [110]. The effect of variant rs7853758 in the *SLC28A3* gene on anthracyclines' transport into cells could be specific for doxorubicin and danorubicin [109]. Besides, it was found that the anthracycline-induced cardiotoxicity was associated with other variants in genes coding for proteins involved in processes known to affect anthracycline ADME, such as *SLC28A1*, *SLC10A2*, and several ATP–binding cassette transporters (*ABCB1*, *ABCB4*, and *ABCC1*) [109]. This study did not confirm previously determined associations of anthracycline-induced cardiotoxicity with the variants, *ABCC2* rs8187694, *CYBA* rs4673, *RAC2* rs13058338, and *NCF4* rs1883112 [111,112], or variant *CBR3* rs1056892 [108]. However, these associations could be different for adult and childhood patients. Additionally, an analysis conducted in a childhood ALL anthracycline-treated cohort of patients did not confirm the previously detected association of antacycline-induced cardiotoxicity with genetic variants in the catalase gene [113].

Another study has confirmed the association of the variants, rs17863783 in the *UGT1A6* (*UGT1A6*4* allele) gene and rs885004 in the *SLC28A3* gene, with anthracycline-induced cardiotoxicity [114]. The

SLC28A3 rs7853758 variant has been associated with a reduced risk of anthracycline-induced cardiotoxicity, i.e., it has a protective role. Furthermore, an effect of rs17583889 and rs17645700 in the histamine N-methyltransferase gene (*HNMT*) was noticed only in children younger than 5 years. Also, the effect of *SULT2B1* rs10426377 was observed in males only. A variant in *ABCB4* (rs4148808) in the promoter region was shown to have an impact on anthracycline-induced cardiotoxicity only in females [114]. These findings need further validation in independent studies.

Further, the same research group revealed two novel variants, rs4982753 in the *SLC22A17* gene and rs4149178 in the *SLC22A7* gene, as predictive markers of anthracycline-induced cardiotoxicity [115]. SLC22A17 (OCT2), an organic cation transporter, is expressed in a variety of tissues, including the heart. It transports naturally occurring nucleosides and nucleotides and several nucleoside-based drugs and, interestingly, shows substrate overlap with concentrative nucleoside transporters, such as SLC28A3, previously related to anthracycline-induced cardiotoxicity [109]. Additional evidence for the association of variants in *SULT2B1* rs10426628 and several antioxidant genes (*CYP2J2, GSTA2, GSTM3, GPX3, SOD2,* and *ABCC9*) was found in this study.

A GWAS using a three-stage genetic association study combined with biological functional analyses identified a nonsynonymous variant in *RARG* (rs2229774, p.Ser427Leu) as being highly associated with anthracycline-induced cardiotoxicity [116]. *RARG* expression has been reported to be particularly high in the heart [117]. RARG has been shown to bind to the *Top2b* promoter [118] and the presence of the rs2229774 variant represses the expression of *Top2b*, finally leading to an anthracycline-induced cardiotoxicity phenotype.

A two-stage study revealed the variant, rs2232228, in the hyaluronan synthase 3 (*HAS3*) gene with a modifying effect on the anthracycline dose-dependent cardiomyopathy risk [119]. Patients who are carriers of the rs2232228 GG genotype did not have any dose-dependent increase of anthracycline-induced cardiomyopathies. However, carriers of the rs2232228 AA genotype were at an increased risk of developing cardiomyopathies when the anthracycline dose was increased. The *HAS3* gene codes for the low-molecular-weight hyaluronan enzyme (HA), an important component of the extracellular matrix, involved in injury processes. Anthracyclines induce apoptosis in heart muscle and injure the cardiomyocytes. Cardiac fibroblasts repair and remodel the heart using the extracellular matrix with accumulated HA as a scaffold [120].

7. Thiopurine Drugs

6-Mercaptopurine and 6-thioguanine are thiopurine drugs used in the treatment of childhood ALL. These drugs are purine analogs, which are metabolically transformed to thioguanine nucleotides (TGN) capable of becoming incorporated into DNA, which leads to cell death.

The thiopurine S-methyltransferase (TPMT) is an enzyme that detoxifies thiopurine drugs by methylation of thiopurine analogs, which interferes with their incorporation into DNA. Patients' TPMT activity depends on variants in the *TPMT* gene and this trait is codominantly inherited: Patients who carry one non-functional allele have intermediate TPMT activity, while patients with two non-functional alleles have very low TPMT activity [121]. Three common variants of the *TPMT* gene (rs1800462, rs1800460, and rs1142345) account for most cases of inherited TPMT deficiency, and their distribution is population specific. In Caucasians and Africans, there is a higher prevalence of non-functional alleles in comparison to East Asian populations. Also, in Caucasians, the most frequent non-functional allele is the *3A (consisting of both rs1800460 and rs1142345 minor variants) allele, while in East Asians, the *3C (rs1142345) allele is the most frequent. Thiopurine dosage and toxicity have been repeatedly and consistently associated with TPMT activity and genetics irrespective of ethnicity or underlying disease. *TPMT* and thiopurines represent one of the first and best documented gene–drug pairs in pharmacogenomics and this knowledge is used for the benefit of patients through therapy individualization [122].

The TPMT enzyme requires S-adenosylmethionine for its activity and this cofactor contributes to TPMT enzyme stability. Intracellular S-adenosylmethionine levels depend on the folate cycle, especially on the activity of the methylenetetrahydrofolate reductase (MTHFR) enzyme. Using a candidate gene approach, TPMT activity and thiopurine toxicity were associated with genetic variants important for the folate cycle [123,124]. To elucidate the genetics of TPMT activity, two large GWAS studies analyzed liver and erythrocyte TPMT enzyme activity in childhood ALL patients and healthy controls. The results showed that TPMT enzyme activity was associated only with variants in the *TPMT* gene, which underlined the utility of *TPMT* genotyping in clinical settings [125,126], but also undermined the role of folate cycle genes for TPMT activity and thiopurine clearance.

Before agnostic approaches using GWAS were available, other candidate gene variants were tested for their associations with thiopurine toxicity. Pharmacogenes that encode transporters and enzymes involved in the clearance of thiopurine drugs have been in the focus, in particular *ITPA* and *ABCC4*. The *ITPA* enzyme catalyzes hydrolysis of the pyrophosphate group from purine analogs triphosphates, which interferes with their incorporation into DNA [127], while the *ABCC4* transporter exports thiopurine drugs and their metabolites [128]. Lower activity variants of *ITPA* and *ABCC4* [129] genes have been associated with a diminished tolerance of thiopurine therapy, however, this is inconsistent [130,131].

A candidate gene approach could not explain all the toxicity of thiopurine drugs, especially in East-Asian patients. Despite having a smaller burden of *TPMT* no-function alleles, East Asians have a lower tolerance of thiopurine drugs compared to other populations [132]. ITPA and ABCC4 deficiencies are more prevalent in East Asians, which served as an explanation for the lower 6-MP tolerance in this population. However, a GWAS involving two large cohorts of childhood ALL patients introduced a new pharmacogene as a major determinant of 6-MP intolerance, which is particularly relevant for East Asians [132]. Variant rs116855232 of the *NUDT15* gene showed both a strong association and clinical importance. Patients with TT and CT genotypes could tolerate only around 10% and 75% of the dose tolerated by patients with the CC genotype. Besides *NUDT15*, the only pharmacogene associated with 6-MP intolerability found by the GWAS study was *TPMT*, which questioned the clinical importance of other pharmacogenes involved in 6-MP clearance. The importance of NUDT15 for thiopurine inactivation and cytotoxicity was subsequently shown both in vitro and in vivo [133]. Also, the association of non-functional *NUDT15* alleles with 6-MP intolerance was corroborated in multiple studies [131,133–135]. Based on overwhelming evidences that emerged in the last 5 years, *NUDT15* testing is now recommended prior to the onset of thiopurine therapy [136].

Protein kinase C and casein kinase substrate in neurons' protein 2 (PACSIN2) was brought into the focus of pharmacogenomics of thiopurine drugs after a GWAS study involving cell lines in which variant rs2413739 showed the highest association with TPMT activity [137]. This result was subsequently corroborated, but only for ALL patients, while in inflammatory bowel disease (IBD) patients and healthy subjects, TPMT activity was not associated with the *PASCIN2* rs2413739 variant [138]. However, the association of *PASCIN2* variants with TPMT enzyme activity was not shown either for ALL patients or for healthy controls in GWAS studies [125,126]. Several studies also dealt with the association of the *PASCIN2* variant with thiopurine toxicity in ALL patients and reported that rs2413739 is a factor of thiopurine-related toxicity [137–139]. Although there are only a few studies on the association of *PACSIN2* gene variants with thiopurine therapy in ALL patients, they included a considerable number of patients and came to similar conclusions. As for non-ALL patients, it was shown that the T allele of the *PACSIN2* rs2413739 variant was not associated with a higher toxicity, although the study was sufficiently powered [140]. Further analyses, optimally including both functional and association studies, are needed to determine whether *PACSIN2* is a factor related to thiopurine intolerance.

Another genetic determinant of thiopurine therapy came into focus after two GWAS studies concurrently and independently associated somatic mutations in the 5′-Nucleotidase, Cytosolic II (*NT5C2*) gene with relapse in childhood ALL patients [141,142]. These mutations were also associated with early rather that late relapse, which underlines their deleterious effect for disease progression. Subsequent analyses showed that acquired mutations related to relapse activate NT5C2, an enzyme that dephosphorylates thiopurine nucleotide monophosphates, making them inactive and prone to export from the cell [141,142]. In a latter study, in which deep sequencing of cancer associated genes was carried out, *NT5C2* mutations were also identified among relapse-associated, somatic mutations [143], underlining the importance of *NT5C2* mutations as prognostic biomarkers related to thiopurine therapy in ALL patients.

A candidate transcript approach can also direct the analysis of pharmacogenes' expression signatures to enhance the prediction of drug toxicity and response. For instance, it was shown that the quantity of *TPMT* transcript can be modulated by variants in the gene promoter, particularly a variable number of tandem repeats (VNTR) [144,145]. However, the impact of the *TPMT* expression profile on thiopurine effects in pediatric ALL patients is scarcely investigated. In one study, it was shown that the *TPMT* expression level was significantly higher during the maintenance phase of therapy than on diagnosis, being the highest in the early stage of the maintenance phase. Also, carriers of specific VNTRs differ in *TPMT* expression levels, which could be important to consider before the onset of maintenance therapy [146].

Many microarray studies have been focused on the expression signatures of ALL relapse [147–151], however, studies dealing specifically with transcriptome of thiopurine or methotrexate in vivo resistance are limited. Zaza and colleagues investigated the correlation of gene expression profiles with the level of thioguanine nucleotides in pediatric ALL patients at diagnosis after initial treatment with 6-MP alone or the combination of 6-MP and MTX. The study identified 60 genes (31 positively and 29 negatively correlated) in 6-MP and 75 genes (50 positively and 25 negatively correlated) in 6-MP + MTX treatment that were significantly associated with TGN accumulation. These two sets of genes did not overlap, indicating different pathways involved in these two therapeutic approaches as well as the fact that the effects of combination therapy are not additive. In the 6-MP treatment, the most associated genes with TGN levels were xanthine oxidase (*XDH*), solute carrier family 29 member 1 (*SLC29A1*), adenosine deaminase (*ADA*), and other genes related to cell proliferation and apoptosis (*CASP7, TOPBP1, ANAPC5, CCT4*) [152]. Xanthine oxidase is, besides the TPMT enzyme, involved in the inactivation of 6-MP and it is the main target of allopurinol, which is used in combination with azathioprine to increase the shunting of 6-MP down the pathway of producing active metabolites. However, compared to TPMT, little attention has been given to this oxidation pathway [153]. The SLC29A1 influx transporter has been positively correlated with the cytotoxicity of nucleoside analogs in human cancer cell lines [154]. In addition to previous results, Zaza and colleagues demonstrated that the inhibition of the SLC29A1 transporter led to approximately a 40% reduction of thioguanines [152]. Contrary to 6-MP alone, the 6-MP + MTX combination yielded genes involved in adenosine triphosphate synthesis, such as *SLC25A3, ATP50, COX5B*, and *COX7A2L*, and other genes implicated in protein synthesis (*RPS19, RPL18, RPS25, RPL23*) and translation factors (*EEF1G, EIF3S5, eIF3k*) [152].

The study of Hogan and colleagues, which examined pediatric B-ALL patients' paired samples taken at diagnosis and relapse, showed that relapse timing (early or late) was associated with distinct gene expression signatures. Particularly, late relapse was associated with the up-regulation of genes involved in nucleotide biosynthesis and folate metabolism, such as *PAICS, TYMS, CAD, ATIC*, and *GART*, which is interesting given that 6-MP and MTX are crucial for maintenance therapy [149]. Also, somatic deletion and consequently decreased expression of the *MSH6* gene, which is involved in the mismatch repair mechanism and was previously associated with thiopurine resistance, has also been detected at the time of relapse [149,151].

Besides identifying pharmacogenes involved in drug response, pharmacotranscriptomic data can be useful in designing predictive algorithms of patient clinical outcomes. Beesley and colleagues used gene expression data of 15 T-ALL cell lines and their sensitivity to 10 therapeutics commonly used in ALL treatment to generate a model which could predict in vivo resistance and therefore patient outcomes. The designed model was validated on the microarray data of three independent pediatric T-ALL cohorts, showing the clinical relevance of identified drug–gene signatures. Moreover, it has been demonstrated that the expression signatures most useful for the accurate prediction of relapse were associated to 6-MP resistance. Genes whose expression was associated to thiopurine resistance were mostly involved in biological pathways, such as gene expression, differentiation/development, cell growth and proliferation, and cell death. Among these, novel associations with the thiopurine drug response were observed for sulfite oxidase (*SUOX*) and multidrug resistance protein (*ABCC1* or *MRP1*) genes. Interestingly, *SUOX* belong to the same family of oxotransferases as xanthine oxidase (XO) and the activity of both relies on molybdenum metabolites from a common biosynthetic pathway. Thus, it is possible that the altered expression of *SUOX* could influence XO activity by modifying the level of molybdenum metabolites and indirectly thiopurines' detoxification [155].

Here, we find a good example showing how a wide transcriptome approach is more useful than a candidate transcript approach in identifying novel potential expression biomarkers of a poor drug response. Interestingly, no significant association was found for *TPMT* gene expression in either of the aforementioned microarray studies.

8. Methotrexate

Methotrexate is one of the key drugs of ALL treatment, which is given in all phases across different ALL therapy protocols, either systemically or locally. Methotrexate enters cells primarily via the solute carrier family 19 member 1 (SLC19A1) transporter, followed by its polyglutamination catalyzed by the folylpolyglutamate synthase (FPGS) enzyme, which further activates the drug and hinders its clearance. MTX and MTX polyglutamates (MTX-PG) inhibit dihydrofolate reductase (DHFR), a key enzyme in the folate cycle essential for the replenishment of active folate forms used in nucleotide synthesis and methylation reactions. MTX-PG also inhibits the thymidylate synthase (TYMS) enzyme, necessary for the synthesis of tymidine nucleotides. Another important enzyme indirectly impacted by MTX is MTHFR, an enzyme which facilitates the synthesis of 5-methyltetrahidrofolate, ultimately used for the methylation reaction at the expense of 5,10 methylentetrahydropholate, necessary for thymidylate synthesis. As a consequence of MTX therapy, important cellular processes, including DNA synthesis and methylation, are tempered, which contributes to MTX anti-cancer effects and MTX-related toxicity.

Response to MTX therapy is associated with the activity of key enzymes and transporters involved in the MTX and folate metabolic pathway. For instance, DHFR upregulation is associated with poor survival of childhood ALL patients [156], while higher intracellular levels of long-chain MTX-PG, correlated with higher FPGS activity, is a factor of improved survival of ALL patients [157]. The complex folate and MTX metabolic pathway allowed for the selection of several candidate pharmacogenes that encode enzymes and transporters involved in MTX anti-cancer effects and clearance. MTX-associated pharmacogenes contain numerous genetic variants that are frequent in human populations and are coupled with functional consequences for the activity of corresponding proteins. For example, one of the most extensively studied variants in the pharmacogenetics of MTX is a common rs1801133 (677C > T) variant in the *MTHFR* gene, which causes amino acid substitution and decreased protein activity. Though several studies conducted on childhood ALL patients showed that the T allele of rs1801133 is associated with toxicity [129,158–160], a few studies showed no association [161,162] or even a protective effect [163]. Two recent meta-analyses tried to settle this dilemma, but they reached opposite conclusions [164,165]. A number of similar studies relying on the candidate gene approach have been carried out in order to find genetic markers of MTX related toxicity and therapy response (recently reviewed by Giletti and colleagues [166]). However, despite extensive analysis of multiple candidate genes, none of the genetic markers so far have been used in MTX therapy protocols due to the lack of a clear association with the response and/or toxicity.

One of the most promising pharmacogenes previously not analyzed in the context of MTX pharmacokinetics, *SLCO1B1*, has emerged following a large GWAS study conducted by Trevino and colleagues in 2009. The results showed that only *SLCO1B1* variants (intronic rs11045879 and rs4149081 tied to functional rs4149056) are associated with MTX clearance and GI toxicity and this result was replicated in an independent cohort [167]. An even larger replication GWAS study, enrolling around 1300 childhood ALL patients, reported essentially the same conclusions reached by Trevino and colleagues [168], associating rs4149081, rs11045879, rs11045821, and functional rs4149056 with MTX clearance. The contribution of functional variants in the *SLCO1B1* gene to MTX clearance variability is around 10% [169]. An association of *SLCO1B1* variants with MTX clearance and toxicity was corroborated using the candidate gene approach [170–172]. *SLCO1B1* variants were also associated with the event-free survival of ALL patients [173], however, another study did not find an association between functional rs4149056 and the risk of relapse [172].

In search of pharmacogenomic markers of MTX therapy, a study by Lopez-Lopez enrolled 151 pediatric B-ALL patients to analyze more than 300 variants in 12 candidate transporter genes related with MTX transport. The results showed that only variants in the *ABCC2* and *ABCC4* gene are in relation with MTX plasma levels [174], which is a surrogate marker of MTX-related toxicity [170]. Variants in the *SLCO1B1* gene did not reach a significant level of association after the correction for multiple testing [174]. None of the two GWAS studies, nor a study focused on MTX transporters, showed significant associations (after the correction for multiple testing) between MTX clearance or MTX plasma levels and variants in the *SLC19A1* gene [167,168,174], by far the most studied MTX transporter encoding pharmacogenes.

Alternations in the expression of candidate genes involved in MTX transport (*SLC19A1*, *ABCC1-4*, *ABCG2*), MTX metabolism (*FPGS*, *FPGH*), as well as MTX target enzyme genes (*DHFR*, *TYMS*) were investigated in relation to MTX resistance [175–177]. Although low *SLC19A1* and *FPGS* as well as high *DHFR* and *TYMS* expression levels have been correlated with poor patient MTX response [157,178–181], some important factors, such as genomic landscape, MTX dosage (high or low), and the subtype of ALL, should be taken into account. Particularly, it was shown that precursor B-cell ALL patients display a higher MTX sensitivity than T-cell ALL patients [157,182,183]. In line with this are results showing higher *FPGS* mRNA expression as well as FPGS enzyme activity in B-cells ALL, and higher levels of *DHFR* and *TYMS* mRNA in T-cells ALL [157,180]. Moreover, children with hyperdiploid ALL (more than 50 chromosomes) showed increased MTX sensitivity, measured by increased MTX-PG accumulation, which was associated with higher *SLC19A1* expression as a result of extra copies of chromosome 21, where the gene is located. However, this effect was seen only if patients were treated with low doses of MTX, during which the main mechanism of the antifolates' entry is via the SLC19A1 [178,184]. In contrast, patients carrying the *E2A-PBX1* and *TEL-AML1* gene fusions displayed a decreased MTX-PG accumulation associated with the diminished expression of *SLC19A1* in *E2A-PBX1* and the elevated expression of *ABCG2* in *TEL-AML1* ALL patients [184]. Additionally, Kager and colleagues established distinct in vivo folate pathway gene expression patterns, which provided an 83% accuracy for correctly assigning the ALL genetic subtype or lineage. These results point out the importance of ALL subtype–specific strategies to overcome MTX drug resistance.

Using a transcriptome wide approach, Sorich and colleagues gave insight into the gene expression signatures of good and poor MTX in vivo responses in de novo pediatric ALL patients, identifying 50 genes (21 positively and 29 negatively) associated specifically with the MTX antileukemic effect [185]. These genes included the ones involved in nucleotide metabolism (*TYMS* and *CTPS*), cell proliferation and apoptosis (*BCL3*, *CDC20*, *CENPF*, and *FAIM3*), and DNA replication or repair (*POLD3*, *RPA3*, *RNASEH2A*, *RPM1*, and *H2AFX*). The study also showed that a low expression of the *DHFR*, *TYMS*, and *CTPS* genes was associated with poor therapeutic response and prognosis A lower expression of these genes is associated with decreased processes of DNA synthesis and cell proliferation, making cells less susceptible to the effects of MTX drugs [185]. As indicated, this is not in contrast to previous results showing that a higher expression of *TYMS* and *DHFR*, due to promoter variants, leads to a worse prognosis, which could have an effect once remission is achieved [156,186,187]. In the microarray study of Kager and colleagues, a significant correlation was demonstrated between *TYMS*, *MTHFD1*, and *RUVBL2* expression and MTXPG accumulation in B-ALL not carrying cytogenetic abnormalities whereas *MTHFD2*, *PPAT*, and *RUVBL2* expression was associated with MTXPG accumulation within T-ALL. A significant correlation between *ABCG2*, *ABCC4*, and *TYMS* expression and the cytotoxic effects of MTX in ALL B-cells not carrying cytogenetic abnormalities has also been found [184].

A list of the pharmacogenomic and pharmacotranscriptomic markers of the drug response or toxicity discovered or validated using high-throughput technologies is summarized in Table 1.

Table 1. Pharmacogenomic and pharmacotranscriptomic markers of the drug response or toxicity discovered or validated using high-throughput technologies. WGS: whole genome sequencing; WES: whole exome sequencing; DEX: dexamethasone; GC: glucocorticoids; 6-MP: 6-mercaptopurine; MTX: methotrexate; EFS: event free survival; OS: overall survival; *: protective role.

Pharmacogene	Variant or RNA	Effect	Methodology	References
Glucocorticoid drugs				
ABCB1, WT 1-AS	rs6007758, rs41488548, rs10264856, rs4728709	Higher clearance of DEX	Microarray	[33]
SERPINA6	rs12589136	Higher plasma cortisol levels	WES	[34]
Intergenic variant	rs10989692	Increased risk of osteonecrosis	WES	[35]
ACP-1	Multiple SNPs	Increased risk of osteonecrosis	Microarray	[36]
hsa-miR-142-3p, hsa-miR-17-5p	miRNA	High correlation with GC resistance	Omni-Search	[40]
EMP1	mRNA	Higher expression in prednisone poor responders	Microarray	[41]
CASP1, NLRP3	mRNA	High expression and subsequent high GC resistance	Microarray	[45]
SMARCA4, ARID1A, SMARCB1	mRNA	Decreased expression is associated with GC resistance	Microarray	[46]
CREBBP	somatic mutations	Presence of damaging mutations leads to GC resistance	Microarray	[12]
Vincristine				
CEP72	rs924607	vincristine-related peripheral neuropathy	Microarray	[58]
ABCC2	rs374006 rs12826	vincristine-related peripheral neuropathy	Targeted DNA sequencing	[63]
SYNE2, MRPL47, BAHD1 *	rs2781377 rs10513762 rs3803357 *	vincristine-related peripheral neuropathy	WES	[64]
COCH	rs1045644 rs7963521	vincristine-related peripheral neuropathy	Microarray	[69]
miR-125b, miR-99a, miR-100	microRNA	resistance to vincristine	microRNA expression study	[72]
miR-300, DROSHA	rs12894467 rs639174	vincristine-related peripheral neuropathy, vomits	Microarray	[74]
miR-3117-3p, miR-4481	rs12402181 rs7896283	vincristine-related peripheral neuropathy	Microarray	[75]
Asparaginase				
MYBBP1A, IL16, SPEF2	rs3809849 rs11556218 rs34708521	allergy, pancreatitis and thrombosis related to asparaginase, EFS, OS	WES	[82]
OPRM1	microRNA	resistance to asparaginase	genome-wide RNAi screening	[87]
PNPLA3	rs738409	elevated alanine transaminase (ALT) levels leading to hepatotoxicity	Microarray	[89]
GRIA1	rs4958351	asparaginase hypersensitivity	Microarray	[91]
HLA-DRB1	HLA-DRB1*07:01	asparaginase hypersensitivity	Microarray	[95]
NFATC2, HLA-DRB1, GRIA1	rs6021191 HLA-DRB1*07:01 rs4958351	asparaginase hypersensitivity	Microarray	[77]
HLADRB1, HLADQ1	HLADRB1*07:01 HLA-DQB1*02:02	asparaginase hypersensitivity	targeted DNA sequencing	[97]
PRSS1-PRSS2 locus NFATC2	rs4726576 rs10273639 rs62228256	asparaginase hypersensitivity, pancreatitis	Microarray	[100]
CNOT3, HLADQA1, TAP2	rs73062673 rs9272131	asparaginase hypersensitivity	Microarray	[101]

Table 1. Cont.

Pharmacogene	Variant or RNA	Effect	Methodology	References
		Anthracyclines		
SLC28A3	rs7853758	anthracycline-induced cardiotoxicity	Microarray	[109]
UGT1A6, SLC28A3	rs17863783 rs885004 rs7853758 *	anthracycline-induced cardiotoxicity	Microarray	[114]
SLC22A17, SLC22A7	rs4982753 rs4149178	anthracycline-induced cardiotoxicity	Microarray	[115]
RARG	rs2229774	anthracycline-induced cardiotoxicity	Microarray	[116]
HAS3	rs2232228	anthracycline-induced cardiotoxicity	Microarray	[119]
		Thiopurine drugs		
TPMT, NUDT15	rs1142345, rs116855232	6-MP dose intensity	WGS	[132]
TPMT	rs1142345	TPMT activity	WGS	[125,126]
PACSIN2	rs2413739, mRNA	TPMT activity	WGS, RNA seq	[137]
NT5C2	somatic mutations	Relapse	WES, RNA seq	[141,142]
XDH, SLC29A1, ADA, CASP7, TOPBP1, ANAPC5, CCT4	mRNA	Level of TGN after initial MP treatment	Microarray	[152]
SLC25A3, ATP5O, COX5B, COX7A2L; RPS19, RPL18, RPS25, RPL23; EEF1G, EIF3S5, eIF3k	mRNA	Level of TGN after initial 6-MP+MTX treatment	Microarray	[152]
PAICS, TYMS, CAD, ATIC, GART, MSH6	mRNA	Late relapse, probably related to 6-MP and MTX	Microarray	[149]
SUOX, ABCC1	mRNA	Thiopurine resistance	Microarray	[155]
		Methotrexate		
SLCO1B1	rs4149081, rs11045879, rs11045821, rs4149056	MTX clearance	WGS	[167,168]
ABCC2, ABCC4	rs3740065, rs9516519	MTX plasma level	Targeted DNA sequencing	[174]
DHFR, TYMS, CTPS; BCL3, CDC20, CENPF, FAIM3; POLD3, RPA3, RNASEH2A, RPM1, 2AFX	mRNA	Reduction of circulating leukemia cells after initial treatment	Microarray	[185]
DHFR, TYMS	mRNA	5-year disease free survival	Microarray	[185]
TYMS, MTHFD1, RUVBL2	mRNA	MTX-PG accumulation after high dose MTX treatment in nonhyperdipoid B-ALL	Microarray	[184]
MTHFD2, PPAT, RUVBL2	mRNA	MTX-PG accumulation after high dose MTX treatment in T-ALL	Microarray	[184]
ABCG2, ABCC4, TYMS	mRNA	MTX cytotoxic effect in nonhyperdipoid B-ALL, as measured by the reduction of circulating ALL cells	Microarray	[184]

9. Conclusions

Pharmacogenomics and pharmacotranscriptomics in childhood ALL are the focus of numerous studies due to the availability of high quality data for the assessment of an association between the genomic and transcriptomic profiles of patients and their response to therapy. Valuable data are accessible because of standardized similar protocols that are used for the treatment of pediatric ALL in many populations, with a similar efficacy and side effects in all of them.

Recent reviews have summarized data related to pharmacogenomics and pharmacotranscriptomics in childhood ALL [188]. In this review, we paid attention to the studies in which high-throughput technologies were used.

We found several reports of studies in the field of pharmacogenomics in childhood ALL using high-throughput technology. In most of them, microarray technology was used, while the reports in which targeted DNA sequencing, WES, or WGS was applied were significantly fewer. It is probably due to the fact that arrays were more cost-effective than sequencing technology. However, at this moment, sequencing technologies are more effective and less expensive and the shift towards sequencing-based studies in this field is obvious. A very small number of studies of somatic mutations relevant for pharmacogenomics in ALL have been conducted. Since a high coverage is required for the detection of somatic mutations in the samples with a large number of subclones, characteristic for leukemia, deep targeted sequencing is indispensable for that type of analysis. Future research should be directed towards association studies of somatic mutations and drug resistance in pediatric ALL.

An even smaller number of studies on pharmacotranscriptomic markers have been performed. RNA seq methodology is used only in a few studies. Studies of regulatory RNA (microRNA of long non-coding RNA) are deficient.

Studies based on high-throughput analyses led to many beneficial discoveries. Since numerous pharmacogenomic/pharmacotranscriptomic studies have found differences in the prevalence of clinically significant variants between populations, propositions of creating databases concerning the pharmacogenetic/pharmacotranscriptomic markers in different populations have sprung up. One of these databases is FINDbase [189], a comprehensive database containing population frequency data of clinically relevant variants. In another pharmacogenomic study [190], significant interpopulation differences have been reported in seven European population concerning seven important pharmacogenomic biomarkers, which change the drug efficacy and/or toxicity of up to 51 treatment modalities. These results could be beneficial in creating accurate population-based preemptive pharmacogenomic testing.

Hypothesis driven studies using a candidate gene approach might be an inefficient way to discover novel pharmacogenomic markers because candidate genes outside the well-studied network of drug absorption, distribution, metabolism, and excretion (ADME) or drug targets are often missed. Besides, the effect of investigated genetic variants is often not clear and functional analyses are often scarce or contradictory. For instance, the effect of the nonsynonimous variant, rs1051266 (SLC19A1 80G > A), on MTX transport efficacy is ambiguous, as it is suggested that the minor A allele has both a higher and lower affinity to MTX, as well as having a marginal functional effect. Nevertheless, a number of candidate gene studies have tried to relate this variant with MTX levels and toxicity, but the results were also inconclusive. Moreover, hypothesis free, high-throughput analyses could not confirm the association of MTX pharmacokinetics and the rs1051266 variant, even though the minor allele frequency is almost 50%. Instead, GWAS studies introduced a novel, SLC19A1 pharmacogene as a factor of MTX, whose significance was later confirmed.

Although high-throughput technology has brought a significant increase of knowledge in pharmacogenomics and pharmacotranscriptomics in childhood ALL, most GWAS/TWAS studies have provided contradictory results. There could be several reasons for this. First, patient cohorts selected for the GWAS/TWAS are usually not uniform. The genetic profile of pediatric ALL is complex and heterogenous, which has led to the treatment of patients according to the stratification principle. A lack of knowledge of the complete biomarker profile at the beginning of the disease could lead to false conclusions at the end. Additionally, the phenotype endpoints should be precisely defined. The time of molecular-genetics analysis is critical and should always be performed in the same phase of the same treatment protocol, especially when expression studies interpret pharmacotranscritomics markers. It is also particularly hard to determine the grade of drug side effects when small children are reporting, for example, the neuropathy pain level. Furthermore, given the complexity of GWAS/TWAS, multiple sources of false positive and false negative errors exist. The inconsistencies in the GWAS/TWAS results are caused either by the design of experiment itself or by the genotype/transcriptome calling process [191].

Many authors consider small sample sizes as being responsible for limited outcomes in pharmacogenomic/pharmacotranscriptomic studies in pediatric ALL. However, some of the studies have included a significant number of patients [69,77,96].

Big data generated in candidate gene/transcripts studies have been enormously expanded due to the implementation of high-throughput technologies. In the last two decades, an accumulation of data in the field of pharmacogenetics/pharmacogenomics has been achieved, reaching more than 20,000 new citations in PubMed. More than 3500 associations between pharmacogenes and pharmacogenomic variants and the efficacy/toxicity of drugs have been validated and can be considered to have strong evidence. More than 200 drugs have drug labels containing information of the mandatory or recommended preemptive pharmacogenomic testing (https://www.fda.gov/Drugs/ScienceResearch/ucm572698.htm).

However, it is necessary to use the available big data in translational research to obtain data that is usable in clinical practice. For that reason, research efforts must be focused on the development of data analysis. Data mining of the current literature and the selection of biomarkers that showed strong evidence for an association with the treatment response and toxicity can be used for the creation of a custom panel for genomic and transcriptomic profiling. Along with patients' clinical data, molecular data obtained via genomic and transcriptomic profiling could be utilized for the design of a prediction model using machine learning algorithms. This form of artificial intelligence requires a training group of ALL patients to learn how selected molecular markers relate to each other to predict specific outcomes, such as patients' drug responses. Also, validation of the model is needed on an independent pediatric ALL cohort to test the model's performance. If the model could predict patients at risk of severe drug related toxicity or poor response with sufficient accuracy, protocol modifications for these patients might be attempted using a randomized clinical trials approach (Figure 1).

A true understanding of the processes leading to disease development and mechanisms of treatment efficacy and toxicity, as well as gaining new knowledge from big data obtained in large omics studies and validation studies from various populations, could be the way to achieve the ultimate goal of all biomedical professionals: Bringing real personalized treatment from the bench to the bedside.

The growing knowledge in pharmacogenomics and pharmacotranscriptomics in pediatric ALL, produced by molecular profiling of patients using high-throughput technology, as well as the development of bioinformatics tools and the implementation of artificial intelligence, are expected to improve the treatment of children with ALL through the individualization of therapy for each patient. The door for personalized medicine is wide-open in the clinical practice of pediatric ALL.

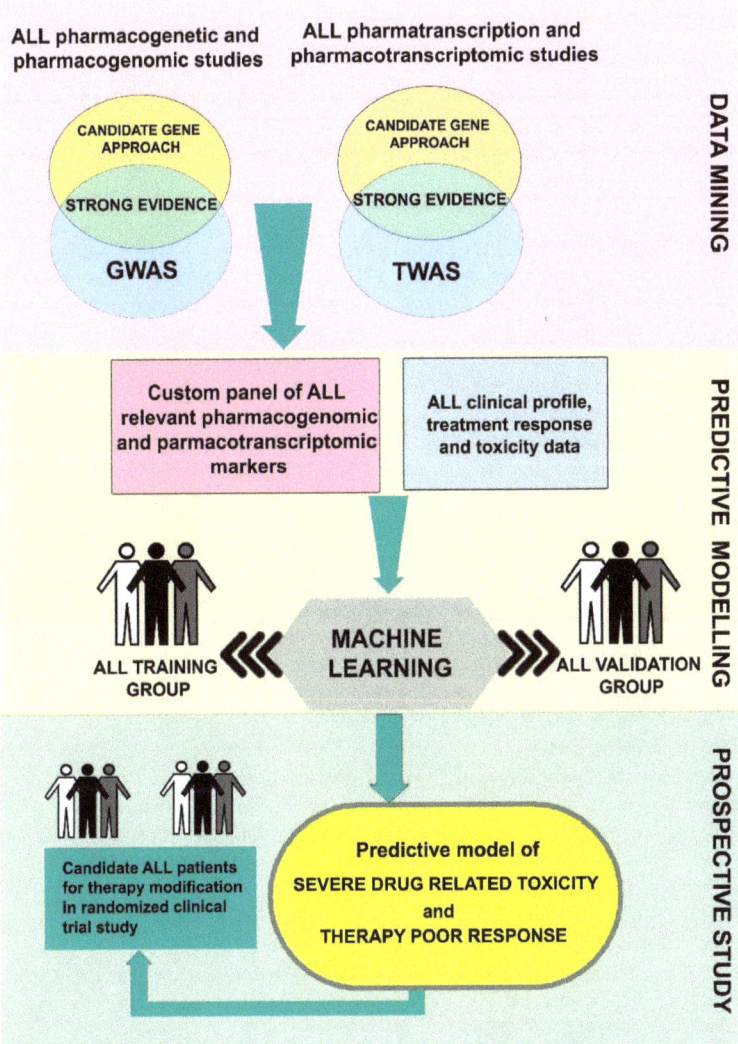

Figure 1. Diagram of the steps in designing a predictive model of childhood acute lymphoblastic leukemia (ALL) patients' drug related toxicity and outcomes using pharmacogenomic and pharmacotranscriptomic data. Data mining of the current literature and the selection of biomarkers that showed strong evidence for an association with the treatment response and toxicity can be used for the creation of a custom panel for genomic and transcriptomic profiling. Along with patients' clinical data, molecular data obtained via pharmacogenomic and pharmacotranscriptomic profiling could be utilized for the design of a prediction model using machine learning algorithms. This form of artificial intelligence requires a training group of pediatric ALL patients to learn how selected molecular markers relate to each other to predict specific outcomes, such as patients' drug responses. Also, validation of the model is needed on an independent ALL cohort to test the model's performance. If the model could predict patients at risk of severe drug related toxicity or poor response with sufficient accuracy, protocol modifications for these patients might be attempted using a randomized clinical trials approach.

Author Contributions: Conceptualization, S.P., N.K., B.S. and B.Z.; Writing—Original Draft Preparation, S.P., N.K., B.S., B.Z., V.G. and L.D.; Writing—Review & Editing, S.P., N.K., B.S., B.Z. and V.G.; Supervision, S.P.

Funding: This research received no external funding.

Acknowledgments: This research has been supported by grant III41004 from the Ministry of Education and Science, Republic of Serbia.

Conflicts of Interest: The authors declare no conflict of interest.

References

1. Geraghty, J.C. 'Omics' and 'Omes'—The Future of Personalised Medicine. Available online: https://www.centogene.com/science/omics-and-omes-the-future-of-personalised-medicine.html (accessed on 2 April 2019).
2. Georgitsi, M.; Zukic, B.; Pavlovic, S.; Patrinos, G.P. Transcriptional regulation and pharmacogenomics. *Pharmacogenomics* **2011**, *12*, 655–673. [CrossRef] [PubMed]
3. Stojiljkovic, M.; P Patrinos, G.; Pavlovic, S. Clinical Applicability of Sequence Variations in Genes Related to Drug Metabolism. *Curr. Drug Metab.* **2011**, *12*, 445–454. [CrossRef] [PubMed]
4. Amos, W.; Driscoll, E.; Hoffman, J.I. Candidate genes versus genome-wide associations: Which are better for detecting genetic susceptibility to infectious disease? *Proc. Biol. Sci.* **2011**, *278*, 1183–1188. [CrossRef] [PubMed]
5. Pui, C.H.; Robison, L.L.; Look, A.T. Acute lymphoblastic leukaemia. *Lancet* **2008**, *371*, 1030–1043. [CrossRef]
6. Greaves, M.F.; Wiemels, J. Origins of chromosome translocations in childhood leukaemia. *Nat. Rev. Cancer* **2003**, *3*, 639–649. [CrossRef] [PubMed]
7. Moricke, A.; Zimmermann, M.; Valsecchi, M.G.; Stanulla, M.; Biondi, A.; Mann, G.; Locatelli, F.; Cazzaniga, G.; Niggli, F.; Arico, M.; et al. Dexamethasone vs prednisone in induction treatment of pediatric ALL: Results of the randomized trial AIEOP-BFM ALL 2000. *Blood* **2016**, *127*, 2101–2112. [CrossRef] [PubMed]
8. Hunger, S.P.; Mullighan, C.G. Acute Lymphoblastic Leukemia in Children. *N. Engl. J. Med.* **2015**, *373*, 1541–1552. [CrossRef] [PubMed]
9. Pui, C.H.; Pei, D.; Sandlund, J.T.; Ribeiro, R.C.; Rubnitz, J.E.; Raimondi, S.C.; Onciu, M.; Campana, D.; Kun, L.E.; Jeha, S.; et al. Long-term results of St Jude Total Therapy Studies 11, 12, 13A, 13B, and 14 for childhood acute lymphoblastic leukemia. *Leukemia* **2010**, *24*, 371–382. [CrossRef] [PubMed]
10. Schrappe, M.; Reiter, A.; Ludwig, W.-D.; Harbott, J.; Zimmermann, M.; Hiddemann, W.; Niemeyer, C.; Henze, G.; Feldges, A.; Zintl, F.; et al. Improved outcome in childhood acute lymphoblastic leukemia despite reduced use of anthracyclines and cranial radiotherapy: Results of trial ALL-BFM 90. *Blood* **2000**, *95*, 3310–3322. [PubMed]
11. Gervasini, G.; Vagace, J.M. Impact of genetic polymorphisms on chemotherapy toxicity in childhood acute lymphoblastic leukemia. *Front Genet* **2012**, *3*, 249. [CrossRef] [PubMed]
12. Mullighan, C.G.; Zhang, J.; Kasper, L.H.; Lerach, S.; Payne-Turner, D.; Phillips, L.A.; Heatley, S.L.; Holmfeldt, L.; Collins-Underwood, J.R.; Ma, J.; et al. CREBBP mutations in relapsed acute lymphoblastic leukaemia. *Nature* **2011**, *471*, 235–239. [CrossRef] [PubMed]
13. Ross, C.J.; Visscher, H.; Rassekh, S.R.; Castro-Pastrana, L.I.; Shereck, E.; Carleton, B.; Hayden, M.R. Pharmacogenomics of serious adverse drug reactions in pediatric oncology. *J. Popul. Ther. Clin. Pharmacol.* **2011**, *18*, e134–e151. [PubMed]
14. Thomas, A. How can we improve on the already impressive results in pediatric ALL? *Hematol. Am. Soc. Hematol. Educ. Program* **2015**, *15*, 414–419. [CrossRef] [PubMed]
15. Mlakar, V.; Huezo-Diaz Curtis, P.; Satyanarayana Uppugunduri, C.R.; Krajinovic, M.; Ansari, M. Pharmacogenomics in Pediatric Oncology: Review of Gene-Drug Associations for Clinical Use. *Int. J. Mol. Sci.* **2016**, *17*, 1502. [CrossRef] [PubMed]
16. Krajinovic, M.; Lemieux-Blanchard, E.; Chiasson, S.; Primeau, M.; Costea, I.; Moghrabi, A. Role of polymorphisms in MTHFR and MTHFD1 genes in the outcome of childhood acute lymphoblastic leukemia. *Pharm. J.* **2004**, *4*, 66–72. [CrossRef] [PubMed]
17. Schmiegelow, K.; Forestier, E.; Kristinsson, J.; Soderhall, S.; Vettenranta, K.; Weinshilboum, R.; Wesenberg, F. Thiopurine methyltransferase activity is related to the risk of relapse of childhood acute lymphoblastic leukemia: Results from the NOPHO ALL-92 study. *Leukemia* **2009**, *23*, 557–564. [CrossRef] [PubMed]

18. Inaba, H.; Pui, C.H. Glucocorticoid use in acute lymphoblastic leukaemia. *Lancet Oncol.* **2010**, *11*, 1096–1106. [CrossRef]
19. Lin, K.T.; Wang, L.H. New dimension of glucocorticoids in cancer treatment. *Steroids* **2016**, *111*, 84–88. [CrossRef] [PubMed]
20. Eipel, O.T.; Nemeth, K.; Torok, D.; Csordas, K.; Hegyi, M.; Ponyi, A.; Ferenczy, A.; Erdelyi, D.J.; Csoka, M.; Kovacs, G.T. The glucocorticoid receptor gene polymorphism N363S predisposes to more severe toxic side effects during pediatric acute lymphoblastic leukemia (ALL) therapy. *Int. J. Hematol.* **2013**, *97*, 216–222. [CrossRef] [PubMed]
21. Tissing, W.J.; Meijerink, J.P.; den Boer, M.L.; Brinkhof, B.; van Rossum, E.F.; van Wering, E.R.; Koper, J.W.; Sonneveld, P.; Pieters, R. Genetic variations in the glucocorticoid receptor gene are not related to glucocorticoid resistance in childhood acute lymphoblastic leukemia. *Clin. Cancer Res.* **2005**, *11*, 6050–6056. [CrossRef] [PubMed]
22. Xue, L.; Li, C.; Wang, Y.; Sun, W.; Ma, C.; He, Y.; Yu, Y.; Cai, L.; Wang, L. Single nucleotide polymorphisms in non-coding region of the glucocorticoid receptor gene and prednisone response in childhood acute lymphoblastic leukemia. *Leuk. Lymphoma* **2015**, *56*, 1704–1709. [CrossRef] [PubMed]
23. Gasic, V.; Zukic, B.; Stankovic, B.; Janic, D.; Dokmanovic, L.; Lazic, J.; Krstovski, N.; Dolzan, V.; Jazbec, J.; Pavlovic, S.; et al. Pharmacogenomic markers of glucocorticoid response in the initial phase of remission induction therapy in childhood acute lymphoblastic leukemia. *Radiol. Oncol.* **2018**, *52*, 296–306. [CrossRef] [PubMed]
24. Zalewski, G.; Wasilewska, A.; Zoch-Zwierz, W.; Chyczewski, L. Response to prednisone in relation to NR3C1 intron B polymorphisms in childhood nephrotic syndrome. *Pediatr. Nephrol.* **2008**, *23*, 1073–1078. [CrossRef] [PubMed]
25. Gregers, J.; Green, H.; Christensen, I.J.; Dalhoff, K.; Schroeder, H.; Carlsen, N.; Rosthoej, S.; Lausen, B.; Schmiegelow, K.; Peterson, C. Polymorphisms in the ABCB1 gene and effect on outcome and toxicity in childhood acute lymphoblastic leukemia. *Pharm. J.* **2015**, *15*, 372–379. [CrossRef] [PubMed]
26. Jamroziak, K.; Mlynarski, W.; Balcerczak, E.; Mistygacz, M.; Trelinska, J.; Mirowski, M.; Bodalski, J.; Robak, T. Functional C3435T polymorphism of MDR1 gene: An impact on genetic susceptibility and clinical outcome of childhood acute lymphoblastic leukaemia. *Eur. J. Haematol.* **2004**, *72*, 314–321. [CrossRef] [PubMed]
27. Marino, S.; Verzegnassi, F.; Tamaro, P.; Stocco, G.; Bartoli, F.; Decorti, G.; Rabusin, M. Response to glucocorticoids and toxicity in childhood acute lymphoblastic leukemia: Role of polymorphisms of genes involved in glucocorticoid response. *Pediatr. Blood Cancer* **2009**, *53*, 984–991. [CrossRef] [PubMed]
28. Anderer, G.; Schrappe, M.; Brechlin, A.M.; Lauten, M.; Muti, P.; Welte, K.; Stanulla, M. Polymorphisms within glutathione S-transferase genes and initial response to glucocorticoids in childhood acute lymphoblastic leukaemia. *Pharmacogenetics* **2000**, *10*, 715–726. [CrossRef] [PubMed]
29. Meissner, B.; Stanulla, M.; Ludwig, W.D.; Harbott, J.; Moricke, A.; Welte, K.; Schrappe, M. The GSTT1 deletion polymorphism is associated with initial response to glucocorticoids in childhood acute lymphoblastic leukemia. *Leukemia* **2004**, *18*, 1920–1923. [CrossRef] [PubMed]
30. Stanulla, M.; Schrappe, M.; Brechlin, A.M.; Zimmermann, M.; Welte, K. Polymorphisms within glutathione S-transferase genes (GSTM1, CSTT1, GSTP1) and risk of relapse in childhood B-cell precursor acute lymphoblastic leukemia: A case-control study. *Blood* **2000**, *95*, 1222. [PubMed]
31. Kamdem, L.K.; Hamilton, L.; Cheng, C.; Liu, W.; Yang, W.; Johnson, J.A.; Pui, C.H.; Relling, M.V. Genetic predictors of glucocorticoid-induced hypertension in children with acute lymphoblastic leukemia. *Pharm. Genom.* **2008**, *18*, 507–514. [CrossRef] [PubMed]
32. Montano, A.; Forero-Castro, M.; Marchena-Mendoza, D.; Benito, R.; Hernandez-Rivas, J.M. New Challenges in Targeting Signaling Pathways in Acute Lymphoblastic Leukemia by NGS Approaches: An Update. *Cancers* **2018**, *10*, 110. [CrossRef] [PubMed]
33. Yang, J.J.; Cheng, C.; Devidas, M.; Cao, X.; Campana, D.; Yang, W.; Fan, Y.; Neale, G.; Cox, N.; Scheet, P.; et al. Genome-wide association study identifies germline polymorphisms associated with relapse of childhood acute lymphoblastic leukemia. *Blood* **2012**, *120*, 4197–4204. [CrossRef] [PubMed]
34. Bolton, J.L.; Hayward, C.; Direk, N.; Lewis, J.G.; Hammond, G.L.; Hill, L.A.; Anderson, A.; Huffman, J.; Wilson, J.F.; Campbell, H.; et al. Genome wide association identifies common variants at the SERPINA6/SERPINA1 locus influencing plasma cortisol and corticosteroid binding globulin. *PLoS Genet.* **2014**, *10*, e1004474. [CrossRef] [PubMed]

35. Karol, S.E.; Yang, W.; Van Driest, S.L.; Chang, T.Y.; Kaste, S.; Bowton, E.; Basford, M.; Bastarache, L.; Roden, D.M.; Denny, J.C.; et al. Genetics of glucocorticoid-associated osteonecrosis in children with acute lymphoblastic leukemia. *Blood* **2015**, *126*, 1770–1776. [CrossRef] [PubMed]
36. Kawedia, J.D.; Kaste, S.C.; Pei, D.; Panetta, J.C.; Cai, X.; Cheng, C.; Neale, G.; Howard, S.C.; Evans, W.E.; Pui, C.H.; et al. Pharmacokinetic, pharmacodynamic, and pharmacogenetic determinants of osteonecrosis in children with acute lymphoblastic leukemia. *Blood* **2011**, *117*, 2340–2347; quiz 2556. [CrossRef] [PubMed]
37. Bottini, N.; MacMurray, J.; Peters, W.; Rostamkhani, M.; Comings, D.E. Association of the acid phosphatase (ACP1) gene with triglyceride levels in obese women. *Mol. Genet. Metab.* **2002**, *77*, 226–229. [CrossRef]
38. Gasic, V.; Stankovic, B.; Zukic, B.; Janic, D.; Dokmanovic, L.; Krstovski, N.; Lazic, J.; Milosevic, G.; Lucafò, M.; Stocco, G.; et al. Expression Pattern of Long Non-Coding RNA Growth Arrest-Specific 5 in the Remission Induction Therapy in Childhood Acute Lymphoblastic Leukemia. *J. Med. Biochem.* **2018**. [CrossRef]
39. Garabedian, M.J.; Logan, S.K. Glucocorticoid receptor DNA binding decoy is a gas. *Sci. Signal* **2010**, *3*, pe5. [CrossRef] [PubMed]
40. Chen, H.; Zhang, D.; Zhang, G.; Li, X.; Liang, Y.; Kasukurthi, M.V.; Li, S.; Borchert, G.M.; Huang, J. A semantics-oriented computational approach to investigate microRNA regulation on glucocorticoid resistance in pediatric acute lymphoblastic leukemia. *BMC Med Inform. Decis. Mak.* **2018**, *18*, 57. [CrossRef] [PubMed]
41. Aries, I.M.; Jerchel, I.S.; van den Dungen, R.E.; van den Berk, L.C.; Boer, J.M.; Horstmann, M.A.; Escherich, G.; Pieters, R.; den Boer, M.L. EMP1, a novel poor prognostic factor in pediatric leukemia regulates prednisolone resistance, cell proliferation, migration and adhesion. *Leukemia* **2014**, *28*, 1828–1837. [CrossRef] [PubMed]
42. Morales, S.A.; Mareninov, S.; Coulam, P.; Wadehra, M.; Goodglick, L.; Braun, J.; Gordon, L.K. Functional consequences of interactions between FAK and epithelial membrane protein 2 (EMP2). *Investig. Ophthalmol. Vis. Sci.* **2009**, *50*, 4949–4956. [CrossRef] [PubMed]
43. Gauld, S.B.; Cambier, J.C. Src-family kinases in B-cell development and signaling. *Oncogene* **2004**, *23*, 8001–8006. [CrossRef] [PubMed]
44. Palacios, E.H.; Weiss, A. Function of the Src-family kinases, Lck and Fyn, in T-cell development and activation. *Oncogene* **2004**, *23*, 7990–8000. [CrossRef] [PubMed]
45. Paugh, S.W.; Bonten, E.J.; Savic, D.; Ramsey, L.B.; Thierfelder, W.E.; Gurung, P.; Malireddi, R.K.; Actis, M.; Mayasundari, A.; Min, J.; et al. NALP3 inflammasome upregulation and CASP1 cleavage of the glucocorticoid receptor cause glucocorticoid resistance in leukemia cells. *Nat. Genet.* **2015**, *47*, 607–614. [CrossRef] [PubMed]
46. Pottier, N.; Yang, W.; Assem, M.; Panetta, J.C.; Pei, D.; Paugh, S.W.; Cheng, C.; Den Boer, M.L.; Relling, M.V.; Pieters, R.; et al. The SWI/SNF chromatin-remodeling complex and glucocorticoid resistance in acute lymphoblastic leukemia. *J. Natl. Cancer Inst.* **2008**, *100*, 1792–1803. [CrossRef] [PubMed]
47. Jordan, M.A.; Wilson, L. Microtubules as a target for anticancer drugs. *Nat. Reviews. Cancer* **2004**, *4*, 253–265. [CrossRef] [PubMed]
48. Ceppi, F.; Langlois-Pelletier, C.; Gagne, V.; Rousseau, J.; Ciolino, C.; De Lorenzo, S.; Kevin, K.M.; Cijov, D.; Sallan, S.E.; Silverman, L.B.; et al. Polymorphisms of the vincristine pathway and response to treatment in children with childhood acute lymphoblastic leukemia. *Pharmacogenomics* **2014**, *15*, 1105–1116. [CrossRef] [PubMed]
49. Egbelakin, A.; Ferguson, M.J.; MacGill, E.A.; Lehmann, A.S.; Topletz, A.R.; Quinney, S.K.; Li, L.; McCammack, K.C.; Hall, S.D.; Renbarger, J.L. Increased risk of vincristine neurotoxicity associated with low CYP3A5 expression genotype in children with acute lymphoblastic leukemia. *Pediatr. Blood Cancer* **2011**, *56*, 361–367. [CrossRef] [PubMed]
50. Hartman, A.; van Schaik, R.H.; van der Heiden, I.P.; Broekhuis, M.J.; Meier, M.; den Boer, M.L.; Pieters, R. Polymorphisms in genes involved in vincristine pharmacokinetics or pharmacodynamics are not related to impaired motor performance in children with leukemia. *Leuk. Res.* **2010**, *34*, 154–159. [CrossRef] [PubMed]
51. Moore, A.S.; Norris, R.; Price, G.; Nguyen, T.; Ni, M.; George, R.; van Breda, K.; Duley, J.; Charles, B.; Pinkerton, R. Vincristine pharmacodynamics and pharmacogenetics in children with cancer: A limited-sampling, population modelling approach. *J. Paediatr. Child Health* **2011**, *47*, 875–882. [CrossRef] [PubMed]
52. Renbarger, J.L.; McCammack, K.C.; Rouse, C.E.; Hall, S.D. Effect of race on vincristine-associated neurotoxicity in pediatric acute lymphoblastic leukemia patients. *Pediatr. Blood Cancer* **2008**, *50*, 769–771. [CrossRef] [PubMed]

53. Aplenc, R.; Glatfelter, W.; Han, P.; Rappaport, E.; La, M.; Cnaan, A.; Blackwood, M.A.; Lange, B.; Rebbeck, T. CYP3A genotypes and treatment response in paediatric acute lymphoblastic leukaemia. *Br. J. Haematol.* **2003**, *122*, 240–244. [CrossRef] [PubMed]
54. Kishi, S.; Cheng, C.; French, D.; Pei, D.; Das, S.; Cook, E.H.; Hijiya, N.; Rizzari, C.; Rosner, G.L.; Frudakis, T.; et al. Ancestry and pharmacogenetics of antileukemic drug toxicity. *Blood* **2007**, *109*, 4151–4157. [CrossRef] [PubMed]
55. Plasschaert, S.L.; Groninger, E.; Boezen, M.; Kema, I.; de Vries, E.G.; Uges, D.; Veerman, A.J.; Kamps, W.A.; Vellenga, E.; de Graaf, S.S.; et al. Influence of functional polymorphisms of the MDR1 gene on vincristine pharmacokinetics in childhood acute lymphoblastic leukemia. *Clin. Pharm.* **2004**, *76*, 220–229. [CrossRef]
56. Dennison, J.B.; Kulanthaivel, P.; Barbuch, R.J.; Renbarger, J.L.; Ehlhardt, W.J.; Hall, S.D. Selective metabolism of vincristine in vitro by CYP3A5. *Drug Metab. Dispos. Biol. Fate Chem.* **2006**, *34*, 1317–1327. [CrossRef] [PubMed]
57. Kuehl, P.; Zhang, J.; Lin, Y.; Lamba, J.; Assem, M.; Schuetz, J.; Watkins, P.B.; Daly, A.; Wrighton, S.A.; Hall, S.D.; et al. Sequence diversity in CYP3A promoters and characterization of the genetic basis of polymorphic CYP3A5 expression. *Nat. Genet.* **2001**, *27*, 383–391. [CrossRef] [PubMed]
58. Diouf, B.; Crews, K.R.; Lew, G.; Pei, D.; Cheng, C.; Bao, J.; Zheng, J.J.; Yang, W.; Fan, Y.; Wheeler, H.E.; et al. Association of an inherited genetic variant with vincristine-related peripheral neuropathy in children with acute lymphoblastic leukemia. *JAMA* **2015**, *313*, 815–823. [CrossRef] [PubMed]
59. Gutierrez-Camino, A.; Martin-Guerrero, I.; Lopez-Lopez, E.; Echebarria-Barona, A.; Zabalza, I.; Ruiz, I.; Guerra-Merino, I.; Garcia-Orad, A. Lack of association of the CEP72 rs924607 TT genotype with vincristine-related peripheral neuropathy during the early phase of pediatric acute lymphoblastic leukemia treatment in a Spanish population. *Pharm. Genom.* **2016**, *26*, 100–102. [CrossRef] [PubMed]
60. Diouf, B.; Crews, K.R.; Evans, W.E. Vincristine pharmacogenomics: 'winner's curse' or a different phenotype? *Pharm. Genom.* **2016**, *26*, 51–52. [CrossRef] [PubMed]
61. Dennison, J.B.; Jones, D.R.; Renbarger, J.L.; Hall, S.D. Effect of CYP3A5 expression on vincristine metabolism with human liver microsomes. *J. Pharmacol. Exp. Ther.* **2007**, *321*, 553–563. [CrossRef] [PubMed]
62. Berg, S.L.; Parsons, D.W. The Pharmacogenomics of Vincristine-Induced Neuropathy: On Pins and Needles. *JAMA Oncol.* **2015**, *1*, 975–976. [CrossRef] [PubMed]
63. Lopez-Lopez, E.; Gutierrez-Camino, A.; Astigarraga, I.; Navajas, A.; Echebarria-Barona, A.; Garcia-Miguel, P.; Garcia de Andoin, N.; Lobo, C.; Guerra-Merino, I.; Martin-Guerrero, I.; et al. Vincristine pharmacokinetics pathway and neurotoxicity during early phases of treatment in pediatric acute lymphoblastic leukemia. *Pharmacogenomics* **2016**, *17*, 731–741. [CrossRef] [PubMed]
64. Abaji, R.; Ceppi, F.; Patel, S.; Gagne, V.; Xu, C.J.; Spinella, J.F.; Colombini, A.; Parasole, R.; Buldini, B.; Basso, G.; et al. Genetic risk factors for VIPN in childhood acute lymphoblastic leukemia patients identified using whole-exome sequencing. *Pharmacogenomics* **2018**, *19*, 1181–1193. [CrossRef] [PubMed]
65. Zhang, X.; Lei, K.; Yuan, X.; Wu, X.; Zhuang, Y.; Xu, T.; Xu, R.; Han, M. SUN1/2 and Syne/Nesprin-1/2 complexes connect centrosome to the nucleus during neurogenesis and neuronal migration in mice. *Neuron* **2009**, *64*, 173–187. [CrossRef] [PubMed]
66. Kenmochi, N.; Suzuki, T.; Uechi, T.; Magoori, M.; Kuniba, M.; Higa, S.; Watanabe, K.; Tanaka, T. The human mitochondrial ribosomal protein genes: Mapping of 54 genes to the chromosomes and implications for human disorders. *Genomics* **2001**, *77*, 65–70. [CrossRef] [PubMed]
67. Zhu, H.; Wan, X.; Li, J.; Han, L.; Bo, X.; Chen, W.; Lu, C.; Shen, Z.; Xu, C.; Chen, L.; et al. Computational Prediction and Validation of BAHD1 as a Novel Molecule for Ulcerative Colitis. *Sci. Rep.* **2015**, *5*, 12227. [CrossRef] [PubMed]
68. Sun, Z.; Wu, Y.; Ordog, T.; Daheti, S.; Nie, J.; Duan, X.; Hojo, K.; Kocher, J.P.; Dyck, P.J.; Klein, C.J. Aberrant signature methylome by DNMT1 hot spot mutation in hereditary sensory and autonomic neuropathy 1E. *Epigenetics* **2014**, *9*, 1184–1193. [CrossRef] [PubMed]
69. Li, L.; Sajdyk, T.; Smith, E.M.L.; Chang, C.W.; Li, C.; Ho, R.H.; Hutchinson, R.; Wells, E.; Skiles, J.L.; Winick, N.; et al. Genetic Variants Associated With Vincristine-Induced Peripheral Neuropathy in Two Populations of Children With Acute Lymphoblastic Leukemia. *Clin. Pharm.* **2018**. [CrossRef] [PubMed]

70. Robertson, N.G.; Cremers, C.W.; Huygen, P.L.; Ikezono, T.; Krastins, B.; Kremer, H.; Kuo, S.F.; Liberman, M.C.; Merchant, S.N.; Miller, C.E.; et al. Cochlin immunostaining of inner ear pathologic deposits and proteomic analysis in DFNA9 deafness and vestibular dysfunction. *Hum. Mol. Genet.* **2006**, *15*, 1071–1085. [CrossRef] [PubMed]
71. Wittamer, V.; Franssen, J.D.; Vulcano, M.; Mirjolet, J.F.; Le Poul, E.; Migeotte, I.; Brezillon, S.; Tyldesley, R.; Blanpain, C.; Detheux, M.; et al. Specific recruitment of antigen-presenting cells by chemerin, a novel processed ligand from human inflammatory fluids. *J. Exp. Med.* **2003**, *198*, 977–985. [CrossRef] [PubMed]
72. Schotte, D.; De Menezes, R.X.; Akbari Moqadam, F.; Khankahdani, L.M.; Lange-Turenhout, E.; Chen, C.; Pieters, R.; Den Boer, M.L. MicroRNA characterize genetic diversity and drug resistance in pediatric acute lymphoblastic leukemia. *Haematologica* **2011**, *96*, 703–711. [CrossRef] [PubMed]
73. Akbari Moqadam, F.; Lange-Turenhout, E.A.; Aries, I.M.; Pieters, R.; den Boer, M.L. MiR-125b, miR-100 and miR-99a co-regulate vincristine resistance in childhood acute lymphoblastic leukemia. *Leuk. Res.* **2013**, *37*, 1315–1321. [CrossRef] [PubMed]
74. Lopez-Lopez, E.; Gutierrez-Camino, A.; Pinan, M.A.; Sanchez-Toledo, J.; Uriz, J.J.; Ballesteros, J.; Garcia-Miguel, P.; Navajas, A.; Garcia-Orad, A. Pharmacogenetics of microRNAs and microRNAs biogenesis machinery in pediatric acute lymphoblastic leukemia. *PLoS ONE* **2014**, *9*, e91261. [CrossRef] [PubMed]
75. Gutierrez-Camino, A.; Umerez, M.; Martin-Guerrero, I.; Garcia de Andoin, N.; Santos, B.; Sastre, A.; Echebarria-Barona, A.; Astigarraga, I.; Navajas, A.; Garcia-Orad, A. Mir-pharmacogenetics of Vincristine and peripheral neurotoxicity in childhood B-cell acute lymphoblastic leukemia. *Pharm. J.* **2018**, *18*, 704–712. [CrossRef] [PubMed]
76. Franca, R.; Rebora, P.; Bertorello, N.; Fagioli, F.; Conter, V.; Biondi, A.; Colombini, A.; Micalizzi, C.; Zecca, M.; Parasole, R.; et al. Pharmacogenetics and induction/consolidation therapy toxicities in acute lymphoblastic leukemia patients treated with AIEOP-BFM ALL 2000 protocol. *Pharm. J.* **2017**, *17*, 4–10. [CrossRef] [PubMed]
77. Fernandez, C.A.; Smith, C.; Yang, W.; Mullighan, C.G.; Qu, C.; Larsen, E.; Bowman, W.P.; Liu, C.; Ramsey, L.B.; Chang, T.; et al. Genome-wide analysis links NFATC2 with asparaginase hypersensitivity. *Blood* **2015**, *126*, 69–75. [CrossRef] [PubMed]
78. Duval, M. Comparison of Escherichia coli-asparaginase with Erwinia-asparaginase in the treatment of childhood lymphoid malignancies: Results of a randomized European Organisation for Research and Treatment of Cancer—Children's Leukemia Group phase 3 trial. *Blood* **2002**, *99*, 2734–2739. [CrossRef] [PubMed]
79. Dinndorf, P.A.; Gootenberg, J.; Cohen, M.H.; Keegan, P.; Pazdur, R. FDA Drug Approval Summary: Pegaspargase (Oncaspar®) for the First-Line Treatment of Children with Acute Lymphoblastic Leukemia (ALL). *oncologist* **2007**, *12*, 991–998. [CrossRef] [PubMed]
80. Rousseau, J.; Gagne, V.; Labuda, M.; Beaubois, C.; Sinnett, D.; Laverdiere, C.; Moghrabi, A.; Sallan, S.E.; Silverman, L.B.; Neuberg, D.; et al. ATF5 polymorphisms influence ATF function and response to treatment in children with childhood acute lymphoblastic leukemia. *Blood* **2011**, *118*, 5883–5890. [CrossRef] [PubMed]
81. Ben Tanfous, M.; Sharif-Askari, B.; Ceppi, F.; Laaribi, H.; Gagne, V.; Rousseau, J.; Labuda, M.; Silverman, L.B.; Sallan, S.E.; Neuberg, D.; et al. Polymorphisms of asparaginase pathway and asparaginase-related complications in children with acute lymphoblastic leukemia. *Clin. Cancer Res.* **2015**, *21*, 329–334. [CrossRef] [PubMed]
82. Abaji, R.; Gagne, V.; Xu, C.J.; Spinella, J.F.; Ceppi, F.; Laverdiere, C.; Leclerc, J.M.; Sallan, S.E.; Neuberg, D.; Kutok, J.L.; et al. Whole-exome sequencing identified genetic risk factors for asparaginase-related complications in childhood ALL patients. *Oncotarget* **2017**, *8*, 43752–43767. [CrossRef] [PubMed]
83. Mori, S.; Bernardi, R.; Laurent, A.; Resnati, M.; Crippa, A.; Gabrieli, A.; Keough, R.; Gonda, T.J.; Blasi, F. Myb-binding protein 1A (MYBBP1A) is essential for early embryonic development, controls cell cycle and mitosis, and acts as a tumor suppressor. *PLoS ONE* **2012**, *7*, e39723. [CrossRef] [PubMed]
84. Owen, H.R.; Elser, M.; Cheung, E.; Gersbach, M.; Kraus, W.L.; Hottiger, M.O. MYBBP1a is a novel repressor of NF-kappaB. *J. Mol. Biol.* **2007**, *366*, 725–736. [CrossRef] [PubMed]
85. Luo, S.X.; Li, S.; Zhang, X.H.; Zhang, J.J.; Long, G.H.; Dong, G.F.; Su, W.; Deng, Y.; Liu, Y.; Zhao, J.M.; et al. Genetic polymorphisms of interleukin-16 and risk of knee osteoarthritis. *PLoS ONE* **2015**, *10*, e0123442. [CrossRef] [PubMed]

86. Lehti, M.S.; Henriksson, H.; Rummukainen, P.; Wang, F.; Uusitalo-Kylmala, L.; Kiviranta, R.; Heino, T.J.; Kotaja, N.; Sironen, A. Cilia-related protein SPEF2 regulates osteoblast differentiation. *Sci. Rep.* **2018**, *8*, 859. [CrossRef] [PubMed]
87. Kang, S.M.; Rosales, J.L.; Meier-Stephenson, V.; Kim, S.; Lee, K.Y.; Narendran, A. Genome-wide loss-of-function genetic screening identifies opioid receptor mu1 as a key regulator of L-asparaginase resistance in pediatric acute lymphoblastic leukemia. *Oncogene* **2017**, *36*, 5910–5913. [CrossRef] [PubMed]
88. Friesen, C.; Roscher, M.; Hormann, I.; Fichtner, I.; Alt, A.; Hilger, R.A.; Debatin, K.M.; Miltner, E. Cell death sensitization of leukemia cells by opioid receptor activation. *Oncotarget* **2013**, *4*, 677–690. [CrossRef] [PubMed]
89. Liu, Y.; Fernandez, C.A.; Smith, C.; Yang, W.; Cheng, C.; Panetta, J.C.; Kornegay, N.; Liu, C.; Ramsey, L.B.; Karol, S.E.; et al. Genome-Wide Study Links PNPLA3 Variant with Elevated Hepatic Transaminase After Acute Lymphoblastic Leukemia Therapy. *Clin. Pharm.* **2017**, *102*, 131–140. [CrossRef] [PubMed]
90. Kienesberger, P.C.; Oberer, M.; Lass, A.; Zechner, R. Mammalian patatin domain containing proteins: A family with diverse lipolytic activities involved in multiple biological functions. *J. Lipid Res.* **2009**, *50*, S63–S68. [CrossRef] [PubMed]
91. Chen, S.H.; Pei, D.; Yang, W.; Cheng, C.; Jeha, S.; Cox, N.J.; Evans, W.E.; Pui, C.H.; Relling, M.V. Genetic variations in GRIA1 on chromosome 5q33 related to asparaginase hypersensitivity. *Clin. Pharm.* **2010**, *88*, 191–196. [CrossRef] [PubMed]
92. Blumenthal, M.N.; Langefeld, C.D.; Beaty, T.H.; Bleecker, E.R.; Ober, C.; Lester, L.; Lange, E.; Barnes, K.C.; Wolf, R.; King, R.A.; et al. A genome-wide search for allergic response (atopy) genes in three ethnic groups: Collaborative Study on the Genetics of Asthma. *Hum. Genet.* **2004**, *114*, 157–164. [CrossRef] [PubMed]
93. Kerner, B.; Jasinska, A.J.; DeYoung, J.; Almonte, M.; Choi, O.W.; Freimer, N.B. Polymorphisms in the GRIA1 gene region in psychotic bipolar disorder. *Am. J. Med Genet. B Neuropsychiatr. Genet.* **2009**, *150B*, 24–32. [CrossRef] [PubMed]
94. Kutszegi, N.; Semsei, A.F.; Gezsi, A.; Sagi, J.C.; Nagy, V.; Csordas, K.; Jakab, Z.; Lautner-Csorba, O.; Gabor, K.M.; Kovacs, G.T.; et al. Subgroups of Paediatric Acute Lymphoblastic Leukaemia Might Differ Significantly in Genetic Predisposition to Asparaginase Hypersensitivity. *PLoS ONE* **2015**, *10*, e0140136. [CrossRef] [PubMed]
95. Rajic, V.; Debeljak, M.; Goricar, K.; Jazbec, J. Polymorphisms in GRIA1 gene are a risk factor for asparaginase hypersensitivity during the treatment of childhood acute lymphoblastic leukemia. *Leuk. Lymphoma* **2015**, *56*, 3103–3108. [CrossRef] [PubMed]
96. Fernandez, C.A.; Smith, C.; Yang, W.; Date, M.; Bashford, D.; Larsen, E.; Bowman, W.P.; Liu, C.; Ramsey, L.B.; Chang, T.; et al. HLA-DRB1*07:01 is associated with a higher risk of asparaginase allergies. *Blood* **2014**, *124*, 1266–1276. [CrossRef] [PubMed]
97. Kutszegi, N.; Yang, X.; Gezsi, A.; Schermann, G.; Erdelyi, D.J.; Semsei, A.F.; Gabor, K.M.; Sagi, J.C.; Kovacs, G.T.; Falus, A.; et al. HLA-DRB1*07:01-HLA-DQA1*02:01-HLA-DQB1*02:02 haplotype is associated with a high risk of asparaginase hypersensitivity in acute lymphoblastic leukemia. *Haematologica* **2017**, *102*, 1578–1586. [CrossRef] [PubMed]
98. Rao, A.; Luo, C.; Hogan, P.G. Transcription factors of the NFAT family: Regulation and function. *Annu. Rev. Immunol.* **1997**, *15*, 707–747. [CrossRef] [PubMed]
99. Xanthoudakis, S.; Viola, J.P.; Shaw, K.T.; Luo, C.; Wallace, J.D.; Bozza, P.T.; Luk, D.C.; Curran, T.; Rao, A. An enhanced immune response in mice lacking the transcription factor NFAT1. *Science* **1996**, *272*, 892–895. [CrossRef] [PubMed]
100. Wolthers, B.O.; Frandsen, T.L.; Patel, C.J.; Abaji, R.; Attarbaschi, A.; Barzilai, S.; Colombini, A.; Escherich, G.; Grosjean, M.; Krajinovic, M.; et al. Trypsin encoding PRSS1-PRSS2 variation influence the risk of asparaginase-associated pancreatitis in children with acute lymphoblastic leukemia: A Ponte di Legno toxicity working group report. *Haematologica* **2018**. [CrossRef] [PubMed]
101. Hojfeldt, S.G.; Wolthers, B.O.; Tulstrup, M.; Abrahamsson, J.; Gupta, R.; Harila-Saari, A.; Heyman, M.; Henriksen, L.T.; Jonsson, O.G.; Lahteenmaki, P.M.; et al. Genetic predisposition to PEG-asparaginase hypersensitivity in children treated according to NOPHO ALL2008. *Br. J. Haematol.* **2019**, *184*, 405–417. [CrossRef] [PubMed]

102. Rodriguez-Gil, A.; Ritter, O.; Saul, V.V.; Wilhelm, J.; Yang, C.Y.; Grosschedl, R.; Imai, Y.; Kuba, K.; Kracht, M.; Schmitz, M.L. The CCR4-NOT complex contributes to repression of Major Histocompatibility Complex class II transcription. *Sci. Rep.* **2017**, *7*, 3547. [CrossRef] [PubMed]
103. Steinke, J.W.; Borish, L.; Rosenwasser, L.J. 5. Genetics of hypersensitivity. *J. Allergy Clin. Immunol.* **2003**, *111*, S495–S501. [CrossRef] [PubMed]
104. Di Marco, A.; Cassinelli, G.; Arcamone, F. The discovery of daunorubicin. *Cancer Treat. Rep.* **1981**, *65* (Suppl. 4), 3–8.
105. Champoux, J.J. DNA topoisomerases: Structure, function, and mechanism. *Annu. Rev. Biochem.* **2001**, *70*, 369–413. [CrossRef] [PubMed]
106. Gewirtz, D.A. A critical evaluation of the mechanisms of action proposed for the antitumor effects of the anthracycline antibiotics adriamycin and daunorubicin. *Biochem. Pharmacol.* **1999**, *57*, 727–741. [CrossRef]
107. Armenian, S.; Bhatia, S. Predicting and Preventing Anthracycline-Related Cardiotoxicity. *Am. Soc. Clin. Oncol. Educ. Book. Am. Soc. Clin. Oncology. Annu. Meet.* **2018**. [CrossRef] [PubMed]
108. Blanco, J.G.; Leisenring, W.M.; Gonzalez-Covarrubias, V.M.; Kawashima, T.I.; Davies, S.M.; Relling, M.V.; Robison, L.L.; Sklar, C.A.; Stovall, M.; Bhatia, S. Genetic polymorphisms in the carbonyl reductase 3 gene CBR3 and the NAD(P)H:quinone oxidoreductase 1 gene NQO1 in patients who developed anthracycline-related congestive heart failure after childhood cancer. *Cancer* **2008**, *112*, 2789–2795. [CrossRef] [PubMed]
109. Visscher, H.; Ross, C.J.; Rassekh, S.R.; Barhdadi, A.; Dube, M.P.; Al-Saloos, H.; Sandor, G.S.; Caron, H.N.; van Dalen, E.C.; Kremer, L.C.; et al. Pharmacogenomic prediction of anthracycline-induced cardiotoxicity in children. *J. Clin. Oncol.* **2012**, *30*, 1422–1428. [CrossRef] [PubMed]
110. Nagasawa, K.; Nagai, K.; Ohnishi, N.; Yokoyama, T.; Fujimoto, S. Contribution of Specific Transport Systems to Anthracycline Transport in Tumor and Normal Cells. *Curr. Drug Metab.* **2001**, *2*, 355–366. [CrossRef] [PubMed]
111. Rossi, D.; Rasi, S.; Franceschetti, S.; Capello, D.; Castelli, A.; De Paoli, L.; Ramponi, A.; Chiappella, A.; Pogliani, E.M.; Vitolo, U.; et al. Analysis of the host pharmacogenetic background for prediction of outcome and toxicity in diffuse large B-cell lymphoma treated with R-CHOP21. *Leukemia* **2009**, *23*, 1118–1126. [CrossRef] [PubMed]
112. Wojnowski, L.; Kulle, B.; Schirmer, M.; Schluter, G.; Schmidt, A.; Rosenberger, A.; Vonhof, S.; Bickeboller, H.; Toliat, M.R.; Suk, E.K.; et al. NAD(P)H oxidase and multidrug resistance protein genetic polymorphisms are associated with doxorubicin-induced cardiotoxicity. *Circulation* **2005**, *112*, 3754–3762. [CrossRef] [PubMed]
113. Rajic, V.; Aplenc, R.; Debeljak, M.; Prestor, V.V.; Karas-Kuzelicki, N.; Mlinaric-Rascan, I.; Jazbec, J. Influence of the polymorphism in candidate genes on late cardiac damage in patients treated due to acute leukemia in childhood. *Leuk. Lymphoma* **2009**, *50*, 1693–1698. [CrossRef] [PubMed]
114. Visscher, H.; Ross, C.J.; Rassekh, S.R.; Sandor, G.S.; Caron, H.N.; van Dalen, E.C.; Kremer, L.C.; van der Pal, H.J.; Rogers, P.C.; Rieder, M.J.; et al. Validation of variants in SLC28A3 and UGT1A6 as genetic markers predictive of anthracycline-induced cardiotoxicity in children. *Pediatr. Blood Cancer* **2013**, *60*, 1375–1381. [CrossRef] [PubMed]
115. Visscher, H.; Rassekh, S.R.; Sandor, G.S.; Caron, H.N.; van Dalen, E.C.; Kremer, L.C.; van der Pal, H.J.; Rogers, P.C.; Rieder, M.J.; Carleton, B.C.; et al. Genetic variants in SLC22A17 and SLC22A7 are associated with anthracycline-induced cardiotoxicity in children. *Pharmacogenomics* **2015**, *16*, 1065–1076. [CrossRef] [PubMed]
116. Aminkeng, F.; Bhavsar, A.P.; Visscher, H.; Rassekh, S.R.; Li, Y.; Lee, J.W.; Brunham, L.R.; Caron, H.N.; van Dalen, E.C.; Kremer, L.C.; et al. A coding variant in RARG confers susceptibility to anthracycline-induced cardiotoxicity in childhood cancer. *Nat. Genet.* **2015**, *47*, 1079–1084. [CrossRef] [PubMed]
117. Bilbija, D.; Haugen, F.; Sagave, J.; Baysa, A.; Bastani, N.; Levy, F.O.; Sirsjo, A.; Blomhoff, R.; Valen, G. Retinoic acid signalling is activated in the postischemic heart and may influence remodelling. *PLoS ONE* **2012**, *7*, e44740. [CrossRef] [PubMed]
118. Delacroix, L.; Moutier, E.; Altobelli, G.; Legras, S.; Poch, O.; Choukrallah, M.A.; Bertin, I.; Jost, B.; Davidson, I. Cell-specific interaction of retinoic acid receptors with target genes in mouse embryonic fibroblasts and embryonic stem cells. *Mol. Cell Biol.* **2010**, *30*, 231–244. [CrossRef] [PubMed]

119. Wang, X.; Liu, W.; Sun, C.L.; Armenian, S.H.; Hakonarson, H.; Hageman, L.; Ding, Y.; Landier, W.; Blanco, J.G.; Chen, L.; et al. Hyaluronan synthase 3 variant and anthracycline-related cardiomyopathy: A report from the children's oncology group. *J. Clin. Oncol.* **2014**, *32*, 647–653. [CrossRef] [PubMed]
120. Perik, P.J.; de Vries, E.G.; Gietema, J.A.; van der Graaf, W.T.; Sleijfer, D.T.; Suurmeijer, A.J.; van Veldhuisen, D.J. The dilemma of the strive for apoptosis in oncology: Mind the heart. *Crit. Rev. Oncol. Hematol.* **2005**, *53*, 101–113. [CrossRef] [PubMed]
121. Weinshilboum, R.M.; Sladek, S.L. Mercaptopurine pharmacogenetics: Monogenic inheritance of erythrocyte thiopurine methyltransferase activity. *Am. J. Hum. Genet.* **1980**, *32*, 651–662. [PubMed]
122. Relling, M.V.; Gardner, E.E.; Sandborn, W.J.; Schmiegelow, K.; Pui, C.H.; Yee, S.W.; Stein, C.M.; Carrillo, M.; Evans, W.E.; Klein, T.E.; et al. Clinical Pharmacogenetics Implementation Consortium guidelines for thiopurine methyltransferase genotype and thiopurine dosing. *Clin. Pharm.* **2011**, *89*, 387–391. [CrossRef] [PubMed]
123. Karas-Kuzelicki, N.; Jazbec, J.; Milek, M.; Mlinaric-Rascan, I. Heterozygosity at the TPMT gene locus, augmented by mutated MTHFR gene, predisposes to 6-MP related toxicities in childhood ALL patients. *Leukemia* **2008**, *23*, 971. [CrossRef] [PubMed]
124. Karas-Kuzelicki, N.; Milek, M.; Mlinaric-Rascan, I. MTHFR and TYMS genotypes influence TPMT activity and its differential modulation in males and females. *Clin. Biochem.* **2010**, *43*, 37–42. [CrossRef] [PubMed]
125. Liu, C.; Yang, W.; Pei, D.; Cheng, C.; Smith, C.; Landier, W.; Hageman, L.; Chen, Y.; Yang, J.J.; Crews, K.R.; et al. Genomewide Approach Validates Thiopurine Methyltransferase Activity Is a Monogenic Pharmacogenomic Trait. *Clin. Pharm.* **2017**, *101*, 373–381. [CrossRef] [PubMed]
126. Tamm, R.; Magi, R.; Tremmel, R.; Winter, S.; Mihailov, E.; Smid, A.; Moricke, A.; Klein, K.; Schrappe, M.; Stanulla, M.; et al. Polymorphic variation in TPMT is the principal determinant of TPMT phenotype: A meta-analysis of three genome-wide association studies. *Clin. Pharm.* **2017**, *101*, 684–695. [CrossRef] [PubMed]
127. Gerbek, T.; Ebbesen, M.; Nersting, J.; Frandsen, T.L.; Appell, M.L.; Schmiegelow, K. Role of TPMT and ITPA variants in mercaptopurine disposition. *Cancer Chemother. Pharm.* **2018**, *81*, 579–586. [CrossRef] [PubMed]
128. Liu, C.; Janke, L.J.; Yang, J.J.; Evans, W.E.; Schuetz, J.D.; Relling, M.V. Differential effects of thiopurine methyltransferase (TPMT) and multidrug resistance-associated protein gene 4 (MRP4) on mercaptopurine toxicity. *Cancer Chemother. Pharm.* **2017**, *80*, 287–293. [CrossRef] [PubMed]
129. Tanaka, Y.; Manabe, A.; Fukushima, H.; Suzuki, R.; Nakadate, H.; Kondoh, K.; Nakamura, K.; Koh, K.; Fukushima, T.; Tsuchida, M.; et al. Multidrug resistance protein 4 (MRP4) polymorphisms impact the 6-mercaptopurine dose tolerance during maintenance therapy in Japanese childhood acute lymphoblastic leukemia. *Pharm. J.* **2015**, *15*, 380–384. [CrossRef] [PubMed]
130. Milosevic, G.; Kotur, N.; Krstovski, N.; Lazic, J.; Zukic, B.; Stankovic, B.; Janic, D.; Katsila, T.; Patrinos, G.P.; Pavlovic, S.; et al. Variants in TPMT, ITPA, ABCC4 and ABCB1 Genes as Predictors of 6-mercaptopurine Induced Toxicity in Children with Acute Lymphoblastic Leukemia. *J. Med. Biochem.* **2018**, *37*, 320–327. [CrossRef] [PubMed]
131. Zhou, H.; Li, L.; Yang, P.; Yang, L.; Zheng, J.E.; Zhou, Y.; Han, Y. Optimal predictor for 6-mercaptopurine intolerance in Chinese children with acute lymphoblastic leukemia: NUDT15, TPMT, or ITPA genetic variants? *BMC Cancer* **2018**, *18*, 516. [CrossRef] [PubMed]
132. Yang, J.J.; Landier, W.; Yang, W.; Liu, C.; Hageman, L.; Cheng, C.; Pei, D.; Chen, Y.; Crews, K.R.; Kornegay, N.; et al. Inherited NUDT15 variant is a genetic determinant of mercaptopurine intolerance in children with acute lymphoblastic leukemia. *J. Clin. Oncol.* **2015**, *33*, 1235–1242. [CrossRef] [PubMed]
133. Moriyama, T.; Nishii, R.; Perez-Andreu, V.; Yang, W.; Klussmann, F.A.; Zhao, X.; Lin, T.N.; Hoshitsuki, K.; Nersting, J.; Kihira, K.; et al. NUDT15 polymorphisms alter thiopurine metabolism and hematopoietic toxicity. *Nat. Genet.* **2016**, *48*, 367–373. [CrossRef] [PubMed]
134. Liang, D.C.; Yang, C.P.; Liu, H.C.; Jaing, T.H.; Chen, S.H.; Hung, I.J.; Yeh, T.C.; Lin, T.H.; Lai, C.L.; Lai, C.Y.; et al. NUDT15 gene polymorphism related to mercaptopurine intolerance in Taiwan Chinese children with acute lymphoblastic leukemia. *Pharm. J.* **2016**, *16*, 536–539. [CrossRef] [PubMed]
135. Moriyama, T.; Yang, Y.L.; Nishii, R.; Ariffin, H.; Liu, C.; Lin, T.N.; Yang, W.; Lin, D.T.; Yu, C.H.; Kham, S.; et al. Novel variants in NUDT15 and thiopurine intolerance in children with acute lymphoblastic leukemia from diverse ancestry. *Blood* **2017**, *130*, 1209–1212. [CrossRef] [PubMed]

136. Relling, M.V.; Schwab, M.; Whirl-Carrillo, M.; Suarez-Kurtz, G.; Pui, C.H.; Stein, C.M.; Moyer, A.M.; Evans, W.E.; Klein, T.E.; Antillon-Klussmann, F.G.; et al. Clinical Pharmacogenetics Implementation Consortium Guideline for Thiopurine Dosing Based on TPMT and NUDT15 Genotypes: 2018 Update. *Clin. Pharm.* **2018**. [CrossRef] [PubMed]

137. Stocco, G.; Yang, W.; Crews, K.R.; Thierfelder, W.E.; Decorti, G.; Londero, M.; Franca, R.; Rabusin, M.; Valsecchi, M.G.; Pei, D.; et al. PACSIN2 polymorphism influences TPMT activity and mercaptopurine-related gastrointestinal toxicity. *Hum. Mol. Genet.* **2012**, *21*, 4793–4804. [CrossRef] [PubMed]

138. Stocco, G.; Franca, R.; Favretto, D.; Giurici, N.; Ventura, A.; Decorti, G.; Vinti, L.; Colombini, A.; Brivio, E.; Bettini, L.R.; et al. PACSIN2 rs2413739 Polymorphism and Thiopurine Pharmacokinetics: Validation Studies in Pediatric Patients. *Blood* **2017**, *130*, 4999.

139. Smid, A.; Karas-Kuzelicki, N.; Jazbec, J.; Mlinaric-Rascan, I. PACSIN2 polymorphism is associated with thiopurine-induced hematological toxicity in children with acute lymphoblastic leukaemia undergoing maintenance therapy. *Sci. Rep.* **2016**, *6*, 30244. [CrossRef] [PubMed]

140. Roberts, R.L.; Wallace, M.C.; Seinen, M.L.; Krishnaprasad, K.; Chew, A.; Lawrance, I.; Prosser, R.; Bampton, P.; Grafton, R.; Simms, L.; et al. PACSIN2 does not influence thiopurine-related toxicity in patients with inflammatory bowel disease. *Am. J. Gastroenterol.* **2014**, *109*, 925–927. [CrossRef] [PubMed]

141. Meyer, J.A.; Wang, J.; Hogan, L.E.; Yang, J.J.; Dandekar, S.; Patel, J.P.; Tang, Z.; Zumbo, P.; Li, S.; Zavadil, J.; et al. Relapse-specific mutations in NT5C2 in childhood acute lymphoblastic leukemia. *Nat. Genet.* **2013**, *45*, 290–294. [CrossRef] [PubMed]

142. Tzoneva, G.; Perez-Garcia, A.; Carpenter, Z.; Khiabanian, H.; Tosello, V.; Allegretta, M.; Paietta, E.; Racevskis, J.; Rowe, J.M.; Tallman, M.S.; et al. Activating mutations in the NT5C2 nucleotidase gene drive chemotherapy resistance in relapsed ALL. *Nat. Med.* **2013**, *19*, 368–371. [CrossRef] [PubMed]

143. Lindqvist, C.M.; Lundmark, A.; Nordlund, J.; Freyhult, E.; Ekman, D.; Carlsson Almlof, J.; Raine, A.; Overnas, E.; Abrahamsson, J.; Frost, B.M.; et al. Deep targeted sequencing in pediatric acute lymphoblastic leukemia unveils distinct mutational patterns between genetic subtypes and novel relapse-associated genes. *Oncotarget* **2016**, *7*, 64071–64088. [CrossRef] [PubMed]

144. Kotur, N.; Stankovic, B.; Kassela, K.; Georgitsi, M.; Vicha, A.; Leontari, I.; Dokmanovic, L.; Janic, D.; Krstovski, N.; Klaassen, K.; et al. 6-mercaptopurine influences TPMT gene transcription in a TPMT gene promoter variable number of tandem repeats-dependent manner. *Pharmacogenomics* **2012**, *13*, 283–295. [CrossRef] [PubMed]

145. Zukic, B.; Radmilovic, M.; Stojiljkovic, M.; Tosic, N.; Pourfarzad, F.; Dokmanovic, L.; Janic, D.; Colovic, N.; Philipsen, S.; Patrinos, G.P.; et al. Functional analysis of the role of the TPMT gene promoter VNTR polymorphism in TPMT gene transcription. *Pharmacogenomics* **2010**, *11*, 547–557. [CrossRef] [PubMed]

146. Kotur, N.; Dokmanovic, L.; Janic, D.; Stankovic, B.; Krstovski, N.; Tosic, N.; Katsila, T.; Patrinos, G.P.; Zukic, B.; Pavlovic, S. TPMT gene expression is increased during maintenance therapy in childhood acute lymphoblastic leukemia patients in a TPMT gene promoter variable number of tandem repeat-dependent manner. *Pharmacogenomics* **2015**, *16*, 1701–1712. [CrossRef] [PubMed]

147. Beesley, A.H.; Cummings, A.J.; Freitas, J.R.; Hoffmann, K.; Firth, M.J.; Ford, J.; de Klerk, N.H.; Kees, U.R. The gene expression signature of relapse in paediatric acute lymphoblastic leukaemia: Implications for mechanisms of therapy failure. *Br. J. Haematol.* **2005**, *131*, 447–456. [CrossRef] [PubMed]

148. Bhojwani, D.; Kang, H.; Moskowitz, N.P.; Min, D.J.; Lee, H.; Potter, J.W.; Davidson, G.; Willman, C.L.; Borowitz, M.J.; Belitskaya-Levy, I.; et al. Biologic pathways associated with relapse in childhood acute lymphoblastic leukemia: A Children's Oncology Group study. *Blood* **2006**, *108*, 711–717. [CrossRef] [PubMed]

149. Hogan, L.E.; Meyer, J.A.; Yang, J.; Wang, J.; Wong, N.; Yang, W.; Condos, G.; Hunger, S.P.; Raetz, E.; Saffery, R.; et al. Integrated genomic analysis of relapsed childhood acute lymphoblastic leukemia reveals therapeutic strategies. *Blood* **2011**, *118*, 5218–5226. [CrossRef] [PubMed]

150. Staal, F.J.T.; de Ridder, D.; Szczepanski, T.; Schonewille, T.; van der Linden, E.C.E.; van Wering, E.R.; van der Velden, V.H.J.; van Dongen, J.J.M. Genome-wide expression analysis of paired diagnosis–relapse samples in ALL indicates involvement of pathways related to DNA replication, cell cycle and DNA repair, independent of immune phenotype. *Leukemia* **2010**, *24*, 491. [CrossRef] [PubMed]

151. Yang, J.J.; Bhojwani, D.; Yang, W.; Cai, X.; Stocco, G.; Crews, K.; Wang, J.; Morrison, D.; Devidas, M.; Hunger, S.P.; et al. Genome-wide copy number profiling reveals molecular evolution from diagnosis to relapse in childhood acute lymphoblastic leukemia. *Blood* **2008**, *112*, 4178–4183. [CrossRef] [PubMed]

152. Zaza, G.; Cheok, M.; Yang, W.; Panetta, J.C.; Pui, C.H.; Relling, M.V.; Evans, W.E. Gene expression and thioguanine nucleotide disposition in acute lymphoblastic leukemia after in vivo mercaptopurine treatment. *Blood* **2005**, *106*, 1778–1785. [CrossRef] [PubMed]

153. Ansari, A.; Aslam, Z.; De Sica, A.; Smith, M.; Gilshenan, K.; Fairbanks, L.; Marinaki, A.; Sanderson, J.; Duley, J. Influence of xanthine oxidase on thiopurine metabolism in Crohn's disease. *Aliment. Pharmacol. Ther.* **2008**, *28*, 749–757. [CrossRef] [PubMed]

154. Huang, Y.; Anderle, P.; Bussey, K.J.; Barbacioru, C.; Shankavaram, U.; Dai, Z.; Reinhold, W.C.; Papp, A.; Weinstein, J.N.; Sadee, W. Membrane transporters and channels: Role of the transportome in cancer chemosensitivity and chemoresistance. *Cancer Res.* **2004**, *64*, 4294–4301. [CrossRef] [PubMed]

155. Beesley, A.H.; Firth, M.J.; Anderson, D.; Samuels, A.L.; Ford, J.; Kees, U.R. Drug-gene modeling in pediatric T-cell acute lymphoblastic leukemia highlights importance of 6-mercaptopurine for outcome. *Cancer Res.* **2013**, *73*, 2749–2759. [CrossRef] [PubMed]

156. Organista-Nava, J.; Gomez-Gomez, Y.; Illades-Aguiar, B.; Rivera-Ramirez, A.B.; Saavedra-Herrera, M.V.; Leyva-Vazquez, M.A. Overexpression of dihydrofolate reductase is a factor of poor survival in acute lymphoblastic leukemia. *Oncol. Lett.* **2018**, *15*, 8405–8411. [CrossRef] [PubMed]

157. Wojtuszkiewicz, A.; Peters, G.J.; van Woerden, N.L.; Dubbelman, B.; Escherich, G.; Schmiegelow, K.; Sonneveld, E.; Pieters, R.; van de Ven, P.M.; Jansen, G.; et al. Methotrexate resistance in relation to treatment outcome in childhood acute lymphoblastic leukemia. *J. Hematol. Oncol.* **2015**, *8*, 61. [CrossRef] [PubMed]

158. Kaluzna, E.; Strauss, E.; Zajac-Spychala, O.; Gowin, E.; Swiatek-Koscielna, B.; Nowak, J.; Fichna, M.; Mankowski, P.; Januszkiewicz-Lewandowska, D. Functional variants of gene encoding folate metabolizing enzyme and methotrexate-related toxicity in children with acute lymphoblastic leukemia. *Eur. J. Pharm.* **2015**, *769*, 93–99. [CrossRef] [PubMed]

159. Roy Moulik, N.; Kumar, A.; Agrawal, S.; Awasthi, S.; Mahdi, A.A.; Kumar, A. Role of folate status and methylenetetrahydrofolate reductase genotype on the toxicity and outcome of induction chemotherapy in children with acute lymphoblastic leukemia. *Leuk. Lymphoma* **2015**, *56*, 1379–1384. [CrossRef] [PubMed]

160. Araoz, H.V.; D'Aloi, K.; Foncuberta, M.E.; Sanchez La Rosa, C.G.; Alonso, C.N.; Chertkoff, L.; Felice, M. Pharmacogenetic studies in children with acute lymphoblastic leukemia in Argentina. *Leuk. Lymphoma* **2015**, *56*, 1370–1378. [CrossRef] [PubMed]

161. Finkelstein, Y.; Blonquist, T.M.; Vijayanathan, V.; Stevenson, K.E.; Neuberg, D.S.; Silverman, L.B.; Vrooman, L.M.; Sallan, S.E.; Cole, P.D. A thymidylate synthase polymorphism is associated with increased risk for bone toxicity among children treated for acute lymphoblastic leukemia. *Pediatr. Blood Cancer* **2017**, *64*, e26393. [CrossRef] [PubMed]

162. Yazicioglu, B.; Kaya, Z.; Guntekin Ergun, S.; Percin, F.; Kocak, U.; Yenicesu, I.; Gursel, T. Influence of Folate-Related Gene Polymorphisms on High-Dose Methotrexate-Related Toxicity and Prognosis in Turkish Children with Acute Lymphoblastic Leukemia. *Turk. J. Haematol.* **2017**, *34*, 143–150. [CrossRef] [PubMed]

163. Lazic, J.; Kotur, N.; Krstovski, N.; Dokmanovic, L.; Zukic, B.; Predojevic-Samardzic, J.; Zivotic, M.; Milosevic, G.; Djoric, M.; Janic, D.; et al. Importance of pharmacogenetic markers in the methylenetetrahydrofolate reductase gene during methotrexate treatment in pediatric patients with acute lymphoblastic leukemia. *Arch. Biol. Sci.* **2017**, *69*, 239–246. [CrossRef]

164. Yao, P.; He, X.; Zhang, R.; Tong, R.; Xiao, H. The influence of MTHFR genetic polymorphisms on adverse reactions after methotrexate in patients with hematological malignancies: A meta-analysis. *Hematology* **2019**, *24*, 10–19. [CrossRef] [PubMed]

165. Zhu, C.; Liu, Y.W.; Wang, S.Z.; Li, X.L.; Nie, X.L.; Yu, X.T.; Zhao, L.B.; Wang, X.L. Associations between the C677T and A1298C polymorphisms of MTHFR and the toxicity of methotrexate in childhood malignancies: A meta-analysis. *Pharm. J.* **2018**, *18*, 450–459. [CrossRef] [PubMed]

166. Giletti, A.; Esperon, P. Genetic markers in methotrexate treatments. *Pharm. J.* **2018**, *18*, 689–703. [CrossRef] [PubMed]

167. Trevino, L.R.; Shimasaki, N.; Yang, W.; Panetta, J.C.; Cheng, C.; Pei, D.; Chan, D.; Sparreboom, A.; Giacomini, K.M.; Pui, C.H.; et al. Germline genetic variation in an organic anion transporter polypeptide associated with methotrexate pharmacokinetics and clinical effects. *J. Clin. Oncol.* **2009**, *27*, 5972–5978. [CrossRef] [PubMed]

168. Ramsey, L.B.; Panetta, J.C.; Smith, C.; Yang, W.; Fan, Y.; Winick, N.J.; Martin, P.L.; Cheng, C.; Devidas, M.; Pui, C.H.; et al. Genome-wide study of methotrexate clearance replicates SLCO1B1. *Blood* **2013**, *121*, 898–904. [CrossRef] [PubMed]
169. Ramsey, L.B.; Bruun, G.H.; Yang, W.; Trevino, L.R.; Vattathil, S.; Scheet, P.; Cheng, C.; Rosner, G.L.; Giacomini, K.M.; Fan, Y.; et al. Rare versus common variants in pharmacogenetics: SLCO1B1 variation and methotrexate disposition. *Genome Res.* **2012**, *22*, 1–8. [CrossRef] [PubMed]
170. Lopez-Lopez, E.; Martin-Guerrero, I.; Ballesteros, J.; Pinan, M.A.; Garcia-Miguel, P.; Navajas, A.; Garcia-Orad, A. Polymorphisms of the SLCO1B1 gene predict methotrexate-related toxicity in childhood acute lymphoblastic leukemia. *Pediatr. Blood Cancer* **2011**, *57*, 612–619. [CrossRef] [PubMed]
171. Radtke, S.; Zolk, O.; Renner, B.; Paulides, M.; Zimmermann, M.; Moricke, A.; Stanulla, M.; Schrappe, M.; Langer, T. Germline genetic variations in methotrexate candidate genes are associated with pharmacokinetics, toxicity, and outcome in childhood acute lymphoblastic leukemia. *Blood* **2013**, *121*, 5145–5153. [CrossRef] [PubMed]
172. Zhang, H.N.; He, X.L.; Wang, C.; Wang, Y.; Chen, Y.J.; Li, J.X.; Niu, C.H.; Gao, P. Impact of SLCO1B1 521T > C variant on leucovorin rescue and risk of relapse in childhood acute lymphoblastic leukemia treated with high-dose methotrexate. *Pediatr. Blood Cancer* **2014**, *61*, 2203–2207. [CrossRef] [PubMed]
173. Liu, S.G.; Gao, C.; Zhang, R.D.; Zhao, X.X.; Cui, L.; Li, W.J.; Chen, Z.P.; Yue, Z.X.; Zhang, Y.Y.; Wu, M.Y.; et al. Polymorphisms in methotrexate transporters and their relationship to plasma methotrexate levels, toxicity of high-dose methotrexate, and outcome of pediatric acute lymphoblastic leukemia. *Oncotarget* **2017**, *8*, 37761–37772. [CrossRef] [PubMed]
174. Lopez-Lopez, E.; Ballesteros, J.; Pinan, M.A.; Sanchez de Toledo, J.; Garcia de Andoin, N.; Garcia-Miguel, P.; Navajas, A.; Garcia-Orad, A. Polymorphisms in the methotrexate transport pathway: A new tool for MTX plasma level prediction in pediatric acute lymphoblastic leukemia. *Pharm. Genom.* **2013**, *23*, 53–61. [CrossRef] [PubMed]
175. Assaraf, Y.G. Molecular basis of antifolate resistance. *Cancer Metastasis Rev.* **2007**, *26*, 153–181. [CrossRef] [PubMed]
176. Cheok, M.H.; Evans, W.E. Acute lymphoblastic leukaemia: A model for the pharmacogenomics of cancer therapy. *Nat. Rev. Cancer* **2006**, *6*, 117–129. [CrossRef] [PubMed]
177. Wijdeven, R.H.; Pang, B.; Assaraf, Y.G.; Neefjes, J. Old drugs, novel ways out: Drug resistance toward cytotoxic chemotherapeutics. *Drug Resist. Updates Rev. Comment. Antimicrob. Anticancer Chemother.* **2016**, *28*, 65–81. [CrossRef] [PubMed]
178. Belkov, V.M.; Krynetski, E.Y.; Schuetz, J.D.; Yanishevski, Y.; Masson, E.; Mathew, S.; Raimondi, S.; Pui, C.-H.; Relling, M.V.; Evans, W.E. Reduced Folate Carrier Expression in Acute Lymphoblastic Leukemia: A Mechanism for Ploidy but not Lineage Differences in Methotrexate Accumulation. *Blood* **1999**, *93*, 1643. [PubMed]
179. Gorlick, R.; Goker, E.; Trippett, T.; Steinherz, P.; Elisseyeff, Y.; Mazumdar, M.; Flintoff, W.F.; Bertino, J.R. Defective Transport Is a Common Mechanism of Acquired Methotrexate Resistance in Acute Lymphocytic Leukemia and Is Associated With Decreased Reduced Folate Carrier Expression. *Blood* **1997**, *89*, 1013. [PubMed]
180. Rots, M.G.; Willey, J.C.; Jansen, G.; Van Zantwijk, C.H.; Noordhuis, P.; DeMuth, J.P.; Kuiper, E.; Veerman, A.J.P.; Pieters, R.; Peters, G.J. mRNA expression levels of methotrexate resistance-related proteins in childhood leukemia as determined by a standardized competitive template-based RT-PCR method. *Leukemia* **2000**, *14*, 2166–2175. [CrossRef] [PubMed]
181. Levy, A.S.; Sather, H.N.; Steinherz, P.G.; Sowers, R.; La, M.; Moscow, J.A.; Gaynon, P.S.; Uckun, F.M.; Bertino, J.R.; Gorlick, R. Reduced Folate Carrier and Dihydrofolate Reductase Expression in Acute Lymphocytic Leukemia May Predict Outcome: A Children's Cancer Group Study. *J. Pediatr. Hematol. Oncol.* **2003**, *25*, 688–695. [CrossRef] [PubMed]
182. Galpin, A.J.; Schuetz, J.D.; Masson, E.; Yanishevski, Y.; Synold, T.W.; Barredo, J.C.; Pui, C.H.; Relling, M.V.; Evans, W.E. Differences in folylpolyglutamate synthetase and dihydrofolate reductase expression in human B-lineage versus T-lineage leukemic lymphoblasts: Mechanisms for lineage differences in methotrexate polyglutamylation and cytotoxicity. *Mol. Pharm.* **1997**, *52*, 155–163. [CrossRef]

183. Rots, M.G.; Pieters, R.; Kaspers, G.-J.L.; van Zantwijk, C.H.; Noordhuis, P.; Mauritz, R.; Veerman, A.J.P.; Jansen, G.; Peters, G.J. Differential Methotrexate Resistance in Childhood T- Versus Common/PreB-Acute Lymphoblastic Leukemia Can Be Measured by an In Situ Thymidylate Synthase Inhibition Assay, But Not by the MTT Assay. *Blood* **1999**, *93*, 1067. [PubMed]
184. Kager, L.; Cheok, M.; Yang, W.; Zaza, G.; Cheng, Q.; Panetta, J.C.; Pui, C.H.; Downing, J.R.; Relling, M.V.; Evans, W.E. Folate pathway gene expression differs in subtypes of acute lymphoblastic leukemia and influences methotrexate pharmacodynamics. *J. Clin. Invest.* **2005**, *115*, 110–117. [CrossRef] [PubMed]
185. Sorich, M.J.; Pottier, N.; Pei, D.; Yang, W.; Kager, L.; Stocco, G.; Cheng, C.; Panetta, J.C.; Pui, C.H.; Relling, M.V.; et al. In vivo response to methotrexate forecasts outcome of acute lymphoblastic leukemia and has a distinct gene expression profile. *PLoS Med.* **2008**, *5*, e83. [CrossRef] [PubMed]
186. Dulucq, S.; St-Onge, G.; Gagne, V.; Ansari, M.; Sinnett, D.; Labuda, D.; Moghrabi, A.; Krajinovic, M. DNA variants in the dihydrofolate reductase gene and outcome in childhood ALL. *Blood* **2008**, *111*, 3692–3700. [CrossRef] [PubMed]
187. Rocha, J.C.; Cheng, C.; Liu, W.; Kishi, S.; Das, S.; Cook, E.H.; Sandlund, J.T.; Rubnitz, J.; Ribeiro, R.; Campana, D.; et al. Pharmacogenetics of outcome in children with acute lymphoblastic leukemia. *Blood* **2005**, *105*, 4752–4758. [CrossRef] [PubMed]
188. Al-Mahayri, Z.N.; Patrinos, G.P.; Ali, B.R. Pharmacogenomics in pediatric acute lymphoblastic leukemia: Promises and limitations. *Pharmacogenomics* **2017**, *18*, 687–699. [CrossRef] [PubMed]
189. Viennas, E.; Komianou, A.; Mizzi, C.; Stojiljkovic, M.; Mitropoulou, C.; Muilu, J.; Vihinen, M.; Grypioti, P.; Papadaki, S.; Pavlidis, C.; et al. Expanded national database collection and data coverage in the FINDbase worldwide database for clinically relevant genomic variation allele frequencies. *Nucleic Acids Res.* **2017**, *45*, D846–D853. [CrossRef] [PubMed]
190. Mizzi, C.; Dalabira, E.; Kumuthini, J.; Dzimiri, N.; Balogh, I.; Basak, N.; Bohm, R.; Borg, J.; Borgiani, P.; Bozina, N.; et al. A European Spectrum of Pharmacogenomic Biomarkers: Implications for Clinical Pharmacogenomics. *PLoS ONE* **2016**, *11*, e0162866. [CrossRef] [PubMed]
191. Hong, H.; Xu, L.; Su, Z.; Liu, J.; Ge, W.; Shen, J.; Fang, H.; Perkins, R.; Shi, L.; Tong, W. Pitfall of genome-wide association studies: Sources of inconsistency in genotypes and their effects. *J. Biomed. Sci. Eng.* **2012**, *5*, 557–573. [CrossRef]

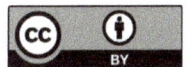

© 2019 by the authors. Licensee MDPI, Basel, Switzerland. This article is an open access article distributed under the terms and conditions of the Creative Commons Attribution (CC BY) license (http://creativecommons.org/licenses/by/4.0/).

MDPI
St. Alban-Anlage 66
4052 Basel
Switzerland
Tel. +41 61 683 77 34
Fax +41 61 302 89 18
www.mdpi.com

Genes Editorial Office
E-mail: genes@mdpi.com
www.mdpi.com/journal/genes

www.ingramcontent.com/pod-product-compliance
Lightning Source LLC
LaVergne TN
LVHW070734100526
838202LV00013B/1236